Psychosocial Intervention in Schizophrenia

An International View

Edited by
H. Stierlin L. C. Wynne M. Wirsching

With 26 Figures
12 of them in Color

Springer-Verlag Berlin Heidelberg GmbH 1983

Professor Dr. med. et phil. Helm Stierlin
Psychosomatische Klinik, Abt. für psychoanalytische
Grundlagenforschung und Familientherapie
Mönchhofstraße 15a, D-6900 Heidelberg 1

Professor Dr. Dr. Lyman C. Wynne
University of Rochester, Dept. of Psychiatry
300 Crittenden Boulevard, Rochester, N.Y. 14642, USA

Professor Dr. med. Michael Wirsching
Zentrum für Psychosomatische Medizin
Friedrichstraße 28, D-6300 Gießen

ISBN 978-3-642-68968-0 ISBN 978-3-642-68966-6 (eBook)
DOI 10.1007/978-3-642-68966-6

Library of Congress Cataloging in Publication Data
Main entry under title:
Psychosocial intervention in schizophrenia.
Includes bibliographical references.
1. Schizophrenia. I. Stierlin, Helm.
II. Wirsching, M. (Michael) III. Wynne, Lyman C.
[DNLM: 1. Schizophrenia–Therapy. WM 203 P9738]
RC514.P7189 1983 616.89'8206 83-4713
ISBN 978-3-642-68968-0

Typesetting: Elsner & Behrens, Oftersheim

2119/3140-543210

Authors, Co-authors, and Discussants

Alanen, Yrjö, Prof., Dept. of Psychiatry, University of Turku, Kurjenmäentie 4, SF-20700 Turku 70, Finland

Anderson, Carol M., Ph.D., Prof., University of Pittsburgh, Western Psychiatric Institute, 3811 O'Hara Street, Pittsburgh, Pa. 15261, USA

Benedetti, Gaetano, Prof. Dr. med., Kantonspital Basel, Psychiatrische Universitätsklinik, Petersgraben 4, CH-4031 Basel, Switzerland

Boscolo, Luigi, M.D., Centro per lo Studio della Famiglia, Via Leopardi 19, I-20123 Milano, Italy

Boström, Christina, M.A., Dept. of Psychiatry, Oulu University, SF-90210 Oulu 21, Finland

Cancro, Robert, M.D., Prof., New York University, Medical Center, 550 First Avenue, New York, N. Y. 10016, USA

Carroll, Alexander, McLean Hospital, 115 Mill Street, Belmont, Mass. 02178, USA

Cecchin, Gianfranco, M.D., Centro per lo Studio della Famiglia, Via Leopardi 19, I-20123 Milano, Italy

Ciompi, Luc, Prof., Dr. med., Sozialpsychiatrische Universitätsklinik, Murtenstr. 21, CH-3010 Bern, Switzerland

Cole, Robert E., University of Rochester, Dept. of Psychiatry, 300 Crittenden Boulevard, Rochester, N.Y. 14642, USA

Fleck, Stephen, M.D., Prof., Yale University, Dept. of Psychiatry, 25 Park Street, New Haven, Conn. 06519, USA

Frank, Arlene, Ph.D., McLean Hospital, 115 Mill Street, Belmont, Mass. 02178, USA

Frosch, James P., M.D., McLean Hospital, 115 Mill Street, Belmont, Mass. 02178, USA

Goldstein, Michael J., Ph.D., Prof., University of California, Dept. of Psychology, Los Angeles, Ca. 90024, USA

Gunderson, John G., M.D., Prof., McLean Hospital, 115 Mill Street, Belmont, Mass. 02178, USA

Järvi, Ritva, M.D., Dept. of Psychiatry, University of Turku, Kurjenmäentie 4, SF-20700 Turku 70, Finland

Kafka, John S., M.D., 7834 Aberdeen Road, Bethesda, Md. 20014, USA

Kaufmann, Luc, Prof. Dr. med., Hôpital de Cery, CH-1008 Prilly, Switzerland

Laakso, Juhani, M.D., Dept. of Psychiatry, University of Turku, Kurjenmäentie 4, SF-20700 Turku 70, Finland

Lahti, Ilpo, M.D., Dept. of Psychiatry, Oulu University, SF-90210 Oulu 21, Finland

Matussek, Paul, Prof. Dr. med. et phil., Max-Planck-Institut für Psychopathologie und Psychotherapie, Montsalvatstr. 19, D-8000 München 40, Germany

Menn, Alma Z., M.S.W., A.C.S.W., MRI/ETC, 555 Middlefield Road, Palo Alto, Ca. 94301, USA
Mosher, Loren R., M.D., Prof., Dept. of Psychiatry, Room C 1 066, University of the Health Sciences, 4301 Jones Bridge Road, Bethesda, Md. 20014, USA
Müller, Christian, Prof., Dr. med., Hôpital de Cery, CH-1008 Prilly, Switzerland
Naarala, Mikko, M.D., Dept. of Psychiatry, Oulu University, SF-90210 Oulu 21, Finland
Paul, Norman L., M.D., Harrington Park, Suite 6, 394 Lowell Street, Lexington, Massachusetts 02173
Prata, Giuliana, M.D., Centro per lo Studio della Famiglia, Via Veneto 12, I-20124 Milano, Italy
Prohjola, Jukka, M.D., Dept. of Psychiatry, Oulu University, SF-90210 Oulu 21, Finland
Räkköläinen, Viljo, M.D., Dept. of Psychiatry, University of Turku, Kurjenmäentie 4, SF-20700 Turku 70, Finland
Rasimus, Riitta, M.D., Dept. of Psychiatry, University of Turku, Kurjenmäentie 4, SF-20700 Turku 70, Finland
Schwartz, Daniel P., M.D., Austen Riggs Center, Stockbridge, Mass. 01262, USA
Selvini-Palazzoli, Mara, M.D., Prof., Centro per lo Studio della Famiglia, Via Veneto 12, I-20124 Milano, Italy
Serra, Paolo, M.D., Via dell'Agnolo 37, I-50100 Firenze, Italy
Siirala, Martti, M.D., Oulunkgläntic 29, SF-00600 Helsinki 60, Finland
Sorri, Anneli, M.D., Dept. of Psychiatry, Oulu University, SF-90210 Oulu 21, Finland
Stierlin, Helm, Prof. Dr. med. et phil., Psychosomatische Klinik, Abt. für psychoanalytische Grundlagenforschung und Familientherapie, Mönchhofstr. 15a, D-6900 Heidelberg 1, Germany
Tienari, Pekka, M.D., Prof., Dept. of Psychiatry, Oulu University, SF-90210 Oulu 21, Finland
Tranchina, Paolo, M.D., Via dell'Agnolo 37, I-50100 Firenze, Italy
Wahlberg, Karl-Erik, M.A., Dept. of Psychiatry, Oulu University, SF-90210 Oulu 21, Finland
Watzlawick, Paul, M.D., Prof., Mental Research Institute, 555 Middlefield Road, Palo Alto, CA. 94301, USA
Weiss, Roger, M. D., McLean Hospital, 115 Mill Street, Belmont, Mass. 02178, USA
Wirsching, Michael, Prof. Dr. med., Zentrum für Psychosomatische Medizin, Friedrichstr. 28, D-6300 Gießen
Wynne, Lyman C., M.D., Ph.D., Prof., University of Rochester, Dept. of Psychiatry, 300 Crittenden Boulevard, Rochester, N.Y. 14642, USA

Table of Contents

General Introduction

Today, more than 70 years after Eugen Bleuler introduced the term schizophrenia, the human condition so labeled continues to pose a formidable challenge to the helping professions. In recent years it may seem that this challenge can be met most successfully by biologically oriented researchers and therapists: All over the world neuroleptic drugs have made it possible to control disturbing symptoms and shorten hospital stays. Ever more refined technologies permit study of intricate neurophysiological and pharmacological processes that seem to underlie, if not contribute to, schizophrenic disorders. Most recently, the discovery of the endorphins promises a new therapeutic breakthrough. At the same time, a vast and growing research literature confirms the importance, if not primacy, of hereditary and neurophysiological factors in the etiopathogenesis of these disorders.

And yet, as Loren Mosher notes in this volume, after 2 decades of almost universal usage of neuroleptics, it is now clear that they do not cure schizophrenia. It is also clear that they have serious, sometimes irreversible toxicities, that recovery may be impaired by them in at least some schizophrenics, and that they have little effect on long-term psychosocial adjustment.

At the same time, evidence is accumulating that relational and communication styles and patterns existing in certain families can powerfully predict whether hospitalized patients with a schizophrenic disturbance will, after an initial improvement, relapse or not. And finally, there is a growing body of research, partly described in this volume, that attests to the power of a given social environment – and especially of a family environment – to foster or counteract the development of schizophrenic disturbances.

In fact, as editors of this volume, we are convinced that there is at present throughout the Western world a new and vital interest in psychosocial interventions in schizophrenia. The contributions in this volume support that conviction. They were drawn from a large number of papers presented by internationally known experts at the 7th International Symposium on the Psychotherapy of Schizophrenia held in Heidelberg from September 30 through October 2, 1981. They present a diversity of assumptions and models about schizophrenia and, accordingly, a diversity of treatment approaches. This might be somewhat unsettling to all those who expect simple guidelines for treatment and further research. We, however, would like to emphasize the positive side in this state of affairs, i.e., the challenge to find out how the various approaches are compatible or incompatible with one other. This requires that we listen to, and learn from, each other, and that we can endure, for a while at least, a possibly "salutary confusion."

Helm Stierlin, Lyman C. Wynne, and Michael Wirsching

I. Family Research

Introduction

Although research on psychosocial environment, including the family, was highly prominent in studies of schizophrenia during the late 1950s and the 1960s, such research has not been so visible in publications in more recent years. A major reason has been that a new research strategy emerged for examining familial and other psychosocial factors longitudinally, and the findings of these studies are only now reaching a point where significant published work is becoming possible. In the papers in this section, three significant programs are reported that illustrate the new thrust of family research on schizophrenia. Just as one must view biologic and psychopharmacologic studies with caution when initial results are reported, so must one view these current reports as preliminary and not definitive at this stage. Nevertheless, such work is generating a new wave of interest, even enthusiasm, both because of the potential contributions to scientific understanding of schizophrenia and its context and also because of direct and quite obvious applications to prevention and treatment.

Goldstein's chapter is noteworthy because of its integrative approach to the family's role in a developmental concept of schizophrenia, both preceding the onset of manifest symptoms and continuing during the course of the disorder. In earlier years, so-called etiologic studies on the precursors of schizophrenia and treatment studies on factors affecting later relapse have had little methodologic overlap. In contrast, the studies reported by Goldstein link (1) the UCLA longitudinal studies of the families of adolescents at risk for later schizophrenia spectrum disorders and (2) the studies of Expressed Emotion (begun in the United Kingdom) in which a longitudinal approach to the families of diagnosed schizophrenics is followed. Goldstein emphasizes poor premorbid adjustment as interactive with family overemotional involvement; this finding illustrates a detailed association between pre-onset and post-illness developmental factors. Also, the UCLA work under Goldstein is starting to untangle how diverse role structures in families, e.g., whether mother or father is the focus of family interaction, function differently depending upon the presence of communication deviance in the family. Other studies in this program are evaluating methodologic issues such as how well methods of studying direct interaction within families correlate with psychological test methods for studying parental communication. The samples in these studies are still small and will require replication, but the work provides numerous leads for scientifically sound and exciting new directions in family research.

A quite different approach to psychosocial factors in schizophrenia is presented by the Finnish group under Pekka Tienari. After results from the Danish adoption studies were first published in a preliminary way in 1968 (Rosenthal et al. 1968), there was a rather uncritical, widespread belief that the genetic basis for schizophrenia had been established. Actually, what was claimed by the authors was no more than a *con-*

tributing genetic factor to a predisposition for at least some schizophrenics. Furthermore, as the data were analyzed more fully and the methodology assessed, even these earlier conclusions have emerged as less clear than was originally believed (Lidz et al. 1981). One of the serious shortcomings in the Danish studies was the failure to study directly the communication and relationships in the adoptive, rearing families. Because of this shortcoming, the Danish studies could not satisfactorily examine the interaction of environment (adoptive family) and genetics (biologic parents). The research group under Tienari has been assembling a very large sample of adopted-away offspring of schizophrenics and controls, with studies of their family relationships and communication that are partly innovative in method and partly replicative of American family research methods. In the latter respect, they have used the Consensus Family Rorschach and test studies of parental communication deviance. The preliminary Finnish data support the Danish evidence for a contributory genetic factor, but, as a new and significant finding, they provide data indicating that this vulnerability becomes expressed in symptomatic schizophrenia only when the adoptive, rearing family has been highly disturbed.

The chapter by Wynne and Cole from Rochester, New York, serves to illustrate a class of family research studies in the so-called high-risk field (see Watt et al. 1982). While most risk research emphasizes the individual vulnerabilities of the growing child and the risk associated with parental diagnosis of schizophrenia, the Rochester program reported by Wynne and Cole includes these two sets of variables and adds detailed studies of family transactions. As in the Finnish adoption study, the Rochester data support the concept of significant and independent contributions to the risk for the offspring that is associated *both* with parental diagnosis and with family relationship patterns. Healthy family functioning, despite the adversity of parental illness, stands out as a hopeful lead that may be relevant to future efforts at prevention and early intervention through more effective tapping of the resources and assets of these families.

A refreshing theme in recent research on psychosocial factors of schizophrenia is an explicit readiness to examine interaction of psychosocial and biologic factors. No longer is there an implicit tendency to ignore genetic and other biologic considerations. It is to be hoped that future research beginning from a biologic perspective will show a similar open-mindedness and willingness to examine psychosocial factors.

References

Lidz T, Blatt S, Cook B (1981) Critique of the Danish-American studies of the adopted-away offspring of schizophrenic parents. Am J Psychiatry 138:1063–1068

Rosenthal D, Wender PH, Kety SS, Schulsinger F, Welner J, Østergaard L (1968) Schizophrenics' offspring reared in adoptive homes. J Psychiatric Res 6 (Suppl 1):377–391

Watt NF, Anthony EJ, Wynne LC, Rolf J (eds) (1983) Children at risk for schizophrenia: A longitudinal perspective. Cambridge University Press, New York

Lyman C. Wynne

Family Interaction: Patterns Predictive of the Onset and Course of Schizophrenia

Michael J. Goldstein[1]

Recent years have witnessed a rekindling of interest in the role of the family in schizophrenia. While it is not possible to specify a single stimulus to this renewed interest, a number of factors seem significant. First, the trend towards deinstitutionalization of schizophrenic patients and the emphasis upon community-based care often places patients back in some sort of family environment. Examination of these family environments has revealed that some families cope well with this newly assigned caretaker role but that many experience considerable difficulty reabsorbing a family member who frequently manifests a number of residual symptoms. Concern with the nature of the family environment and its impact on the newly discharged schizophrenic patient has revived interest in the family's role in schizophrenia in general.

Secondly, the work by Brown and his colleagues (1972) and later by Vaughn and Leff (1976) in Great Britain provided empirical evidence that deleterious aspects of the family environment could be specified and measured with standardized procedures. Their work on *expressed emotion* (EE) revealed that indices of overinvolvement, hostility, and critical comments made by the patient's relatives (usually the parents) in the course of a standardized interview, the Camberwell Family Interview (CFI), administered around the time the patient was admitted to the hospital, possessed powerful prognostic information concerning the likelihood of relapse over a 9-month follow-up period. The EE variable, assumed to reflect on-going intrafamilial attitudes and processes, suggested a particular sensitivity of the schizophrenic patient to discriminable attributes of the family emotional environment.

Thirdly, the past 10 years have witnessed a number of research programs concerned with the developmental antecedents of adult schizophrenia (Garmezy 1974). These studies have focused on populations believed at greater than average risk for schizophrenia, which are identified and studied prior to the onset of the clinical form of the disorder or its prodromal phases. These samples are then followed from some earlier life period until they enter the risk period for adult schizophrenia. Several of these projects have included measures of intrafamilial characteristics in their early assessments

1 The research reported in this chapter was supported by grants MH08744 and MH30911 from the U.S. National Institute of Mental Health. Special appreciation is due Jeri A. Doane, PhD, Julia M. Lewis, PhD, and David Miklowitz, MA, for their generous contributions to the research program and for permitting aspects of their data to be reproduced in this chapter. Ian Falloon, MD, has been most generous in sharing data from his intervention projects with families containing schizophrenic offspring.

so that the value of familial predictors of the likelihood of the onset of a schizophrenic episode can be evaluated. These studies have involved a high level of sophistication in the assessment of family relationships and more precise specification of family parameters than was the case in earlier family research. Some of the variables measured have been derived from these earlier studies of families containing adult schizophrenic offspring, as for example, the Wynne-Singer concept of communication deviance (1977). Others have been derived from the work on family factors associated with the course of schizophrenia involving interpersonal derivatives of the expressed emotion dimensions.

It is sometimes implied that current interest in the family's role in the course of schizophrenia has little bearing on etiological issues. In one sense, this is entirely correct. However, in another sense it represents a false distinction between family factors which are associated with onset and those which relate to course. Both types of research actually deal with issues of life course – one from an ostensibly illness-free period to the first appearance of a schizophrenic disorder, and the other from a period of overt, symptomatic manifestation of the disorder to a relatively illness-free period. While this is an issue ultimately answered by empirical data, it is difficult for the present author to view family life as so discontinuous across the life span that those attributes of the family environment related to the onset of schizophrenia do not overlap with those associated with differential course after an initial episode.

Family Factors Related to the Onset of Schizophrenia

Are there definable aspects of intrafamilial relationships which precede the onset of schizophrenia or its prodromal signs? A recent study carried out at the University of California at Los Angeles (UCLA) by my research group (Doane et al. 1981) provides evidence that family attributes measured during adolescence are associated with the *subsequent* presence of schizophrenia or schizophrenia-related disorders in the offspring once they entered young adulthood. A cohort of 65 nonpsychotically disturbed adolescents and their families participated in this prospective longitudinal study. At the time of the first 5-year follow-up, a measure of communication deviance as defined and measured by the Singer-Wynne criteria was available for 37 of the cases and predicted the presence of disorders on the extended schizophrenia spectrum (Wender et al. 1968). Very briefly, a measure of parental communication deviance (CD) developed by Jones (1977) was obtained from Thematic Apperception Test (TAT) data obtained at the time of the original assessment. Examples of this measure included such things as lack of commitment to ideas or percepts, unclear or idiosyncratic communication of themes or ideas, language anomalies, disruptive speech, and closure problems. It can be seen in Table 1 that offspring of parents with high levels of parental CD were more likely to have schizophrenia or schizophrenia spectrum disorders at the time of the first 5-year follow-up. However, a number of false-positive errors occurred in which several cases with relatively benign outcomes also had parents with high CD. Low CD in the parents, however, was a good predictor of a relatively benign, nonschizophrenia

Table 1. Relationship between parental communication deviance and outcome diagnosis (N = 37) (Doane et al. 1981)

Parental CD risk rating	Wender scale levels						
		Extended schizophrenia spectrum					
		"Soft" end			"Hard" end		
	1–4	5			6		7
	Normal to mild and marked character neuroses	Drug abuse with antisocial personality	Schizoid personality	Probable borderline	Definite borderline	Probable schizophrenia	Definite schizophrenia
Low or intermediate CD	19	1	0	1	0	0	0
High CD	7[a]	2	0	3	2	1[a]	1

[a] One index young adult in each of these two cells had a sibling who developed definite schizophrenia.

Note: The degree of relationship was determined by a 2 x 3 chi-square test, collapsing the drug abuse with antisocial personality, schizoid, and probable borderline categories and the definite borderline, probable, and definite schizophrenia categories: $\chi^2 = 10.3$, $df = 2$, $P < 0.01$.

Table 2. Parental affective style profile pattern and communication deviance (CD) as combined predictors of outcome diagnosis (N = 37) (Doane et al. 1981)

Parental affective style profile pattern and parental CD risk rating		Wender scale levels						
			Extended schizophrenia spectrum					
			"Soft" end			"Hard" end		
		1–4	5			6		7
		Normal to mild and marked character neurosis	Drug abuse with antisocial personality	Schizoid personality	Probable borderline	Definite borderline	Probable schizophrenia	Definite schizophrenia
Low CD	Benign AS	9	0	0	0	0	0	0
	Negative AS	10	1	0	1	0	0	0
High CD	Benign AS	7[a]	0	0	1	0	0	0
	Negative AS	0	2	0	2	2	1[a]	1

[a] One index young adult in each of these two cells had a sibling in whom definite schizophrenia developed.

Note: The degree of relationship was determined by a 3 x 4 χ^2 test collapsing the drug abuse with antisocial personality, schizoid personality, and probable borderline categories and the definite borderline, probable schizophrenia, and definite schizophrenia categories ($\chi^2 = 27.9$, $df = 6$, $P < 0.001$).

spectrum disorder. Thus, the CD index alone did not allow precise identification of those cases destined to develop schizophrenic and related disorders.

Next, a measure somewhat similar to EE, called affective style (AS) was used to determine whether this attribute would enhance the prediction of the onset of schizophrenia in this sample of disturbed adolescents once they reached young adulthood. Certain key components of this affective style index (such as criticism, guilt inducement, and intrusiveness), derived from directly observed family interactions, can be construed as interpersonal analogues of certain dimensions of the EE construct. Doane et al. (1981) found that indeed when a measure of affective style [obtained from a modified Strodtbeck (1954) direct interaction task involving all family members] was added to the CD index, remarkably precise prediction resulted. In Table 2 we see that all cases whose parents exhibited both high CD and negative AS manifested schizophrenia spectrum disorders at the 5-year follow-up. Only two cases received spectrum diagnoses who did not reveal this parental pattern, and both received soft spectrum diagnoses. It should be emphasized that while both of these parental characteristics were measured at least 5 years prior to the onset of overt schizophrenic symptomatology and therefore clearly not reactive to the presence of psychosis in offspring, one cannot assume from these results that they play an etiological role in the development of schizophrenia. Data which will become available shortly from the 15-year follow-up of these cases will provide even clearer evidence for the predictive value of these and other family characteristics.

Interactional Correlates of Communication Deviance

The measure of communication deviance clearly serves as an important marker of parental attributes associated with subsequent schizophrenia spectrum disorders in offspring. However, unlike the AS index which is derived from directly observed interaction between parent and teenager, CD is based upon transactions between a parent and a tester during the administration of a projective test, the TAT. But, what does this index reveal about actual ongoing family interaction? Researchers from our group have previously reported on some correlates of CD (Goldstein et al. 1978) which reveal that in the triadic interactions, high CD parents manifested significantly more nonacknowledging behavior than parents classified as intermediate or low, particularly when responding to the offspring. Also, Lieber (1977) found that high CD parents, when observed in a structured discussion of video tapes of their own triadic interaction, were less likely than other parents to use task-focusing comments when the discussion drifted away from the requested structure. Both of these studies support the idea that high CD parents, when actively involved in a three-way emotionally charged discussion with their disturbed teenager, have difficulty maintaining an effective focus of discussion.

A recent study by Lewis (1979) pursued this issue in more detail as she examined aspects of role structure, communication drift, and nonverbal behavior in these triadic family discussions. Her role structure estimates were based on speaking patterns of *who* talks and *who* is the recipient of others' remarks. Using a profile approach, she was able to characterize families as (a) father central, (b) mother central, (c) dual pa-

Table 3. Parental role structure versus communication deviance ($N = 47$) (Lewis et al. 1981)[a]

Level of communication deviance	Parental role structure			
	Father-central	Mother-central	Dual parental focus	Mixed patterns
Low	10	2	0	0
Intermediate	5	2	0	8
High	5	8	6	1

Chi square, 30.96; $P < 0.0001$.

[a] 47 of 65 cases had both communication deviance ratings and ratable interaction transcripts.

rental focus, and (d) mixed. Father and mother central are self-explanatory as each contains a single parent who is the primary speaker and recipient of the other two family members' remarks. Dual parental focus characterizes a triadic interaction in which both parents are equally active and direct the majority of their comments to the teenager. In the mixed pattern either the parents speak only to one another, or one parent talks to the child, who in turn addresses the other parent, who in turn addresses another speaker, a ronde if you will. Lewis predicted, based on research in families containing a schizophrenic offspring, that the father-central pattern would be less common in the high CD family units. These results are presented in Table 3. Here we see that the prediction is indeed confirmed although the rates for high and intermediate CD groups are the same. In addition, we see that other patterns are noted in high CD family units, particularly mother–central and dual parental focus, are rarely noted in intermediate or low CD family units. Obviously, there is more heterogeneity in the role structure patterns of high CD than the other two CD groups, but father-central occurs much less frequently than in low CD families. The discrepancy between high and low CD families is particularly noteworthy for the mother-central and dual parental focus family structures.

The heterogeneity in the high CD groups may explain why previous attempts to compare families containing schizophrenic offspring with other groups on similar measures may have produced a "now you see it, now you don't" pattern of results. These have all looked for a single pattern, such as maternal or paternal dominance, when in fact Lewis' data (1979) strongly suggests that there may be a number of distorted role patterns in preschizophrenic families which are lost when simple averages are used to contrast groups. These data are also congruent with the observations of Lidz and Fleck (1965) who observed a number of different role structure patterns in their sample of families of schizophrenics, all of which were disordered in some fashion. It appears that as with the Lidz et al. data that preschizophrenic families share a common feature of disordered communication and affective style, but vary in the precise formal organization in which these processes are expressed.

Lewis went one step further in attempting to account for the hererogeneity in role patterns. She hypothesized that they may reflect different types or patterns of CD in the parents. The criteria developed by Jones for the high CD classification utilized the multifactorial nature of the index. Jones (1977) found that when a single parent scored

Table 4. Parental communication deviance inclusion criteria and role structure pattern ($N = 20$)

Communication deviance factor pattern	Role structure		
	Father-central	Dual parental focus	Mother-central
Father high (2, 6) *or* both parents (2, 6)	4	1	2
Both parents high (1, 3, 4, or 5)	0	4	2
Mother only high (2, 6)	1	1	5

high (T score $\geqq$ 60) on Factor 2 (misperceptions) or Factor 6 (major closure problems) that the probability of offspring schizophrenia was high. Therefore, he classified a parental unit as high CD if either parent manifested a high score on Factors 2 or 6 independent of the other parent's score. For the remaining CD factors, Jones found that T scores greater than 60 were required from *both* parents for offspring schizophrenia risk to be high. Therefore, another group in the UCLA sample was classified as high CD only when *both* parents manifested T scores above 60.

Lewis next grouped the high CD parents on the basis of the different criteria suggested by Jones for entry into the high CD group (e.g., single or dual parent requirement). In Table 4 one can see that there is a close correspondence between these criteria and role structure pattern. Where father was high CD on the basis of the 2, 6 factor pattern (regardless of mother's pattern), we see the father-central structural pattern; where mother was classified as high CD on the basis of the 2, 6 pattern, we see a mother-central pattern and where *both* parents manifested high CD on the remaining factors, the dual parental focus pattern is noted. Thus, not only was Lewis able to demonstrate parallelism between CD criteria and role structure, but she found that the parent or parents who actually have the high CD deficit are central in the triadic family discussion. This means that such parents are actively involved in family relationships and may, in fact, dominate the family environment. Were this not the case, a theoretical embarrassment would exist. If the high CD parent was relatively inactive or ignored, then we would have to explain the mechanism by which the CD index translates into pathological family relationships. The notable activity level of the parent or parental unit manifesting the high CD projective test pattern suggests that high CD parent(s) are very significant in setting the form and probably the intensity of family discussions.

In order to better understand what type of tone is set within these parental structures, Lewis investigated the two other dimensions of communication drift and nonverbal affect display. Communication drift was measured with regard to two factors: adherence to the topic and shared expression of feelings. Failures to adhere to the topic were indexed by one of two patterns: drift away from the problem assigned for discussion or such rigid adherence to the topic as defined that meaningful discussion was precluded. For sharing feelings, two parallel deviations were excessive outpouring of feelings or rigid suppression of all feelings. High CD families ($P < 0.04$) generally avoided sharing feelings with each other and they were more likely to show distorted communication of the assigned topic, but surprisingly the tendency was toward the rigid adherence to the topic rather than the drifting disorganized style. However, the relationship between

Table 5. Nonverbal behaviors versus communication deviance ($N = 34$) (Lewis et al. 1981)[a]

Level of communication deviance	Nonverbal behavior		
	Nonavoidant and relaxed	Nonavoidant and rigid	Avoidant and rigid
Low	8	0	2
Intermediate	2	6	1
High	2	4	9

Chi square, 20.12; $P < 0.0005$.

[a] Only 34 families had communication deviance ratings and usable videotapes for rating facial expression and body position.

CD and communication drift was not as sharp as was noted for the previously mentioned role structure measures.

Where notable rigidity and avoidance of feelings were both observed, it was most common in father-central family units. This was an important difference between father-central families in the high and low CD groups. In the low CD groups, high father activity was associated with clear communication and affect sharing. In the high CD group, the same role structure was associated with rigid adherence to the topic and avoidance of affect sharing. Thus, in the high CD families of this subgroup, paternal activity blocks rather than facilitates family communication. Simply categorizing families as father- or mother-central, as has been done in prior family research, would lose this qualitative difference and lead to the erroneous conclusion that schizophrenic and nonschizophrenic families are similar.

The third correlate of CD explored by Lewis was nonverbal aspects of parental behavior noted during the triadic discussion. The components were: eye contact, facial expression, and voice tone. Voice tone did not relate to the other nonverbal measures but did relate strongly ($P < 0.01$) to the Affective Style Index which was derived from content analysis of verbal transcripts only. The eye contact and facial expression measures were combined into profile groupings as follows: (a) avoidant eye contact, rigid facial expression; (b) nonavoidant eye contact, rigid facial expression; and (c) nonavoidant eye contact, relaxed facial expression. In Table 5, we can see that high CD is associated with parental avoidance of eye contact with the adolescent and a rigid unchanging facial expression, while the other CD groups show less avoidance behavior and emotional rigidity.

We can see that two broad constructs, CD and affective style, are valuable in predicting offspring diagnostic status at the time of the 5-year follow-up. Communication deviance, as measured by an individual projective test administered to the parents clearly indexes more than its name would imply and reveals family units generally lacking in effective paternal participation, which are poorly organized to deal with emotional material, and which show signs of marked interpersonal tension between parent and teenager. The affect measures, which are most parsimoniously thought of as measures of an affective evaluation of the teenager expressed in words and tone of voice, appear orthogonal – or at least oblique – to the interpersonal correlates of the CD index. Further, they are an important ingredient for accounting for the variation in early adult outcomes. Poorly organized and tense family structures lacking negative evaluative attitudes (criticism, guilt induction, or intrusiveness) do not contain early onset, definite, or probable schizophrenia, or borderline personality disorders. Whether the evidence from the longer term follow-up supports this two factor model or indicates that it may only be relevant for early onset cases remains to be seen.

Family Factors Associated with the Course of Schizophrenia

A second body of research is currently underway which is addressing the role of family factors in the course of schizophrenia, once it has been diagnosed. As mentioned earlier, the work by Brown et al. (1972) showed patients returning to a high EE family environment were much more likely to relapse during the 9 months following hospitalization. Vaughn and Leff (1976) replicated their initial findings and the combined data from these studies revealed the following relapse rates: 51% of the high EE group had relapsed within 9 months of hospital release versus 13% of the low EE group (Leff 1976).

While the work on EE has been very stimulating, it has raised as many questions as it has answered. Several important issues are highlighted by this work and are currently being addressed in a number of studies: (a) Can this finding be replicated in other settings? (b) Is the construct valid? Do people displaying critical or overinvolved attitudes on the CFI also convey these attitudes during actual interactions with the patient? (c) Are EE attitudes in the family members independent of patient characteristics such as premorbid status or quality or severity of symptomatology, as suggested by the original investigators? (d) How does EE relate to other familial attributes, such as communication deviance, shown in previous research to be associated with families of schizophrenics? (e) Is the relationship between EE and relapse rates equally valid for other cultural or subcultural groups?

Replication Studies

A recent replication study by Vaughn et al. (to be published) at UCLA and Camarillo State Hospital reports remarkably similar relapse rates for a sample of 54 schizophrenics of low and high EE families. These investigators found that 57% of the high EE cases relapsed within 9 months in contrast to only 17% of the low EE group. Other replication studies are currently underway in this country as well as in Denmark, England, and India (Day 1982).

Construct Validity Issues

While replication studies are important in any scientific endeavor, equally crucial are issues involving the validity of the findings. If we take EE, for example, we can ask what exactly does this measure reflect? Presumably EE attitudes, as conveyed to interviewer during the CFI, are reflective and perhaps even characteristic of how the relative relates to the patient in the interpersonal situations and discussions of everyday life. This issue has not been put to empirical test as yet, however. In short, does high EE status indicate discriminable, characteristic negative interpersonal modes of relating to the patient, or does it reflect more of an attitudinal position, not manifested in actual behavior?

Two recent studies provide some indirect evidence for the construct validity of EE. Tarrier et al. (1979) recently reported that in the home setting, low EE and high EE patients both displayed a high degree of arousal, measured as a high frequency of spontaneous fluctuations in skin conductance, when the target relative was *not* present in the room. However, when the target relative had entered the room, the low EE patients rapidly habituated while the high EE patients did not. This finding was replicated in a recent report by Sturgeon et al. (1981) who found very similar results. These studies suggest that there is indeed something relatively more soothing or less noxious about the low EE relatives. What exactly the high EE relatives do differently, however, remains unexamined.

An obvious hypothesis is that the high EE relative actually *behaves* in a highly critical, hostile, or overinvolved fashion when interacting with the patient. The measure of affective style cited previously (Doane et al. 1981) is being used to examine this question in two projects currently underway in Los Angeles. In a project directed by Dr. Ian Falloon of the University of Southern California, 40 high EE families are randomly assigned to family therapy or individual therapy (Falloon et al. 1981).

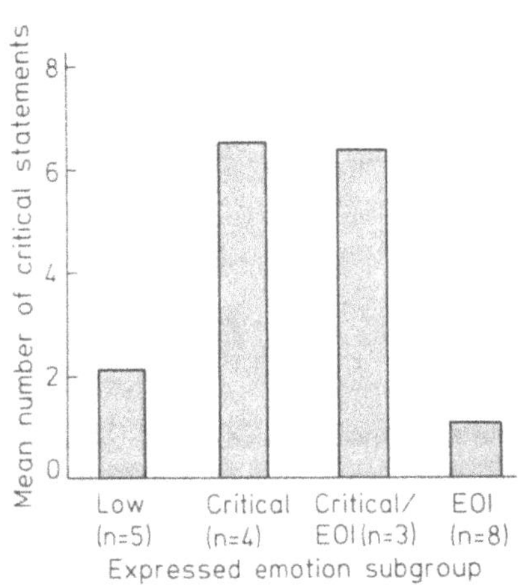

Fig. 1. Number of critical statements expressed in direct interaction by mothers in different EE subgroups

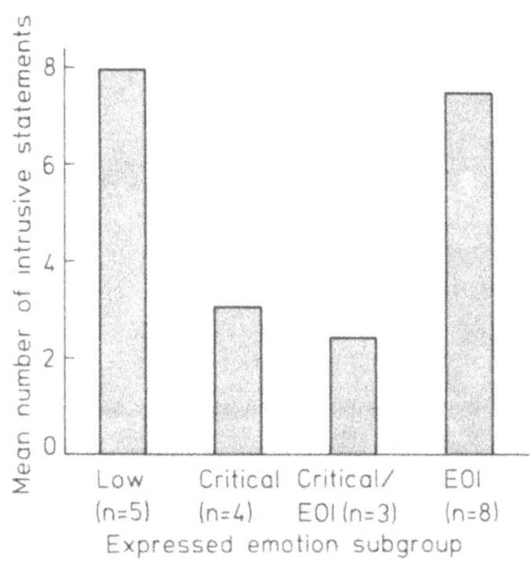

Fig. 2. Number of intrusive statements expressed in direct interaction by mothers in different EE subgroups

Among the data collected in this project are EE ratings of criticism, hostility, and overinvolvement derived from the CFI, and two directly observed family interaction tasks, similar in format to those used in the UCLA longitudinal study mentioned earlier (Doane et al. 1981). Preliminary analyses on a pilot sample of 15 high and 5 low EE families indicate that measures of Doane's affective style in the family discussion tasks are associated with corresponding attitudes conveyed during the CFI. Note that the high EE families have been subdivided into three groups: critical ($N = 4$), critical plus emotional overinvolvement (EOI) ($N = 3$), and EOI only ($N = 8$). This classification was based on the pattern manifested by the relative on the CFI. Results presented in Fig. 1 indicate that high EE parents so designated because of an excess number of critical comments also use significantly more critical remarks in the direct interaction task, while those designated as high EE because of noncritical but overinvolved attitudes, (as indicated in Fig. 2) display less criticism but significantly more intrusive remarks such as telling the patient how he or she thinks or feels and what motivates him or her. It is important to note that subdividing the high EE relatives into those who were predominantly critical, predominantly overinvolved, or those with both characteristics, resulted in significant relationships to the affective style measure. This strategy is in sharp contrast to the dichotomous categorization employed in the British predictive studies. It may be that perhaps the dichotomous grouping is sufficient for prediction of relapse, while further subcategorization of high EE is more useful for analyzing its relationship to other variables.

Expressed Emotion Status and Patient Characteristics

Vaughn and Leff (1976) originally reported that high or low EE status of the relatives could not be explained by patient characteristics such as severe symptomatology or premorbid status. This area is being further explored in a number of ongoing research projects studying the impact of EE on the course of schizophrenia. A pilot analysis by Miklowitz (1981) of data from the Falloon study, however, suggests this issue is more complex than originally suggested by Vaughn and Leff. Of 33 cases, patients from families where the mothers displayed emotionally overinvolved attitudes on the CFI were rated as significantly poorer in premorbid adjustment on the UCLA Social Attainment Scale (Goldstein 1978) than patients whose mothers were highly critical or low EE. These data are presented in Fig. 3 in which a lower score reflects poorer preillness social adjustment. If this finding is sustained for the larger sample, it raises the issue of whether emotional overinvolvement results from having to care for an individual with a long-term history of limited psychosocial competence or whether it in fact contributes to the development of a poor premorbid history.

Further, Miklowitz found that patients categorized as either from low or high EE family environments could not be discriminated in form or severity of schizophrenic symptomatology at admission or shortly following discharge. However, when the high EE cases were subdivided, those from environments designated as high EE solely on the basis of emotional overinvolvement were significantly more symptomatic at discharge than those coming from high EE environments defined by excess criticism as

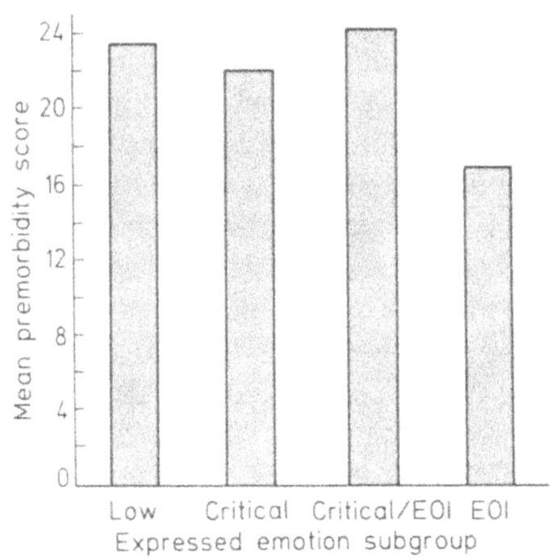

Fig. 3. Relationship between premorbid adjustment scores on the UCLA Social Attainment Scale and parental EE subgroup

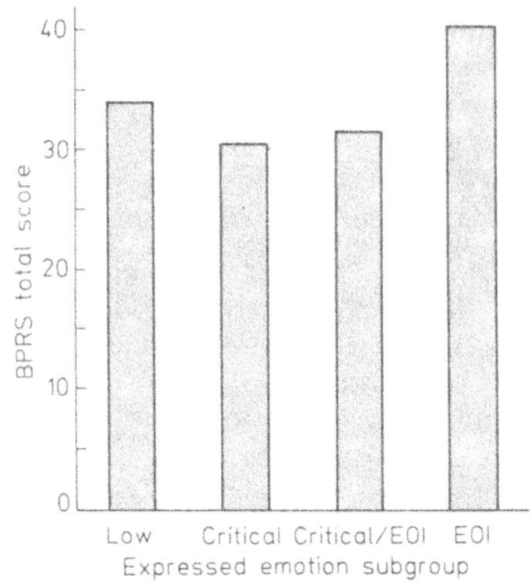

Fig. 4. BPRS scores following discharge and parental EE subgroup

can be seen in Fig. 4. Thus, in this area, as well as in the study on affective style previously mentioned, the strategy of breaking down the high EE construct into substyles has proved fruitful, while the dichotomous grouping of low versus high EE does not always reveal major differences.

Expressed Emotion and Other Parent Characteristics

A fourth area of interest to family researchers in schizophrenia concerns the relationship of EE to other parental attributes shown in previous research to be associated with families of schizophrenics.

Parental communication deviance has been shown in a number of studies to be associated with offspring diagnosed as schizophrenic (Wynne et al. 1976; Jones 1977; Singer 1967; Wild et al. 1975; Wild et al. 1965; Wynne et al. 1975). In the report of the prospective study cited earlier, Doane et al. (1981) found that both communication deviance and a measure similar to EE were independently predictive of the subsequent onset of schizophrenia spectrum disorders in disturbed adolescents. This finding raises the possibility that adding a measure of communication deviance to the EE variable might improve the prediction of relapse in already diagnosed schizophrenics. Currently, several studies are underway which will examine this issue (Falloon et al. 1981; Vaughn et al., to be published).

Cross-cultural Validity of Expressed Emotion

Another very important issue concerning the family's role in the course of schizophrenia is the question of whether findings employing measures such as EE or communication deviance are equally valid for cultural or subcultural groups other than the British and American cohorts studied to date.

In a study currently in progress at UCLA, Karno (1981, personal communication) is attempting to replicate the findings on EE and relapse rate in a sample of Spanish-speaking Mexican-American families of schizophrenics. He has found that the CFI, administered in the household setting, is well accepted and responded to by the population. Preliminary trends from a pilot study of 19 families, suggest a very striking difference in the incidence of low EE relatives in this population from that observed in the studies carried out with Anglo populations. Of the 19 cases whose relatives were administered the CFI in this pilot study, only four cases (or 21% of the families) were categorized as high EE on the basis of Vaughn and Leff's criteria (1976). This is in sharp contrast to the prevalence rate of approximately 67% in the studies by Liberman and by Falloon mentioned earlier. If this finding persists for the larger sample, it raises the very important issue of whether the criteria used for defining high EE in Anglo cultures is appropriate for use in other cultural groups. Low rate of high EE might suggest that Anglo-American criteria used for rating high EE might need to be recalibrated for other cultural settings. Alternatively, however, a lower prevalence rate of high EE cases may be reflective of different familial tolerance levels and response patterns to psychopathology, which might in turn be associated with lower relapse rates.

Very preliminary findings from the World Health Organization collaborative group studying EE and relapse in Chandigar, India also indicate a very low incidence of high EE relatives compared to those found in British and American samples (Day 1982). These two pilot reports suggest that the EE construct is a complex one and perhaps best understood in the context of the socio-ecological parameters of the culture in which it is measured.

Comment

The data reviewed in this paper indicate that recent research on the role of the family in schizophrenia is characterized by a closer attention to methodology and to a more precise specification of family parameters investigated. There appears to be a reasonable congruence between those variables found before the onset of a schizophrenic episode and those which relate to the subsequent course of the disorder once it appears. The strongest evidence for continuity from the prepsychotic to the postpsychotic family environment is for the affective climate of the family as reflected in the interview measure of EE or the interactional coding of AS. Families in which significant others, usually parents, express strongly critical and/or emotional overinvolved (intrusive) attitudes are at higher risk for *onset of* and *relapse for* schizophrenia. The data from the prospective sample indicate that these affective attitudes predict schizophrenia only when associated with high levels of communication deviance. Thus, affective style appears to be a potentiator of life course from a disturbed adolescence to early adult schizophrenia or schizophrenia-like disorders. It does not appear to be uniquely linked to a life course directed towards schizophrenia as numerous other outcomes can be noted when a negative affective style is associated with low levels of parental communication deviance.

The data with regard to the course of schizophrenia also reveal the significant role of parental affective evaluations in predicting relapse. It is not so clear how a family attribute such as communication deviance, which is so significant for predicting onset, relates to relapse. If communication deviance is a necessary family property for the onset of schizophrenia, then it should bear at least a limited relationship to course as all families should manifest the attribute. On the other hand, there are different styles of communication deviance, as we indicated earlier, as well as variation in quantity even in those families designated as high CD. Possibly, form and/or quantitative level of CD can provide additional information about the family environment of the newly released schizophrenic patient which can further aid us in understanding how some environments foster recovery and other potentiate relapse.

References

Brown GW, Birley JLT, Wing JF (1972) Influence of family life on the course of schizophrenic disorders: A replication. Br J Psychiatry 121:241–258

Day R (1982) Research on the course and outcome of schizophrenia in traditional cultures: Some potential implications for psychiatry in the developed countries. In: Goldstein MJ (ed) Preventive Interventions in Schizophrenia: Are We Ready? U.S. Government Printing Office, Washington, D.C.

Doane JA, West KL, Goldstein MJ et al. (1981) Parental communication deviance and affective style: Predictors of subsequent schizophrenic spectrum disorders in vulnerable adolescents. Arch Gen Psychiatry 38:679–685

Falloon IRH, Boyd JL, McGill CW et al. (1981) Family management training in the community care of schizophrenia. In: Goldstein MJ (ed) New Developments in Interventions with Families of Schizophrenics. Jossey-Bass, San Francisco

Garmezy N (1974) Children at risk: The search for the antecedents of schizophrenia. Part II: Ongoing research programs, issues and interventions. Schizophr Bull 9:55–125

Goldstein MJ (1978) Further data concerning the relation between premorbid adjustment and paranoid symptomatology. Schizophr Bull 4:236–243

Goldstein MJ, Rodnick EH, Jones JE, McPherson SR, West KL (1978) Familial precursors of schizophrenia-spectrum disorders. In: Wynne LC, Cromwell RL, Matthysse S (eds) The nature of schizophrenia. John Wiley & Sons, New York, pp 487–498

Jones JE (1977) Patterns of transactional style deviance in the TATs of parents of schizophrenics. Fam Process 16:327–337

Jones JE, Wynne LC, Al-Khayyal M et al. (to be published) Predicting current school competence of high-risk children with a cross-situational measure of parental communication deviance. In: Watt N et al. (eds) Children at Risk for Schizophrenia. Cambridge University Press, New York

Miklowitz DJ (1981) Familial and symptomatic characteristics of schizophrenics living in high and low EE home environments. Master Thesis, University of California, Los Angeles

Leff JP (1976) Schizophrenia and sensitivity to the family environment. Schizophr Bull 2:566–574

Lewis JM (1979) Family interaction behaviors associated with a communication disorder index of risk for schizophrenia. Doctoral dissertation, University of California, Los Angeles

Lewis JM, Rodnick EH, Goldstein MJ (1981) Intrafamilial Interactive Behavior, Parental Communication Deviance and Risk for Schizophrenia. J Abnorm Psychol, vol 49, 5:448–457

Lidz T, Fleck S, Cornelison A (1965) Schizophrenia and the family. International University Press, New York

Lieber DJ (1977) Parental focus of attention in a videotape feedback task as a function of hypothesized risk for offspring schizophrenia. Fam Process 16:467–475

Singer M (1967) Family transactions and schizophrenia: I. Recent research findings. In: Romano J (ed) The origins of schizophrenia: Proceedings of the First Rochester International Conference in Schizophrenia. Excerpta Medica, Amsterdam

Strodtbeck FL (1954) The family as a three-person group. Am Social Rev 19:23–29

Sturgeon D, Kuipers L, Berkowitz R et al. (1981) Psychophysiological responses of schizophrenic patients to high and low expressed emotion relatives. Br J Psychiatry 138:40–45

Tarrier N, Vaughn C, Lader M et al. (1979) Bodily reaction to people and events in schizophrenics. Arch Gen Psychiatry 36:311–315

Vaughn CE, Leff JP (1976) The influence of family and social factors on the course of psychiatric illness: A comparison of schizophrenic and depressed neurotic patients. Br J Psychiatry 129: 125–137

Vaughn C, Snyder KS, Liberman RP et al. (to be published) Family factors in schizophrenic relapse: A replication. Schizophr Bull

Wender PH, Rosenthal D, Kety SS (1968) A psychiatric assessment of the adoptive parents of schizophrenics. In: Rosenthal D, Kety SS (eds) The Transmission of Schizophrenia. Pergamon Press, New York

Wild C, Shapiro L, Golderberg L (1975) Transactional communication disturbances in families of male schizophrenics. Fam Process 14:131–160

Wild C, Singer M, Rosman B et al. (1965) Measuring disordered styles of thinking using the object sorting test on parents of schizophrenic patients. Arch Gen Psychiatry 13:471–476

Wynne L, Singer M, Bartko J et al. (1977) Schizophrenics and their families: Research on parental communication, in psychiatric research. In: Tanner JM (ed) Developments in psychiatric research. Hodder and Stoughton, pp 254–286

Wynne L, Singer M, Toohey M (1975) Communication of the adoptive parents of schizophrenics. In: Jørstad J (ed) Schizophrenia 75: Psychotherapy, Family Studies Research. Universitetsforlaget, Oslo

The Finnish Adoptive Family Study: Adopted-Away Offspring of Schizophrenic Mothers

Pekka Tienari, Anneli Sorri, Mikko Naarala, Ilpo Lahti, Jukka Pohjola, Christina Boström, and Karl-Erik Wahlberg

One limitation of the information obtained from traditional genetic and family-dynamic research has been the fact that the children of disturbed parents have grown up together with their parents. In contrast, when the child is separated from his/her biologic parents at an early age and placed in an adoptive family, discrimination between the hereditary and environmental factors is possible, because the adoptive children receive their genetic characteristics from the biologic parents and their family environment from the adoptive parents. This gives an opportunity to investigate heredity and environment.

Heston and Denny (1968) and Rosenthal et al. (1971) reported more schizophrenia and other psychopathology in the offspring of schizophrenics adopted away as compared with the offspring of nonschizophrenic parents. Lidz et al. (1981) discussed this topic recently and maintained that, on the basis of the findings reported thus far, Rosenthal's Danish study does not provide even the modest evidence of a genetic factor that the authors claim; rather, the results are inconclusive. In contrast to the design of the Finnish study to be described here, the biologic parents have not been interviewed in the Danish study; the diagnostic classifications were based on summaries from hospital records. In addition, no adoption study of schizophrenia has thus far reported data using direct family relationship measures. Rosenthal et al. (1975) indirectly assessed the quality of the relationship between the child and his adoptive parents on the basis of the individual interview data of the children. The degree of psychopathological disorder in the child was then correlated with the quality of the parent-child relationship. Wender et al. (1968, 1974, 1977) tried to investigate the role of parental psychopathology as an environmental variable. Wynne et al. (1976) reported a blind assessment of the individual parental Rorschach protocols obtained from Wender's study (1968). They found that all the 16 parental pairs with a schizophrenic child (regardless of whether they were biologic parents who had reared a schizophrenic child or adoptive parents who had adopted and reared a child who later became schizophrenic) were perfectly separable from the nine adoptive parental pairs in the normal control group.

Methods

Sample Collection

In Finland, as in most countries, the intimacy of adoption is officially protected, which ordinarily prevents one from obtaining information on the biologic parents who have given over their child to be adopted, and on the family that has adopted the child. While planning this project in 1967–1968, we began several negotiatory discussions with various governmental and private organizations. We do not have a national adoption register in Finland. (Most adoptions in Finland take place through a private organization, Pelastakaa Lapset r.y. – "Save the Children Association", with a smaller number of cases adopted through community social boards). It appeared that the best starting point was the patient records of the hospitals and thereafter gradually trying to find a sufficient number of children given over to adoption. Upon this basis, the project was launched in several different stages, expanding until we have now collected a national sample covering the whole of Finland.

First Sample. In 1969–1972, it proved possible to collect records for a total of 9,832 women hospitalized because of schizophrenia. The series thus covered over three million Finns, while about 1.5 million of the population of Finland were excluded (six hospital districts were unable to cooperate at this phase). All the women undergoing hospital therapy in these hospitals on 1 January, 1960, were included in the series. Patient records older than these were omitted because random tests showed that the data in the older records were too vague to yield adequately reliable diagnostic information. In addition, all the women hospitalized between 1 January, 1960, and 30 April, 1970, were included in the series. Both of these groups only included patients whose diagnosis during the hospital therapy had been schizophrenia or paranoid psychosis. The years of birth 1910–1954 were selected as the sample range for the mothers in order to avoid difficulties involved in classification of subjects over 60 years of age when hospitalized for the first time because of schizophrenia.

Information supplied by civil and parish population registers showed which of these women had had a baby and given it over for adoption. Separate inquiry from every parish or register in which the subject in question had been recorded during the course of her life was necessary. The inquiry had to be sent to each register because the information is only entered in the register in which the mother is recorded at the time when the baby is born. The information does not follow the mother as she moves to another locality. Thus, after correspondence with the registers continued for 10 years, we eventually found in this sample 122 children given over for adoption by schizophrenic mothers, 93 of them during the first 4 years of life. In addition to these, 59 children had been given to foster parents without formal adoption, and about 820 children had remained to live with their father after either parental divorce or the mother's death.

Second Sample. We felt that an expansion of the material was necessary for several reasons. One of these was that we wanted the series to represent the whole of Finland. Also, the smallness of the first sample had made it necessary to include for later field study those children adopted away as late as age four; we questioned their suitability for a study separating genetics and environment. We deemed it important that the series include a sufficient number of children adopted away earlier. For these reasons, in the summer of 1978 a request was sent to the six hospital districts in which the collection of material had not been successful in the early 1970s; their inclusion was now possible. Also, the time period for consecutive admissions was extended to 1979. In the second sample, when all the resident population on 1 January, 1960, and the consecutive admissions from 1 January, 1960–1979 were considered, a total of 9,615 new schizophrenic women were found. For both samples, the names and relevant demographic data for 19,447 women were collected. The population registers have been checked in order to find out which of these women, after giving birth to a child, had later on given the child away for adoption. This work has not yet been finished. Since the information of a possible child given away for adoption does not follow the mother if she moves from a given locality, several mothers still have periods in their lives in which our survey does not cover, but each woman has been checked for at least part of her life. We do not expect to find very many children any more, but several thousand inquiries remain to be sent.

We have by now found a total of 274 adopted-away children of schizophrenic mothers. One hundred and eighty-eight of them were placed in the adoptive family during their first 4 years of life, and 26 later than that. In addition, 28 have been adopted abroad and 32 by relatives. The figures have changed slightly during the years because it has sometimes been possible to find out from the registers that the child has been placed in care of relatives or that the adoptive family has moved abroad after the adoption.

Matched Controls. Initially, we picked two control adoptive cases from the files of Pelastakaa Lapset r.y. for each index child. The matching was made by people outside our clinic who were given the criteria and who carried out the procedure quite independently. Because we very soon realized that not all the index cases had been placed through Pelastakaa Lapset r.y., we went on to collect control cases from the community social boards as well. Later, when the number of index children had increased, we decided that it was unnecessary and impractical to identify and investigate a *double* number of controls.

The matched controls have been made comparable with the index group as follows: The age of the adoptive control child and the index child differs by a year at the most; the age of the adoptive parents differs by 10 years at the most; the sex of the child is the same; the age of placement in the family (or the age of adoption) differs by 6 months at the most in such a way that the children in the two series have been placed within the age periods of 0–6 months, 6–12 months, 12–18 months, 18–24 months, 24–30 months, 30–36 months, 36–42 months, 42–48 months, or 48–60 months. The two series are further comparable with regard to social status, the residence of the family (town/country), and the structure of the family (mother + father, only mother or father). The research and control series are numbered at random in such a way that the psychiatrists performing the personal examination are not aware to which group the adoptive family belongs.

Biologic Parents. The identity of the biologic father has been established from records in about half of the cases. Their morbidity data have been obtained, as have the morbidity data of the biologic mothers in the control series. Only if some of the biologic parents have been treated because of psychosis have they been excluded from the control series. Hence some of the biologic parents in the control series have needed psychiatric help for reasons other than psychosis.

The patient records of the biologic mothers have been obtained and copied. Their diagnoses will be confirmed by several psychiatrists performing the classification independently of each other. The final criteria for inclusion or exclusion have not been decided because we believe that an international diagnostic system must be used. Also, we will interview personally as many of the biologic parents as possible. One of our raters has now reviewed the hospital records for 107 mothers (who have given away altogether 115 children). Ninety-five of these mothers have been considered schizophrenic, either definitively or probably, and in 12 cases the diagnosis of schizophrenia seems unlikely.

Field Work with Adoptive Families

In the practical field work, we must examine the index and control families scattered in different parts of Finland. The examination of each family usually takes 2 days (14–16 h). Each family is investigated intensively through family and spouse interviews. The list of questions has been designed to serve as a semistructured interview. The list is made separately for family interview and spouse interview. The total family interview material was used for rating the overall mental health of the families as units.

In addition, the Consensus Rorschach (Loveland et al. 1963) and Interpersonal Perception Method (Laing et al. 1966) tests are given. The Consensus Rorschach is conducted in two parts: the Spouse Rorschach with the parents together is followed by the Family Rorschach in which the parents interact with the child about the task before the whole family attempts to reach consensus. Through this procedure, we hope to get an impression of how the parents teach tasks and interpret ideas to the child. We also believe that it is useful to examine first the relation of the spouses and then the effect of the child's presence on the interspousal relation. The examination procedure is described in more detail elsewhere (Tienari et al. 1981).

Both the parents and the children also are interviewed personally and given individual Rorschach tests after the Consensus Rorschach. The MMPI test is only taken by the adoptive children. An abbreviated version of the WAIS test is used with the adoptees for screening gross intellectual deficiencies, serious visual and other perceptive disorders, and obvious organic differences.

Obviously, investigation with so many field procedures creates practical difficulties, especially as the sample has enlarged. An aid in analysis is that all the interviews and most of the experimental examinations are tape recorded. This makes it possible to carry out comparative blind ratings and reclassifications later on.

The hospital records of the schizophrenic mothers will be reviewed by several psychiatrists independently. In 1982, we will initiate the personal interviews of the biologic parents, both in the index group and in the control group.

Preliminary Results

We have by now investigated most of the first sample of cases collected in 1970–1972 and their matched controls. As to the second sample (collected in 1978–1979), we have focused thus far on those children who were placed in the adoptive families before they were $2^1/_2$ years old. Drawing upon the two samples together, by September 1981 we had contacted about 200 families for fieldwork, of which 180 had been preliminarily scored (of the children, only 178).

Family Mental Health Rating. An illustration of these preliminary data is shown in Table 1, which gives the distribution of the overall ratings of family mental health. Here we present ratings on a scale from 1 to 5. The categories 1 and 2 include "healthy families in the clinical sense," while categories 3, 4 and 5 are "disordered." Category 5 subsumes categories 5–7 that were previously differentiated (Tienari et al. 1981).

1. "*Healthy*": Usually families where anxiety is very slight and the individual boundaries are clearly distinct. Primitive defenses are not significantly used and interaction is unambiguous. There is no open or chronic conflict in the family.
2. "*Mildly disturbed family*": There sometimes is a conflict and observable mild anxiety or depression. Primitive defenses are seldom used. The reality testing in the family is good.
3. "*Neurotic family*": There exist an unresolved conflict of mild or moderate severity. The interactional patterns in the family are restricted. The members easily develop symptoms. Rigid defenses are used. Reality testing is good.
4. "*Rigid, family-syntonic family*": Analogously to the ego-syntonic functioning of individuals, the family that is syntonic itself feels its way of coping to be adequate, but the environment sees it as symptomatic. The homeostasis is rigid. There exists a major chronic unresolved conflict in the family. The level of anxiety is usually low. The external boundaries of the family are strikingly clear.
5. "*Severely disturbed family*": There are boundary function problems for both the individual family members and for the family unit. Primitive defenses are widely

Table 1. The distribution of the mental health ratings of the adoptive families

	Number	Percent
1. "Healthy"	23	13
2. "Mild disturbance"	63	35
3. "Neurotic"	39	22
4. "Rigid family syntonic"	33	18
5. "Severely disturbed"	22	12
Total	180	100
"Mean score"[a]	2.82	

[a] See footnote on p. 26.

Table 2. The distribution of the mental health ratings of the offspring

	Number	Percent
1. Healthy	16	9.0
2. Mild disturbance	86	48.3
3. Neurotic	48	27.0
4. Character disorder	15	8.4
5. Borderline	9	5.1
6. Psychotic	4	2.2
Total	178	100.0
"Mean score"[a]	2.59	

[a] See footnote below.

used. The level of anxiety is high and basic trust low. Reality testing is disturbed for prolonged periods.

The above features are an attempt to describe the most common characteristics of the families in different ratings. We consider the following factors to contribute most significantly to our ratings: Anxiety and its level, boundary functions, quality of interaction, flexibility of homeostasis, "transactional defenses" (Alanen 1980), conflicts, empathy, power relations, reality testing, and basic trust.

From Table 1, we can see that about half (86 out of 180) of the families investigated so far have been rated "healthy in the clinical sense," while the other half (94) is "disordered." The "mean score"[1] of the family ratings is 2.8.

Mental Health Ratings of Adoptive Offspring. The distribution of the mental health ratings of the offspring is presented in Table 2. Each individual is rated on a scale from 1 to 6, where 1 and 2 mean "healthy in the clinical sense" and 3–6 refer to "clinical cases." In this sample, character disorder is mainly descriptive of ego-syntonic cases. The borderline cases have been classified in accordance with Kernberg (1975). In "higher level" borderline states, there are neurotic as well as the borderline features. "Lower level" borderline states are much closer to psychosis, with a virtual absence of stable neurotic defenses and of relatively advanced ego development. Of the 178 children rated so far, 102 (57%) have been rated healthy and 76 (43%) clinically disturbed; 28 of them (16%) have been classified as more severely ill than neurotic. The number of clinical cases is higher than in ordinary population surveys, which is quite understandable. The early environment of the children often has been unusual. The children may have experienced the knowledge that their own parents have not been able (or willing) to take care of them as a narcissistic trauma.

Table 3 shows the mental health ratings of the offspring separately in the index group and in the control group for the first 54 pairs in which both the index cases and

1 The mean scores presented in Table 1 (and in the following tables) should not be regarded as statistical concepts, but rather as illustrative of the figures presented.

Table 3. The mental health ratings of the offspring (54 index cases and their matched controls)

	Offspring of schizophrenics	Offspring of controls
1. Healthy	3	7
2. Mild disturbance	28	21
3. Neurotic	11	20
4. Character disorder	6	4
5. Borderline	3	2
6. Psychotic	3	–
Total	54	54
"Mean score"[a]	2.76	2.50

[a] See footnote on p. 26.

Table 4. The mental health ratings of the adoptive families (54 index cases and their matched controls)

	Offspring of schizophrenics	Offspring of controls
1. "Healthy"	5	9
2. "Mildly disturbed"	23	17
3. "Neurotic"	11	12
4. "Rigid, family-syntonic"	8	13
5. "Severely disturbed"	7	3
Total	54	54
"Mean score"[a]	2.8	2.7

[a] See footnote on p. 26.

their matched controls have been investigated. Twelve of the 54 index cases (22%) have been classified as more severely ill than neurotic, compared with 6 (11%) in the control group. The "mean scores" are 2.8 and 2.5 respectively.

In Table 4, the mental health ratings of the adoptive families in the index group and in the control group have been presented separately. The "severely disturbed families" are slightly overrepresented in the index group.

As can be seen from Table 5, the two groups of offspring have almost the same ratings both in "normal" and in "neurotic" families, whereas in the "more disturbed families" ("rigidly syntonic" and "severely disturbed") there is a clear-cut difference between the index group and the control group. This might mean that the offspring of schizophrenic mothers are more vulnerable when they have been reared in disturbed families.

Table 5. Mental health ratings of offspring in relation to the ratings of their adoptive families (54 index cases and their matched controls)

The rating of the family	Offspring of schizophrenics		Offspring of controls		Total	
	Number	"Mean score"[a]	Number	"Mean score"[a]	Number	"Mean score"[a]
"Healthy" (1–2)	28	2.04	26	2.12	54	2.07
"Neurotic" (3)	10	2.80	12	2.75	22	2.77
"Severe" (4–5)	16	4.00	16	2.94	32	3.47
Total	54	–	54		108	
"Mean score"[a]		2.76		2.50		2.63

[a] See footnote on p. 26.

Table 6. The assessment of offspring in relation to the ratings of their adoptive mothers and fathers

The ratings of the offspring	Adoptive mother		Adoptive father	
	Healthy	Disturbed	Healthy	Disturbed
1. Healthy	13	3	9	5
2. Mild disturbance	54	30	46	34
3. Neurotic	17	30	22	20
4. Character disorder	5	10	2	12
5. Borderline	2	7	2	6
6. Psychotic	2	2	2	1
Total	93	82	83	78
"Mean score"[a]	2.30	2.93	2.37	2.78

[a] See footnote on p. 26.

Both of the parents have been rated individually, using the same scale from 1 to 6 as was used in rating the offspring. If both the mothers and the fathers are divided into two groups, "healthy" (1 and 2) and "disturbed" (3 to 6), the offspring of "healthy" mothers have received a mean score of 2.30 as compared with 2.93 of the offspring of "disturbed" mothers. The difference is less conspicuous in comparison with the fathers – the mean scores are 2.37 and 2.78, respectively. The psychotic cases are evenly distributed, whereas the borderline cases mostly have grown up with disturbed parents. If we consider the two parents together, there is no clear difference between the cases where both the parents are rated "healthy" (2.27) and those where one of them is "disturbed" and the other "healthy" (2.43). But if both of the parents are "disturbed," the offspring have been rated higher (mean score 3.15). Thus, it seems that one "healthy" parent can greatly compensate for the situation.

Table 7. The assessment of offspring in relation to the ratings of their adoptive parents combined

The ratings of the offspring	Both healthy	One disturbed, the other healthy	Both disturbed
1. Healthy	8	5	1
2. Mild disturbance	32	32	14
3. Neurotic	12	16	15
4. Character disorder	2	3	9
5. Borderline	1	–	7
6. Psychotic	1	2	–
Total	56	58	46
"Mean score"[a]	2.27	2.43	3.15

[a] See footnote on p. 26.

Table 8. The mental health ratings of offspring in relation to their age

Age	Offspring of schizophrenics		Offspring of controls	
	Number	"Mean score"[a]	Number	"Mean score"[a]
10–14	6	2.17	13	2.08
15–19	20	2.45	32	2.25
20–24	20	3.05	17	2.65
25–29	11	2.27	23	2.57
30–34	13	3.31	6	2.83
35–39	4	3.50	3	2.67
40–	3	3.33	7	2.57
Total	77		101	
"Mean score"[a]		2.79		2.44

[a] See footnote on p. 26.

Problems and Possible Biases in Our Study

1. Of the 180 offspring investigated so far, 109 (60%) were under 25 years old when interviewed. The mean age of all is 23.3 years. Hence, many of them have not yet passed the age of risk for schizophrenia. Follow-up is therefore necessary. On the other hand, this prospective aspect provides an opportunity to evaluate the families before the offspring's disorder possibly manifests itself. It can be seen from Table 8 that there is a slight tendency for the index children to receive higher ratings at older ages.

2. Another problem concerns the period before the child was placed in the adoptive family. This is really difficult to evaluate. We hope that the interviews of the biologic mothers can give some illumination on this point. The younger group may be

Table 9. The mental health ratings of offspring in relation to their age at adoption

Age at adoption (months)	Offspring of Schizophrenics		Offspring of controls	
	Number	"Mean score"[a]	Number	"Mean score"[a]
0–6	22	3.14	30	2.57
7–18	28	2.68	35	2.49
>18	27	2.63	36	2.28
	77	2.79	101	2.44

[a] See footnote on p. 26.

Table 10. The mental health ratings of offspring in relation to their age at adoption

Age at adoption (months)	Healthy families				Disturbed families			
	Sch[a]		Contr[b]		Sch[a]		Contr[b]	
	N	"Mean score[c]	*N*	"Mean score"[c]	*N*	"Mean score"[c]	*N*	"Mean score"[c]
0–6	9	2.00	12	2.17	13	3.92	18	2.83
7–18	16	2.31	10	2.00	12	3.17	23	2.74
>18	15	2.13	24	1.92	12	3.25	14	2.86
	40	2.18	46	2.00	37	3.46	55	2.80

[a] Offspring of schizophrenics.
[b] Offspring of controls.
[c] See footnote on p. 26.

easier to check somehow through other sources (including information from institutions).

One might perhaps expect that the age of placement into the adoptive home would correlate with the mental health ratings in such a way that late placement correlates with higher scores. As Table 9 shows, this seems not to be the case. In both groups, the children placed into the adoptive family before the age of 6 months score slightly higher (worse) than those placed at the age of 6–18 months; these latter children, in turn, score a bit higher than those who have been placed after 18 months. Thus, the correlation is just the opposite from what we expected.

Table 10 shows that for all ages of adoption, the offspring is more disturbed if reared in a disturbed adoptive family than in a healthy family. The greatest difference is seen between the offspring of schizophrenics adopted early (before 6 months) and placed in disturbed families, as compared with those placed early in healthy families (mean offspring health ratings of 3.92 versus 2.00).

3. The next problem is the fact that the families have been actively contacted instead of their seeking help. We have felt them to be less guilty and less ashamed than the families with an "identified" patient. On the other hand, adoptive families generally seem to have a greater need to explain how they have tried best and how "good" they have been as parents. They feel that their competence and success also is being evaluated.

What probably is more important is that the families are interviewed in their homes and not in an office or in a laboratory. We feel that they are more natural, relaxed, and enthusiastic than they would be in a clinic setting, for example. On the other hand, the interviewer may also be more exposed. Their vigilance may be more variable because of long traveling and often late appointments.

4. Perhaps the biggest problem lies in the fact that one and the same psychiatrist has interviewed and assessed both the families and the individuals. We were not allowed to let more than one person see each family. It is therefore quite natural that someone might suspect that the family ratings have influenced the later ratings of the offspring. We do not believe this to be the case, but have tape-recorded all the interviews, making possible future blind, comparative ratings. Also, all the tests (individual Rorschach, MMPI, Family Rorschach, and Interpersonal Perception Method) are being scored independently and blindly.

Tables 11 and 12 illustrate that the MMPI ratings of the offspring follow the same patterns as the ratings based on interviews. Despite the fact that the ratings of MMPI have been made blindly by a psychologist who was unaware of the clinical data on the families or the individuals, most offspring classified as severely disturbed have been brought up in disturbed adoptive families.

Table 13 illustrates the distribution of the ratings of the offspring (1–6) in relation to the ratings of the families (1–5). As one can see, there is a wide distribution in every group. The child mean scores naturally follow more or less the severity of the ratings of the families. The wide distribution in the table gives an impression that the danger of contamination is not necessarily big. It is interesting that most psychotic cases have grown up in "rigid syntonic families," whereas most of the borderline cases come from "severely disturbed families." This might support the clinical experience suggesting that a rigid and syntonic family only gives the child its own model, a kind

Table 11. The MMPI ratings of the offspring

	Offspring of schizophrenics	Offspring of controls
1. Healthy	25	41
2. Mild disturbance	9	14
3. Severe disturbance	7	3
Total	41	58
"Mean score"[a]	1.56	1.34

[a] See footnote on p. 26.

Table 12. The MMPI ratings of offspring in relation to the ratings of their adoptive families

MMPI	Healthy families		Disturbed families	
	Sch[a]	Contr[b]	Sch[a]	Contr[b]
1. Healthy	14	21	11	20
2. Mild disturbance	6	6	3	8
3. Severe disturbance	1	1	6	2
Total	21	28	20	30
"Mean score"[c]	1.38	1.29	1.75	1.40

[a] Offspring of schizophrenics.
[b] Offspring of controls.
[c] See footnote on p. 26.

Table 13. Distribution of the mental health ratings of the offspring in relation to the ratings of the families (total sample, experimental, and control)

Ratings of the offspring	Ratings of the families[a]				
	1	2	3	4	5
1. Healthy	7	5	3	1	–
2. Mild disturbance	13	44	17	9	3
3. Neurotic	3	13	15	10	7
4. Character disorder	–	–	2	9	4
5. Borderline	–	1	2	–	6
6. Psychotic	–	–	–	3	1
Total	23	63	39	32	21
"Mean score"[b]	1.8	2.2	2.6	3.2	3.8

[a] See Table 1.
[b] See footnote on p. 26.

of family ideal, and that the family prevents any compensatory adult relationships. In more disturbed cases, the children may have better possibilities to distance themselves from their parents' disturbance.

Discussion

If we compare our study with Rosenthal's Danish study from the methodological point of view, we can see that in both studies the interviewer has been blind as to who is the offspring of a schizophrenic and who is the offspring of a control. In Rosenthal's study, the diagnosis of the biologic parents has been based on translated summaries from hospital records. In addition to study of untranslated records, we expect to interview the biologic parents directly. Our sample covers the whole of Finland and is much larger. Most importantly, unlike the Danish study, in the Finnish study the (adoptive) family environment is directly and systematically evaluated.

If we compare our preliminary results with the Danish study, we see that in both studies all the adopted-away offspring who have become schizophrenic have been the biologic offspring of schizophrenics. In our study, 22% (12/54) of the index cases had an illness more severe than neurotic, as compared with 11% (6/54) having a severe disorder in the control cases. In Rosenthal's study, the offspring of definite and possible schizophrenics had a diagnosis of "schizophrenia spectrum" in 26.9% (14/52) as compared to 17.9% (12/67) with all controls. The corresponding figure for the offspring of manic-depressives and those with indefinite diagnoses was 41.6% (10/24) (Lidz 1981).

What seems important in the figures now available is the finding that the index and control groups of offspring do not differ if they have been brought up in relatively undisturbed adoptive families; but if the rearing family is more disturbed, the index adoptees are clearly more disturbed than the control adoptees. Thus, the presumptive genetic vulnerability in the adopted-away offspring appears to interact with the family rearing environment; the preliminary results clearly support a vulnerability/stressor hypothesis.

Summary

A national sample of 274 Finnish, adopted-away offspring of schizophrenic mothers has been identified. Records indicate that 153 of these offspring of 134 mothers were placed in an unrelated Finnish family during their first 4 years of life and are now at age of risk for schizophrenia. They are compared with matched adoptive controls, that is, adopted-away offspring of nonschizophrenic biologic parents. The adoptive families are being investigated thoroughly with family and individual interviews and psychological tests. Preliminary results support the hypothesis that genetic and environmental rearing factors interact in those adoptees who become severely disturbed.

References

Alanen YO (1980) In search of the interactional origin of schizophrenia. In: Hofling CK, Lewis JM (eds) The familiy: evaluation and treatment. Brunner/Mazel, New York, pp 285–314

Heston L, Denney D (1968) Interactions between early life experience and biological factors in schizophrenia. In: Rosenthal D, Kety S (eds) The transmission of schizophrenia. Pergamon, Oxford, pp 363–376

Kernberg O (1975) Borderline conditions and pathological narcissism. Jason Aronson, New York

Laing RD, Philipson H, Lee AR (1966) Interpersonal perception: A theory and a method of research. Tavistock Publications, London

Lidz T, Blatt S, Cook B (1981) Critique of the Danish-American studies of the adopted-away offspring of schizophrenic parents. Am J Psychiat 138(8):1063–1068

Loveland N, Wynne LC, Singer MT (1963) The Family Rorschach: A new method for studying family interaction. Fam Process 2:187–215

Rosenthal D, Wender PH, Kety SS et al. (1971) The adopted-away offspring of schizophrenics. Am J Psychiat 128(3):307–311

Tienari P, Sorri A, Naarala M, Lahti I, Boström C, Wahlberg K-E (1981) The Finnish adoptive family study: Family-dynamic approach on psychosomatics, a preliminary report. Psychiatry Soc Sci 1:107–115

Wender PH, Rosenthal D, Kety SS (1968) A psychiatric assessment of the adoptive parents of schizophrenics. J Psychiat Res 6(suppl 1):235–250

Wender PH, Rosenthal D, Kety SS, Schulsinger F, Welner J (1974) Cross-fostering: A research strategy for clarifying the role of genetic and experiental factors in the etiology of schizophrenia. Arch Gen Psychiat 30:121–128

Wender PH, Rosenthal D, Rainer JD, Greenhill L, Sarlin MB (1977) Schizophrenics' adopting parents: Psychiatric Status. Arch Gen Psychiat 34:777–784

Wynne LC, Singer MT, Toohey ML (1976) Communication of the adoptive parents of schizophrenics. In: Jørstad J, Ugelstad E (eds) Schizophrenia 75: Psychotherapy, family studies, research. Universitetsforlaget, Oslo pp 412–452

The Rochester Risk Research Program: A New Look at Parental Diagnoses and Family Relationships[1]

Lyman C. Wynne and Robert E. Cole

During the past 15 years a major thrust in research on the origins and development of schizophrenia and other mental disorders has been the "risk research" strategy. The rationale and early phases of risk research programs was described most fully by Garmezy (1974) and will be reviewed from a more recent vantage point in a forthcoming volume edited by Watt et al. (in press). Part of the impetus for these programs was dissatisfaction with earlier family studies that began only after an offspring already was mentally ill. Did disturbed family relationships precede or follow the onset of mental disorder in the offspring? To answer this question, there was a growing recognition that prospective longitudinal studies were needed to eliminate retrospective distortions about the sequences in development. On the other hand, studying development of psychopathology longitudinally with random population samples would be prohibitively large and expensive. Therefore, a number of research programs selected samples in which a child was believed to be at increased, preferably "high" risk for later serious difficulties. Because the variety of variables constituting "risk," and the developmental and contextual factors modifying them, are so numerous and interwoven, risk researchers have agreed that a degree of replication across studies, combined with deliberate differences in sampling and in the methods of study used, would accelerate progress optimally. At the University of Rochester Medical Center, a risk research program, begun in 1972, had features in common with other studies and also incorporated a number of distinctive features that need to be identified before one can interpret the findings that are now emerging.

A Model for Risk Research

In most of the risk research programs, a model has been used that emphasizes parental psychopathology as a primary if not sole risk factor. Parental psychopathology, especially schizophrenia, has been assumed to introduce a statistical risk for the offspring both genetically and through the environmental impact upon the children reared with ex-

1 Research reported in this chapter was supported by NIMH grant MH22836, Lyman C. Wynne, Principal Investigator. The authors are indebted for essential contributions to this work by numerous colleagues in the research team, especially Alfred Baldwin, James E Jones, and Patricia Perkins.

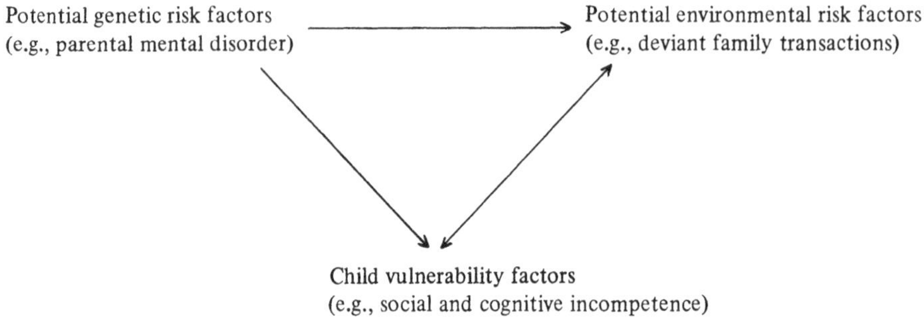

Fig. 1. Model for risk research

posure to the parental illness. As indicated in Fig. 1, the Rochester program included parental psychopathology as one class of risk variable. Additionally, we formally included a hypothesized class of family variables, above and beyond past or current parental psychopathology, namely, the relationships and communication in the family unit (system). Other research has shown that parental psychopathology and parental communication patterns are conceptually and statistically separable (Wynne et al. 1977; Wynne et al. 1976; Johnston and Holzman 1979). Furthermore, it seems obvious that most parent-child relationships over time are not simply a function of parental symptoms and disorder. Such symptoms become part of a matrix to which spouse and offspring contribute – variously ignoring, accentuating, and counteracting what may be only episodic disorder of the diagnosed parent. Therefore, we wished to study family relationships as a class of risk variables, linked to parental diagnosis but also distinctive. In order to minimize biases produced by our interventions, we sought to emphasize procedures in which family members would be interacting directly with one another, without a staff member participating, and with recorded transactions that could be scored by independent investigators.

The UCLA risk research led by Goldstein, Rodnick, and their colleagues (1978) is most similar to the Rochester program in their use of family procedures, but the UCLA study differed by not including parental psychopathology as a risk variable. Thus, the Rochester program has endeavored to examine the interaction of the risk factors of parental psychopathology and family relationships. However, the Rochester program as well as most of the other current studies has not tried to select samples in which risk associated with broader factors such as proverty, race, social, and ethnic differences is studied systematically.

In the model for the Rochester program, the offspring have been studied independently from the parents as well as in transactions with them. Thus, the child measures can be regarded as dependent variables in relation to the predictor, independent variables of parent and family. Although the offspring already may have incipient evidence of vulnerability to later disorder when they are first studied, our research strategy called for selecting a child sample that at least was not under clinical care at the beginning of the study and were in an age group (age 4–10) younger than the age of risk for onset of schizophrenia and major functional psychatric disorders. We gave considerable attention to study of the social and cognitive competence of the children. In addition, psychologic tests and psychophysiologic studies of the children were conducted to identify measures that might prove to be precursors of later disorder. Thus, our strategy called for selecting families with children who might manifest vulnerability to later disorder but who initially would not be seriously ill; the prediction of *later* illness and health in the offspring was a key aspect of the longitudinal design.

In some other risk research programs, offspring have been selected because they were believed to have preschizophrenic clinical symptoms. For example, Fish has selected infants with certain neurologic problems (1975). In the Goldstein-Rodnick UCLA program (1978), 15-year-old adolescents were selected from an outpatient clinic and thus already had some degree of symptomatic disturbance, although not of psychotic proportions. These various distinctions between risk research programs should be carefully noted in order to understand the scope and limitation of the findings.

Sample Selection

In order to obtain reasonably homogeneous grouping for those variables that we regarded as of special interest, we deliberately chose to restrict our sample along certain lines (see Table 1). First, in order to study family communication and transactions directly, we required that the family be intact and available for conjoint meetings, at least at the beginning of the study. Thus the family consisted of at least two parents and an index son, age 4, 7, or 10. Because males and females show psychophysiologic differences and because males tend to show schizophrenic pathology earlier than females, we limited the sample to families with sons. Nearly all of the families also had at least one other offspring who took part in some of the evaluations. Also, in the interest of homogeneity, we limited the samples to Caucasians of social classes I through IV. We assumed that families from the lowest social class (V) would be less able to take part in lengthy research procedures and follow-up and also would introduce many other variables that are undoubtedly important in child development but are presumably not unique to those who develop later serious psychopathology, particularly schizophrenia.

As a risk factor associated with parental psychopathology, we required that at least one parent have a history of hospitalization for psychiatric disorder. Although we

Table 1. University of Rochester child and family study

URCAFS selection criteria (N = 145 families)
1. Intact family available for conjoint meetings a) Two parents b) Index son aged 4, 7, or 10
2. One parent hospitalized in past for psychiatric disorder
3. Caucasian
4. Social classes I–IV

Table 2. Accelerated longitudinal "convergence" design

Ages of index sons "at risk"	
Initially (1972–1976)	At 3-year follow-up
Age 4 →	Age 7
Age 7 →	Age 10
Age 10 →	Age 13

Ages 7 and 10 are convergence points

were especially interested in families with a schizophrenic parent, we assumed that other parental disorders might have similar consequences for the offspring. We hypothesized that a dimensional approach to parental functioning (degrees of severity, chronicity, affectivity, etc.) might be as meaningful, or more so, than typologic psychiatric diagnoses, such as schizophrenia. Thus, we introduced into the study parents with a wide array of hospitalized diagnoses and anticipated, correctly, that these families also would have a wide array of transactional and communicational dysfunctions which then could be defined as risk factors for the offspring.

Another feature of the Rochester program was to try out a "convergence" design for accelerating the construction of a composite, developmental gradient (Bell 1953). Beginning with three cohorts of index sons at ages 4, 7, and 10, we planned to follow them up at ages 7, 10, and 13. Ages 7 and 10 then became points of potential convergence. Thus, in 3 years, the development of the child over an age span of 9 years could be surveyed (see Table 2).

Principal Measures

Parental Psychopathology

Formal diagnoses were obtained for the parents in the study based upon a standardized, structured interview using a modification of the Present State Examination (Wing et al. 1974), as well as a semistructured interview conducted by Dr. John Romano. These interviews provided systematic data permitting diagnosis with alternative criteria as well as ratings on dimensions such as affectivity, paranoid tendencies, and chronicity. Although hospital diagnoses were recorded, diagnoses of the research team have been used in all data analyses, the most recent of these with the final, 1980 DSM-III criteria. Table 3 lists the DSM-III research diagnoses for the 145 index parents in the study. These diagnoses were applicable to the illness during the most recent key hospitalization, but rediagnoses and assessment of current functioning at the time of research evaluation were also carried out. In addition, a considerable series of psychological

Table 3. DSM-III research diagnosis of index parents at key hospitalization

		N[a]
1. Schizophrenia		18 (13)
(N.B.: 63/145 cases given hospital diagnosis of schizophrenia)		
2. "Psychoses not elsewhere classified"		12 (7)
Schizophreniform	2	
Schizoaffective	9 (7)	
Atypical psychosis	1	
3. Bipolar affective disorders		35 (25)
With psychosis	27 (12)	
Without psychosis	8 (3)	
4. Severe unipolar affective disorders		20 (16)
With psychosis	11 (9)	
With melancholia	9 (7)	
5. Personality disorders		30 (15)
Severe (e.g., borderline, schizotypal)	11 (7)	
Moderate (e.g., histrionic)	19 (8)	
6. "Neuroses"		30 (22)
Depression without melancholia	22 (18)	
Anxiety and adjustment disorders	8 (4)	
	Total	145 (98)

[a] The total sample of families was 145. For purposes of data in the present report, *N* was only 98, primarily because this sample excluded families with sons who were 4 years old at initial study and hence did not yet have school ratings.

tests were administered with the parents, including the Rorschach, TAT, WAIS, MMPI, KAS (Katz Adjustment Scales), and a word association test.

A noteworthy point about diagnosis is reflected in the finding that 43% of the 145 index parents had been diagnosed as schizophrenic by DSM-II criteria at the university hospital when they were first seen. However, using DSM-III criteria, only 12% could be diagnosed as schizophrenic, although 35% more received diagnoses of other types of functional psychoses, mostly affective. Because of this remarkable shift in diagnostic categorization, dependent upon the criteria used, it seems necessary to be wary of the meaning of findings based upon vague or unstated diagnostic classifications. That is, what is the significance of alleged genetic or environmental risk from parental schizophrenia when the diagnostic has been obtained with uncertain interview methods and diagnostic criteria?

We have hypothesized that a dimensionalized approach to parental psychopathology may be more illuminating than typologic categories such as those in DSM-III. One dimension in which we have been especially interested is chronicity of illness versus episodic course. Operationally, we have defined this dimension on a six-point scale. For purposes of data analysis in this report, we have simplified the scale to make a distinction between episodic parental illness versus a chronic course, defined as a continuation of symptoms between acute exacerbations or episodes. We also have examined the dimension of affectivity that cuts across diagnostic categories. For the present report we have identified the nonaffective illnesses in our sample as schizophrenia, personality disorders, and anxiety disorders. The affective diagnoses include schizoaffective psychosis, bipolar and unipolar affective disorders (both psychotic and nonpsychotic), and depressive neurosis. Finally, we have classified the sample in terms of psychotic versus nonpsychotic. Here the psychoses include schizophrenia and schizoaffective disorder and a portion of both the bipolar and unipolar affective disorders, while the severe personality disorders and melancholics are among those who have been seriously disturbed but not psychotic.

Family Functioning

Procedures

The Rochester study includes six family interaction and communication procedures (see Table 4). Data from two procedures, the Consensus Rorschach (Loveland et al. 1963) and the Free Play (Baldwin et al. 1982) are available for the present report.

The entire family, at least all those 4 years old and older, participate in the Consensus Rorschach (CR). In this procedure, the parents, and then the whole family, are asked to reach as many agreements as they can about what a Rorschach inkblot looks like to them. The discussion is videotaped with the staff member out of the room. The parents are first presented with the task and do it once without the children present (Spouse Rorschach). They then are asked to explain the task to the children and to reach consensus as a family (Family Rorschach).

Several elements of the task should be noted: (1) There is a specific task – to reach agreement on percepts; (2) an achievement standard is implied – to reach as

Table 4. Rochester family interaction and communication procedures

1. Consensus Rorschach (CR)
   A. Spouse Rorschach (couple alone)
      couple asked to agree
   B. Family Rorschach (whole family)
      1. Parents instruct children in the task
      2. Family tries to reach agreements
2. Free play (FP) 1/2 h with standard toys
   (parents and index son)
3. Clean-up procedure following play
   (whole family)
4. Plan-something-together
   (whole family)
5. How-did-you-meet?
   (couple only)
6. Individual parental Rorschach and TAT
   (interpreted transactionally)

many agreements as possible; (3) limits are imposed – all must sit at a table and participate; (4) responsibility is given to the group for task closure – the family is told to ring the bell when they are done; and (5) certain work is assigned to the parents – they are to instruct the children about the task.

In the Free Play (FP) only the mother, father, and index son participate. No specific task is given; few limits are set; the only request is to ask the family to play as they might at home. A standard set of age-appropriate toys are provided. They are interesting but complicated and difficult enough so that the children might well need parental help, and the parents might be prompted to help. The toys are also interesting to the parents and many parents play alone with them. The parents are not required to play with their children, but no adult pastimes (e.g., magazines, books, etc.) are provided.

Usually, the most active interchange in the Free Play is between father and son. In part, this may be due to the fact that mother most often had been the patient and, understandably, might tend to be less active than the spouse. This would be true of any patient, regardless of the gender. But the father-son interaction may also be due to the family's interpretation of the situation as an age-appropriate opportunity for the father and son to play together. This same pattern occurs in the Free Play of families with sons of comparable age in which there has been no parental mental illness. As a result, we have an opportunity to view, in some detail, the father-child relationships in these families.

Family Measures

For purposes of this program, measures of family functioning were divided into three domains: communication/attention; affect/relationship; and family structure (see Table 5). The applicability of the Consensus Rorschach (CR) and the Free Play (FP) to these various measures of family functioning is indicated in the table. Other domains,

Table 5. Measures of family functioning

1. Domain of communication/attention
   - Communication deviance (CR)
   - Healthy communication (CR)
   - Acknowledgment (CR)
   - Task focus (CR)
2. Domain of affect/relationship
   - Warmth (FP)
   - Positive and negative relationships (CR)
3. Domain of family structure
   - Amount of interaction (CR, FP)
   - "Balance" in role activity (CR, FP)
     - Father/child; mother/child (FP)
     - Parents/children (CR)
     - Husband/wife (FP, CR)

such as family subcultural values and the extrafamilial network, were not studied explicitly except with respect to social class measures.

Communication. Our interest in communication orginates with the work of Singer and Wynne (1966, 1978) regarding communication deviance. We have measures of parental communication deviance from the conjoint family interaction tasks (Doane 1977) as well as from the individual Rorschach sessions (Singer and Wynne 1966), and measures of healthy, constructive communication from both procedures (Al-Khayyal 1980; Schuldberg 1981). Measures of healthy communication are related to, but are not simply the inverse of communication deviance.

Affect. Even in the more critical reviews of the literature describing the relationships between family interaction and individual psychopathology (Jacob 1975), communication and the expression of affect have been regarded as particularly important. The English work on Expressed Emotion (Vaughn and Leff 1976) and the work of Doane et al. (1981) on Affective Style have demonstrated the longitudinal predictive power of measures of family affect. The generalizability of these findings is being intensively studied in centers throughout the world. In our risk research, we use measures of positive and negative affect in the Consensus Rorschach and a measure of positive affect in the Free Play.

Although communication and affect are listed as separate domains, we have found that the measures of communication and affect are related. The correlation in the Family Rorschach between mother's communication deviance and mother's negative affect is 0.31 ($P \leqslant 0.001$, $N = 140$). The correlation for the fathers is 0.35 ($P \leqslant 0.001$). In other studies in which we administer the Camberwell Family Interview (CFI) with the relatives about their schizophrenic children or spouses – from which measures of Expressed Emotion (EE) are taken – communication deviance and critical statements frequently occur not only during the same interview but also during the same passage. We plan to examine how the combination of communication deviance and expressed emotion may compound the developmental impact on the child.

Family Structure. The third domain is family structure. This includes measures of the relative activity and involvement of each of the family members in each task. There are obvious and striking differences between families in the rate and total amount of interaction among family members, in who *initiates* the interaction and to whom the interactions are directed. In one of our procedures, the Free Play, the amount of father-child interaction ranges from two acts per 30 min to over 200 acts, a 100-fold difference, and these differences are quite predictive of child functioning. Thus far, we have focused our attention on the relative activity between or within various family subsystems. In the whole family procedures, we look at the number of speeches made by parents versus children, mother versus father, and each of the children compared to their siblings. In other procedures, we compare the number of mother-to-child initiations with child-to-mother initiations, and father-to-child initiations with child-to-father initiations. The equality, or balance, of parent initiations and child initiations in a task suggest the mutual engagement of parents and children in a relationship in which both share an equal interest, and this relates to the children's cognitive and psychosocial development. For a more detailed description of these measures, see Cole et al. (1982).

Table 6. Measures of child functioning

1. School ratings
   - Teachers — Cognitive
   - Peers — Social-emotional
2. Parental views
   - Global interview ratings
   - Quantified scores
3. Health professional assessments
   - Psychological testing
   - Psychiatric interview
     - Q-sort
     - Global ratings
     - Child diagnosis (if applicable)
4. Psychobiological assessment
   - Obstetrical record review
   - Neurological examination
   - Psychophysiologic and neurophysiologic studies

Child Functioning

Table 6 outlines the four approaches to child assessment in this program: (1) school ratings, by teachers and by peers, (2) parental interview ratings of the child, (3) clinical assessment by psychological testing and psychatric interview, and (4) an array of psychobiological assessments. For purposes of reporting the sample of data here, we shall focus upon the school ratings. These have the special merit of being totally independent of the ratings made from conjoint family interaction and from reports by the parents. The index children were assessed by teachers and peers in comparison with their peers in the same school classroom, without designation of the child as a participant in this study.

Results

Parental Psychopathology

Data about parental psychopathology are important in predicting child school competence, but the significance of such data does not lie in the comparison of schizophrenics versus other diagnostic groups. Viewed across six major diagnostic categories, a simple one-way analysis of variance, listed in Table 3, shows a significant diagnostic effect in the peer ratings [$F(5,95) = 2.59$; $P \leqslant 0.03$] and a near significant effect in the teacher ratings [$F(5,92) = 1.95$; $P \leqslant 0.09$]. However, the children of the schizophrenics do *not* form a unique subset of children; although these children do poorly in school, they are not the only group doing poorly. Indeed, focusing exclusively on any one diagnostic *type* appears relatively uninformative.

Table 7. The relationship between parental illness and children's school functioning

Illness variable	Overall teacher rating[a]	Overall peer rating[a]
Nonaffective (N = 32)	46.1	46.7
Affective (N = 66)	52.1	53.2
	$t = -3.23$	$t = -3.39$
	$P \leqslant 0{,}002$	$P \leqslant 0.001$
Psychotic (N = 51)	51.6	52.2
Nonpsychotic (N = 47)	48.3	49.6
	$t = 1.69$	$t = 1.33$
	$P \leqslant 0.09$	$P \leqslant 0.19$
Chronic (N = 47)	46.5	47.5
Episodic (N = 51)	53.4	54.2
	$t = 4.07$	$t = 3.68$
	$P \leqslant 0.001$	$P \leqslant 0.001$

[a] Teacher and Peer Ratings are constructed so that each child's classroom mean is 50, with a standard deviation of 10. Higher scores reflect better adjustment.

By contrast, categorizing the parental illnesses in dimensional terms is more illuminating. Assessment of an affective-nonaffective dimension and the course of illness as chronic or episodic in the index parent is *highly* correlated with child functioning (see Table 7). Children whose parents have affective and/or episodic illnesses are rated to be performing much better than children whose parents have chronic or nonaffective illnesses. These two effects are independent and additive and together account for 19% [$F(2,95) = 10.95; P \leqslant 0.01$] of the variance in the overall teacher rating, and 16% [$F(2,98) = 8.92; P \leqslant 0.01$] of the variance in the overall peer rating. Strikingly, there are no differences between the children whose parents have had a psychotic versus a nonpsychotic illness.

Family Interaction and Child Functioning

The family interaction variables also are related to the children's functioning. First, both mother's communication deviance and mother's healthy communication in the Family Rorschach are related to the children's school functioning (see Table 8). Second, mother's negative affect in the Family Rorschach and father's positive affect in the Free Play are also related to the children's school ratings.

Third, the measure of activity/balance in the Family Rorschach, i.e., the relative contributions of parents and children, mother and father, and each of the children vis-à-vis their siblings – and the measure of the number and balance of interpersonal initiations between father and child in the Free Play are also related to the children's school ratings.

In summary, the measures of maternal communication and affect from the structured Consensus Rorschach and the measures of paternal warmth and activity/balance

Table 8. Relationship between family interaction and children's school functioning[a]

Consensus Rorschach	Overall teacher rating (N = 98)	Overall peer rating (N = 100)
Mother's healthy communication	0.24 $P \leqslant 0.01$	0.21 $P \leqslant 0.03$
Mother's communication deviance	−0.24 $P \leqslant 0.01$	−0.15 $P \leqslant 0.07$
Mother's negative affect	−0.26 $P \leqslant 0.01$	−0.19 $P \leqslant 0.03$
Parent-child activity/balance	0.23 $P \leqslant 0.01$	0.18 $P \leqslant 0.04$
Free play		
Father's positive affect	0.24 $P \leqslant 0.01$	0.27 $P \leqslant 0.01$
Father-child activity/balance	0.26 $P \leqslant 0.01$	0.31 $P < 0.001$

[a] Pearson product-moments correlations; P values are for one-tailed tests.

in the unstructured Free Play are strongly related to the ratings of the children's school functioning.

We then used a stepwise multiple regression procedure to select the most efficient combination of the six variables listed in Table 8. Variables from each of the three domains of communication, affect, and family structure made independent significant contributions to the prediction of teacher and peer ratings of the children. For the mean teacher's ratings, the composite measure explains 27% [$F(4,90) = 8.30; P \leqslant 0.0001$] of the variance, and also for the mean peer ratings, 27% [$F(3,94) = 11.88; P \leqslant 0.0001$] of the variance was explained. The percentage of variance explained was still higher for the 10-year-old sample compared to the 7-year-olds.

The Combination and Interaction of Parental Psychopathology and Family Interaction

An important question now is: Do these two sets of risk variables, parental illness and family interaction, *each* contribute separately to the children's school functioning, or is knowledge of either one sufficient? It could be hypothesized that because the two sets of risk variables are related, only one set may be sufficient and the other redundant. Our hypothesis, alternatively, was that *both* are important.

To test this hypothesis, we used six variables for the teacher ratings and five for the peer ratings. For assessing parental psychopathology, we used chronic versus episodic course as one variable, and affectivity versus nonaffectivity as the other variable, both previously shown to be predictive of child functioning. Among the family interaction variables in the domain of family structure, we used activity/balance in the father-son interaction in the Free Play procedure. In the affective domain, we used the father-to-son warmth measure from the Free Play and the mother's negative affect statements from the Consensus Rorschach; the latter measure was omitted for the peer ratings because it did not contribute additional variance to the peer-rating prediction. In the communication domain, we used the mother's healthy communication in the Consensus Rorschach.

When the parental and family sets of variables are combined in a stepwise multiple regression, adding the family interaction ratings to the parental psychopathology variables increases the explained variance (R^2) in the teacher ratings of the children from 19% to 34% [$F(6,87) = 7.42; P \leqslant 0.0001$]. In the peer ratings, the explained variance is increased from 16% to 34% [$F(5,91) = 9.18; P \leqslant 0.0001$]. The increase in the explained variance for each set of ratings is significant at $P \leqslant 0.01$. Reversing the procedure and adding the parental psychopathology variables to the family interaction variables increases the explained variance in the teacher and the peer ratings from 27% to 34%. The increase is significant at $P \leqslant 0.02$.

Thus, dimensionalized parental illness variables and family interaction variables *each* contribute significantly and independently to variance in ratings carried out entirely separately in the school by teachers and peers of the index sons in these families.

Discussion and Summary

A number of interesting question remain and are now being investigated. In what way does the parental pathology affect the family interaction in each of the two family procedures? What other factors (SES, family constellation) influence family interaction? What other factors influence the children's functioning (SES, family configuration, the availability of other adults)?

Tentatively, what we are learning, first, is that parental psychopathology appears to be related to child functioning (outside the family in the school setting) in relation to *dimensions* of parental functioning more than to traditional typologic diagnostic categories, such as schizophrenia. Chronicity and a narrow range of affective expression seem to be associated with poor child functioning. In contrast, children of parents who have been ill only episodically and who have a wide range of available affect are more competent.

The advantages of studying an array of parental diagnoses beyond schizophrenia become apparent in this aspect of the study. We should caution, however, that because schizophrenic disorders probably are heterogeneous, some genetically important, severely ill subgroups of schizophrenics may not be represented in this sample of parents. On the other hand, those schizophrenics who are still more impaired are less likely to have become parents, to have produced offspring, and to have contributed to the genetic pool, than are those persons, schizophrenic and otherwise, who are found in this study.

Second, family relationship variables – the presence of healthy communication with a low degree of communication deviance, positive affective relationships, and an age-appropriate balance in interaction between parents and children, with each taking initiative – are associated with favorable or even superior functioning of the children *despite* the risk factor of a parental psychiatric hospitalization. Thus, perhaps the most interesting and important finding to date is the elucidation of family relationship variables that promote health in these families despite the expectable adverse effects of serious parental disorders. On the basis of both genetic and environmental theories, nearly all of these children would be expected to have grim developmental prospects. Instead, the diversity, both positive and negative, in the levels of social and cognitive competence of the children at ages 4, 7, and 10 is striking. This preliminary impression will need to be reexamined in the light of later development of the families and the children. For example, it is quite possible that the impact of affectively labile parents on these children may have consequences in adolescence or later in life, or have genetic relevance at a later age; but such an impact is not yet apparent in the data reported here. Nevertheless, this work should help encourage therapists who view families as constructive resources for psychoeducational and psychotherapeutic programs in which these assets can be tapped to forestall or alleviate developmental impasses and emerging symptomatology.

References

Al-Khayyal M (1980) Healthy parental communcation as a predictor of child competence in families with a schizophrenic and psychiatrically disturbed nonschizophrenic parent. Unpublished Doctoral Dissertation, University of Rochester, Rochester

Baldwin A, Baldwin C, Cole RE (1982) Family free play interaction: setting and methods. In: Baldwin A, Cole RE, Baldwin C (eds) Parent pathology, familiy interaction, and the competence of the child in school. Monographs of the Society for Research in Child Development 47 (No. 4).

Bell RO (1953) Convergence: an accelerated longitudinal approach. Child Development 24:145–152

Cole RE, Baldwin A, Baldwin C, Fisher L (1982) Family interaction in free play and children's social competence. In: Baldwin A, Cole RE, Baldwin C (eds) Parent pathology, family interaction, and the competence of the child in school. Monographs of the Society for Research in Child Development 47 (No. 4)

Doane JA (1977) Parental communication deviance as a predictor of child competence in families with a schizophrenic and nonschizophrenic parent. Unpublished Doctoral Dissertation, University of Rochester, Rochester

Doane JA, Goldstein MJ, Rodnick EH (1981) Parental patterns of affective style and the development of schizophrenia spectrum disorders. Family Process 20:337–349

Fish B (1975) Biologic Antecedents of Psychosis in Children. In: Freedman DX (ed) Biology of the major psychoses: a comparative analysis. Research Publications: Association for Research in Nervous and Mental Disease, vol 54. Raven, New York, pp 49–80

Garmezy N (1974) Children at risk: The search for the antecedents of schizophrenia. Part II: ongoing research programs, issues and interventions. Schizophrenia Bulletin 9:55–125

Goldstein MJ, Rodnick EH, Jones JE, McPherson SR, West KL (1978) Familial precursors of schizophrenia-spectrum disorders. In: Wynne LC, Cromwell RL, Matthysse S (eds) The nature of schizophrenia: New approaches to research and treatment. Wiley, New York, chap 45, pp 487–498

Jacob T (1975) Family interaction in disturbed and normal families: A methodological and substantive review. Psychology Bull 82:33–65

Johnston MH, Holzman PS (1979) Assessing schizophrenic thinking. Jossey-Bass Publishers, San Francisco

Loveland N, Wynne LC, Singer MT (1963) The Family Rorschach: A method for studying family interaction. Family Process 2:187–215

Schuldberg D (1981) Healthy features in the individual rorschach transactions of parents of children at risk for severe mental disorders. Unpublished Doctoral Dissertation, University of California, Berkeley, California

Singer MT, Wynne LC (1966) Principles for scoring communcation defects and deviances in parents of schizophrenics: Rorschach and TAT scoring manuals. Psychiatry 29:260–288

Singer MT, Wynne LC, Toohey ML (1978) Communication disorders and the families of schizophrenics. In: Wynne LC, Cromwell RL, Matthysse S (eds) The nature of schizophrenia: new approaches to research and treatment. Wiley, New York, chap 46, pp 499–511

Vaughn C, Leff J (1976) The influence of family and social factors on the course of psychiatric illness: A comparison of schizophrenic and depressed neurotic parents. Brit J Psychiatry 129: 125–137

Watt NF, Anthony EJ, Wynne LC, Rolf J (eds) (1983) Children at risk for schizophrenia: A longitudinal perspective. Cambridge University Press, New York

Wing JK, Cooper JE, Sartorius N (1974) The description and classification of psychiatric symptoms: An instruction manual for the PSE and CATEGO system. Cambridge University Press, London

Wynne LC, Singer MT, Bartko J, Toohey ML (1977) Schizophrenics and their families: Recent research on parental communication. In: Tanner JM (ed) Developments in psychiatric research. Hodden and Stoughton, London, pp 254–286

Wynne LC, Singer MT, Toohey ML (1976) Communication of the adoptive parents of schizophrenics. In: Jørstad J, Ugelstad E (eds) Schizophrenia 75: psychotherapy, family studies, research. Universitetsforlaget, Oslo, pp 413–452

II. The Treatment Setting

Introduction

The course and outcome of the treatment of schizophrenics depend very much on the context within which patient and therapist meet. The following chapters show how a given view of the problem shapes the treatment strategy and how limited psychotherapeutic resources may be combined in various treatment settings. We learn also that a given treatment model may not be followed despite its proven efficacy and cost efficiency when it runs counter to ruling opinion. We read further how a national change of consciousness and of existing laws may change drastically, not only treatment approaches but also presenting symptomatology.

Ciompi's contribution shows how most treatment approaches to schizophrenics derive either from a one-sided biologic or psychosocial viewpoint. Rather, treatment plans should be individually tailored to a multicausal model of schizophrenia. For this, a multidisciplinary team approach appears necessary. Thus, we may prevent acutely ill patients from being overtaxed by a maximum of psychosocial measures while chronic patients run the risk of obtaining merely custodial care without stimulation for further development.

Alanen presents a complex model for the community-based care of schizophrenic patients. One hundred unselected schizophrenic patients in the Finnish town of Turku were treated by a multidisciplinary team. During the first 2 years of the project 98 were treated with neuroleptics and 81 additionally with various forms of psychotherapy. However, the study shows that the recommendations of the clinical conference which decided on the various treatment approaches could not always be fully realized. Thus, family therapy was carried out only in one-third of the recommended cases, probably due to the fact that at that time the team was not yet acquainted with newer (for example, strategic) approaches. The study shows also that in this multidisciplinary team psychiatric nurses, physicians-in-training, and experienced therapists obtained approximately the same results.

Here is the place to introduce Mosher's well-known Soteria Project which radically abandoned traditional approaches and greatly reduced medication. Rather, the patients lived in a therapeutic community where they were cared for by a nonprofessional staff who had received on-the-job training. Looking back now over 10 years, Mosher finds that their sample of young first admission schizophrenics had better long-term outcomes than a control group from a modern well-equipped psychiatric hospital (criteria: fewer readmissions as in patients and better psychosocial integration). However, this challenge has not been accepted by the decision-making political and psychiatric groups. On the contrary, the project will very likely abandoned for financial reasons.

In contrast, Tranchina and Serra show how in Italy the movement toward a democratic psychiatry has, over the last 20 years, resulted in a change of consciousness. This led in 1975 to a revolution of psychiatric thinking and legislation. Treatment of psychiatric patients was completely handed over to the home and to the community. Inpatient treatments, especially compulsory admissions are no longer possible except in general medical hospitals; psychiatric hospitals are being closed down. This has far-reaching consequences for treatment models and even the phenomenology of psychiatric illness. In addition, this process seems to have had an impact on all medical treatment. Difficulties and resistances in the country are correspondingly great. Patients who for years have been living in psychiatric hospitals can only with great difficulties be reintegrated into the community. Whatever further developments will bring, the authors are probably right when they assume that changes of such magnitude cannot be reversed by new legislation.

Michael Wirsching

How to Improve the Treatment of Schizophrenics: A Multicausal Illness Concept and Its Therapeutic Consequences[1]

Luc Ciompi

The past decades have been marked by significant progress in various fields of schizophrenia research. Drugs, new methods of behavioral, social, and family therapy, as well as modernized psychiatric hospitals have resulted in considerable improvement in the treatment of schizophrenic patients. In addition, a multitude of community-based halfway facilities for flexible crisis intervention and gradual social and vocational rehabilitation have contributed to these favorable developments. Nevertheless, the treatment of schizophrenics still suffers from many serious shortcomings. Many patients are exposed to an appalling discontinuity in long-term treatment by successive teams and institutions or to an often quite antitherapeutic environment or an inappropriate attitude of the professional staff. In our opinion such shortcomings are primarily due to the absence of a differentiated understanding of the disease with adequate integration of the multiple biological and psychosocial factors involved. However, we may be closer to the beginnings of a synthesis than is commonly admitted.

On the basis of a selection of the literature and the author's own contributions, the following chapter endeavors to present various lines of modern thinking and research which seem to converge to form a rather integrative disease concept and open up some promising therapeutic possibilities.

Toward a Multicausal Concept of Schizophrenia

According to practically all modern research – especially genetics research – a great variety of factors must be implicated in the development of schizophrenia. On the somatic and biochemical side, the importance of *genetic influences* has been confirmed by recent studies of families, adoptees, and twins (Gottesman et al. 1976; Kety et al. 1976; Shields 1978; Zerbin-Ruedin 1979). However, is it not yet clear how much of the variance is attributable to genetic factors. In the light of the concordance rates for monozygotic twins as the best currently available indicator, genetic influences seem to be considerably less significant than was suggested some 30 years ago by the well-known Kallmann data (up to 87% concordance) which were distorted by sampling effects (Rosenthal 1969; Kallmann 1976). In their extensive survey, Gottesman and Shields (Gottesman et al. 1976) reported current concordance rates between 14%–50% and

1 Based on a paper published in German in *Der Nervenarzt* 52:506–515, 1981

35%–58% depending on the method of calculation. As they are not completely independent of environmental influences, it seems reasonable to attribute at least half of the variance to nongenetic factors.

The inherited disturbance is generally held to be some specific vulnerability which leads to manifest illness only under certain adverse conditions. The nature of this vulnerability is not clear; *biochemical and psychophysiological defects,* possibly related to synaptic transmission, are often suspected (Iversen 1978). There is also increasing evidence supporting the hypothesis that a higher than average nervous excitability and lability might be important (Spohn et al. 1979). Ongoing longitudinal studies in high-risk children show interesting results as to the predictive values of a variety of neurological, motoric, electrophysiological, and attentional premorbid disorders which might be related to an overall dysfunction of neuroregulatory integration (Mednick et al. 1978; Erlenmeyer-Kimmling et al. 1982). In addition, according to recent research, minimal brain damage caused by *intrauterine and perinatal traumatismes* may play a more significant role than was hitherto admitted (Lempp 1973; Bellak 1979; Keppler et al. 1979). As such trauma occurs more frequently in twins, this factor may contribute to the concordance rates referred to above.

A particular difficulty of schizophrenics – *to handle complex information* – seems to be the common denominator of the multiple *cognitive disorders* which are currently being explored with increasing interest (Broen et al. 1967; Poljakow 1973; Venables 1978; Chapman 1979). These difficulties include maintaining a steady focus of attention, distinguishing between relevant and irrelevant stimuli, forming consistent abstractions and logical classes, and, as a result, difficulties in organizing daily activities in appropriate sequences. According to the concept of "overinclusion" and "response interference," schizophrenics are easily overwhelmed by irrelevant stimuli and suffer therefore from low thresholds of tension, fear, anxiety, emotional lability, and confusion (Mednick 1958; McGhie et al. 1961; Venables et al. 1962; Mirsky et al. 1964; Broen et al. 1967; Brown et al. 1972). This view is fully consistent with modern crisis theory and several interesting, although in part not yet fully confirmed, findings that there is a statistical relationship between acute psychotic breakdowns and psychosocial overstimulation, particularly due to stressful "life events" involving change and readaptation (Birley et al. 1970; Jacobs et al. 1976; Leff 1978; Katschnig 1980; Dohrenwend et al. 1981).

On the other hand, there are also obvious connections between the afore mentioned cognitive disorders and the striking inconsistencies and contradictions in the *intrapsychic organization and in the interpersonal communications of schizophrenics.* These have been described for many years by psychodynamically orientated investigators. They include such phenomena as the inadequate differentiation of the internalized self and object representations, the schizophrenic's failure to distinguish clearly between his own thoughts and feelings and those of others, the excessively permeable ego boundaries, the symbiotic fusional relations with persons playing an important part in their lives (especially with the mother), the marked "blurring of intergenerational boundaries," the "interpersonal enmeshment," and the "emotional overinvolvement" observed in many "families with schizophrenic transactions" (Bateson et al. 1956; Lidz et al. 1957; Haley 1959; Searles 1959; Watzlawick 1969; Hirsch et al. 1975; Stierlin 1975; Minuchin 1977; Selvini-Palazzoli et al. 1977; Goldstein 1978; Singer et al. 1978; Kernberg 1980). These phenomena constitute a fascinating link between organic and psychosocial causes, since they are simultaneously influenced by neurophysiological factors as well as by acquired experience. A link of a similar kind is provided by the as yet barely integrated recent findings regarding the neuronal-dentritic plasticity of the brain under the influence of experience (Cotman 1978). As we have fully developed elsewhere (Ciompi 1982) the best explanation of all these cognitive and communicational disorders is offered by the hypothesis – derived from Piagetian views – that schizophrenics suffer from a partly inherited and partly acquired *defective structuring of the internalized "affective-cognitive system of reference"* that determines our thoughts, feelings, and actions.

Some of our other contributions in this area are mainly concerned with research on the long-term evolution of schizophrenia and on the predictors of successful social and vocational rehabilitation. In the former[2], an initial sample of 1642 narrowly defined schizophrenics, hospitalized in a given catchment area in Switzerland from the beginning of the century to the 1950s, was systematically followed-up into old age and death. Mortality studies on the deceased provided information on the most important selection factors for the 289 survivors who were personally reexamined after an average follow-up of 36.9 years. The following results seem particularly important for the concept of schizophrenia(s):

The enormous variance in long-term evolutions seems incompatible with the idea of a progressive or organic process similarly at work in all cases.

The overall long-term outcome is considerably better than is commonly believed: About one-fourth of the cases evolve to complete remission and an additional one-fourth to one-third to marked improvement; sometimes a favorable development can be observed even after decades of a severe course.

The marked difference between the long-lasting chronic stages with predominantly nonproductive symptoms (affective flatness, passivity, indifference, subdepressivity) on the one hand and the acute productive stages on the other hand suggests possible causal differences.

Among the very few statistically significant predictors, premorbid adaptation and personality structure as well as some possibly related psychopathological features (acuteness of onset and of initial symptomatology) are of particular importance. Surprisingly, genetic factors (as measured by the presence of no, one, or more than one secondary cases in the family) were statistically totally unrelated to long-term outcome.

Very similar results, in particular regarding the low weight of heredity, have been found in the two other major long-term studies that were recently carried out in Europe by Bleuler (1972), and Huber, Gross, and Schüttler (1979). Combined with our own observations, these data suggest that the long-term course of many forms of schizophrenia is more affected by social variables than by "endogenous" disease factors. Our own observations support the outstanding importance of psychosocial variables, as compared to psychopathological ones, in the socioprofessional rehabilitation of chronic schizophrenics (Ciompi et al. 1979). Other findings emphasize the impact environmental influences on the long-term course (effects of social under- and overstimulation,

2 The results of this investigation are published in an untranslated German monograph (Ciompi and Müller 1976). In English, only two brief summaries are available (Ciompi 1980b, c)

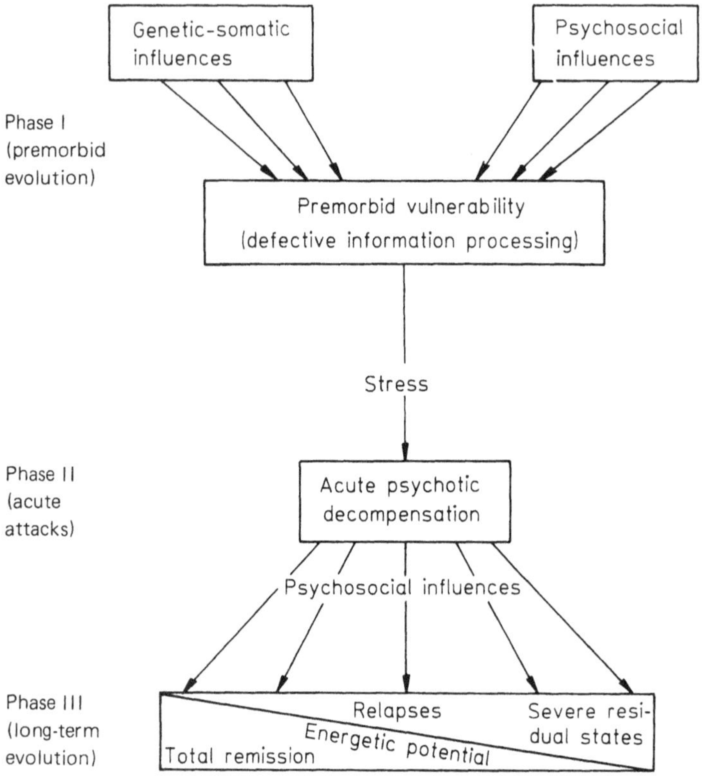

Fig. 1. Three-phase model of schizophrenia

hospital infrastructure and systems of care, family attitudes, and other socioeconomical and cultural factors (Birley et al. 1970; Wing et al. 1970; Brown et al. 1972; Vaughn 1976a, b; Beck 1978; Leff 1978; Sartorius et al. 1978). Thus, "chronic schizophrenia" could even be predominantly a kind of "social artifact" (Ciompi 1980a). The alternative hypothesis would be that the residual states mainly characterized by a massive "reduction of the energetic potential" are caused by an unknown cerebral process, as suggested by the sometimes observed enlargement of the third ventricule (Huber et al. 1979). However, the currently available evidence supporting such a hypothesis seems comparatively weak.

As shown by Fig. 1 [partly derived from Bleuler (1981)], the above considerations and findings can be integrated into a differentiated, *multicausal model of schizophrenia* with three successive phases, possibly induced by quite different clusters of causes.

In the *premorbid phase* variable combinations of genetic, organic, and biochemical factors with psychogenic and sociogenic factors prepare a vulnerable terrain characterized mainly by a particular hypersensitivity and a diminished capacity to handle complex information. In the *acute phase* this vulnerable coping system becomes unbalanced as a result of (relatively) overwhelming demands such as those related to stressful life events, crisis, necessity of change, and adaptation. This entails a gradual increase of tension, agitation, confusion, and ambivalence. Finally, complex biochemical and psychosocial processes lead in vicious circles to the generation of productive psychotic symptoms, such as depersonalization and derealization, cognitive and affective inadequacies, delusions, and hallucinations. After an acute psychotic breakdown, a great variety of possible evolutions – ranging from complete remission and repeated acute relapses to chronic residual states of different degrees – is typical for the *third phase.* The most plausible explanation for this phenomenon is, in our view, the variable pattern of multiple psychosocial influences in interaction with the preexisting impaired coping capacities. Under particularly unfavorable circumstances, including chronic understimulation combined with active defensive withdrawal, a massive reduction of the energetic potential in the sense of severe chronicity and/or institutionalization might occur. Different subgroups of schizophrenia could be characterized by different evolutionary pathways through the mentioned clusters of influences.

General Therapeutic Consequences

As we have pointed out before, this integrative model leads to certain practical conclusions and *general therapeutic principles* whose value has in part already been well confirmed. If the various schizophrenic symptoms are indeed predominantly the result of a reduced capacity to process complex information (in the broad sense, including a whole range of environmental influences which may be summarized as "psychosocial overstimulation or understimulation"), *the simplification on any information input* would appear to be one of the most important general principles in the treatment of schizophrenics. In practice this implies the following:

The utmost simplicity, clarity, and coherence is necessary not only in all interpersonal communcations (e.g., messages about thoughts and feelings, demands, expectations, programs, etc.) but also in the whole physical therapeutic environment (house and room setting, architecture, functioning of the environmental, social, and communication systems).

States mainly characterized by acute productive symptoms require a graded reduction of psychosocial stimuli in the broad sense, including communications, demands, and information, as well as other environmental characteristics.

States mainly characterized by chronic unproductive symptoms call for a cautious, graded increase of psychosocial stimuli, including again interpersonal communications of all types *and* the environmental setting.

We shall now use the initially mentioned critique as a starting point to discuss in greater detail the application of such principles on the basis of recent surveys (Bennet 1978; Goldstein 1978; Wing 1978; Mosher et al. 1980) and of our own experience.

Lack of Coherence in Long-Term Treatment Programs

In spite of considerable local differences it seems justified to maintain that, on the whole, the standard concepts of long-term schizophrenia therapy are not yet as well-defined and consistent as they ought to be in the light of the above principles. Short-term or long-term hospitalizations, drug therapy, occupational or work therapy, and additional activities such as group therapy, behavior therapy, or art therapy are rarely integrated into a long-term program of sufficient coherence to ensure for everybody involved (patients, families, and nursing personnel) the desirable clear-cut and simple global information. In the acute phase patients are, as a rule, exposed to an appalling lack of continuity as far as environment and human contacts are concerned. In the course of a few weeks they may pass through three or four hospital departments, each with its own staff, and in addition be exposed to the incessant coming and going of equally bewildered fellow patients. In other words, the already confused psychotic patient is overwhelmed by new impressions which would be difficult to handle even for a healthy person. Obviously, all this adds to fear, tension, and confusion which then have to be controlled by massive doses of neuroleptics and measures of restraint. The result is a vicious circle which increasingly affects the remaining healthy coping abilities.

When the patient leaves the hospital the lack of continuity is even more pronounced. If any posthospital treatment is provided at all – and that is by no means always the case – it is only very rarely organized as a comprehensive therapeutic program ensuring effective coordination and cooperation with external caseworkers. Often, vocational and social rehabilitation programs do not come into force until the most propitious moment has long passed. Alternating phases of hospitalization and releases contribute to these discontinuities. After several unsuccessful attempts at active escape from the vicious cycle, the most likely and emotionally economical solution consists in resignation and withdrawal into indifference and passivity, i.e., into precisely those defective conditions which are – certainly not by accident – centered on a "reduction of the energetic potential."

What Can Be Done to Change This Situation?

In the first place the situation can be improved by a greater awareness of the afore mentioned shortcomings and their gradual elimination from the daily hospital routine. The next step is the modification of long-term treatment programs and structures in accordance with the principles discussed. The emphasis should be on small and quiet therapeutic units in natural settings with as few staff changes as possible. Such units already exist in small therapeutic communities and sometimes also within traditional hospitals. An example of the former is the exceptionally well-documented Soteria Project which was founded by Mosher et al. Up to now approximately 200 young acute schizophrenics have been successfully treated in this six-patient center with its unconventional setting (Mosher et al. 1975; Mosher 1978). Other authors report similar positive experiences (Mosher et al. 1980). Small group homes have also proved to be an excellent solution for the reintegration of long-term hospital patients into the community (Capstick 1973; Sandall et al. 1975; Ciompi 1978).

According to a recent survey (Mosher et al. 1980), the success of combined psychosocial treatment programs increases with the degree of their structural clarity. In their particularly thorough study Paul and Lentz (Paul et al. 1977) arrived at the following list of the most effective factors:

1. Treatment as „client", not "patient"
2. Induction of specific, positive expectations
3. Structured activities with progressive handing over of responsibility
4. Emphasis on action instead of explanation
5. Organized, structured programs
6. Stable, predictable environment
7. Focusing on concrete skills in household, profession, etc.
8. Establishing of contacts with the community
9. Supportive aftercare

Over a 5-year period such programs were clearly superior to a more traditional treatment, while environmental approaches of the therapeutic community type were of intermediate efficacy. Numerous other findings speak for the importance of a supporting social network (Hogarty et al. 1973; Hogarty et al. 1974; Sartorius et al. 1978). For example, patients in developing countries have significantly better courses in comparison with the evolutions observed in industrialized countries. In the author's own experience (Ciompi 1977, 1979), the most suitable objectives for long-term programs are very concrete social aims that are easily grasped by patients, helpers, and families rather than vague psychopathological or psychodynamic changes. The former can be represented along the following two (combinable) axes of living and working conditions:

Living Axis	*Working Axis*
1. Closed hospital unit	1. No work
2. Open hospital unit	2. Occupational therapy
3. Day or night hospital	3. Work therapy
4. Residential or transitional home	4. Rehabilitation workshop
5. Sheltered group home	5. Sheltered workshop
6. Semisheltered group home	6. Semisheltered work environment
7. Normal living environment	7. Normal work environment

Partial aims are formulated and objectified along both axes, e.g. with reference to social and work behavior scales (Imfeld 1977; Drezdowics-Parizek 1980). Appropriate, clearly conceptualized programs can then be set up accordingly. It is important in this context to be constantly aware of the already mentioned links between psychosocial overstimulation and increased tension on the one hand, and understimulation and increased passivity on the other hand (Wing and Brown 1970). For 81 predominantly schizophrenic long-term patients, we reached 72% success within a year on the living axis (at least grade 5, see above), 36% success on the work axis (at least grade 6), and 26% success simultaneously on both axes (Ciompi et al. 1979). American authors expect 20%–30% work success and a 40%–50% rehospitalisation rate within a year

(Anthony et al. 1972; Anthony et al. 1978). Outpatient aftercare doubled or tripled the relapse-free period (Beard et al. 1978).

Small multidisciplinary teams (e.g., psychiatrist, social worker, nurse) have proved to be effective in *ensuring adequate continuity* in spite of changing places and situations. They accompany the patient through the different stages of his long-term rehabilitation program in which several institutions are involved, and keep in constant contact with the family as well as with the various participating professional workers. This solution is much easier in a sectorized care system where the same team is responsible for inpatient care as well as for outpatient care. Also private psychiatrists or family doctors can play an important role in ensuring continuity. As a rule, long-term helpers and their programs must be placed in a hierarchically higher position than short-term helpers (Parras 1979).

Regarding the place of *pharmacotherapy* in sociotherapeutic programs, it appears from various studies that neuroleptics reduce the frequency of relapses and enhance the results of sociotherapy (Freeman 1978). According to Goldberg et al. (1977), 80% of patients treated with placebo suffered relapses within a period of 2 years compared to only 48% of those treated with neuroleptics. Additional sociotherapy reduced the relapse rate to 37% and significantly improved social adaptation. It is not yet clear, however, how long medication should be continued after a remission. In view of the increase of passivity and the apparently high incidence of irreversible tardive dyskinesias – according to Freeman up to 40% (Freeman 1978) – the well-known findings of Brown et al. (1972) and Vaughn and Leff (1976a, b) are of particular interest: neuroleptics reduce the frequency of relapses predominantly in patients with close contacts to so-called "emotional overinvolvement"-families, while they are practically ineffective in patients living in families with "low expressed emotions". Another important observation is that in a relaxed holding environment agitated schizophrenics can become calm within 2–3 days virtually without medication (Matthews et al. 1979). Neuroleptic drugs are therefore especially indicated when there is a danger of emotional overtaxation. Where this is not the case, they are probably superfluous, in the long run, and sometimes harmful (Gardos et al. 1976; Anthony et al. 1978). Also our own long-term investigations showed many former schizophrenics to have remained free of relapses for decades although they were not on neuroleptics.

Therapeutic Environment and Attitude Toward Schizophrenics

The therapeutic environment of acute schizophrenics is usually characterized by psychosocial overstimulation and therefore inconsistent with the demand for utmost simplicity and clarity throughout the cognitive-affective area. Even when it is divided into small wards, a traditional hospital can never equal the transparent setting of small autonomous treatment units of the Soteria type, for instance. However, it should not be overlooked that *acute cases* are easily overtaxed by therapeutic community activities, for example of the Maxwell Jones type (Spadoni et al. 1969; Goldberg et al. 1977). There are occasions when it is important for patient and co-worker to stay quietly together without doing or saying anything in particular. The concept of a reduced

Table 1. Unfavorable and favorable milieu influences

Pathological milieu (e.g., family, institution)	Psychopathological phenomena	Therapeutic milieu
Overstimulating, tense, agitated, complex, artificial setting with anonymous, unstable large group	Productive psychotic symptoms (tension, anxiety, agitation, confusion, inattention, thought disorders)	Reduction of stimuli; relaxed, small, neutral setting with personified, stable small group interpersonal relations
Symbiotic interpersonal relations, forced consensus, denial of differences, pseudomutuality	Blurred ego-limits, hypersensitivity, incapacity for conflict, negation, denial	Clear demarcation of persons, recognition of differences in opinion, feelings, and behavior
Irrationality, mystification, vagueness, ambiguity	Irrationality, vagueness, distortion	Rationality, clarity, simplicity
Contradictory implicit expectations and communications (double bind)	Ambivalence, derealization, depersonalization, delusions, hallucinations	Unequivocal demands and prohibitions, clear explicit expectations
Distrust, invalidation, intolerance	Distrust and anger, low self–esteem	Trust, validation of thoughts and feelings, tolerance
Lack of understanding and engagement, coldness, indifference	Disappointment, dysphoria, withdrawal	Understanding, warmth, support, engagement, dialogue, explanations
Infantilization, dependency, lack of responsibility	Regression, infantilism, dependency, incompetence	Autonomy, responsibility
Poverty of stimulation, intellectual and affective narrowness, rigidity, stereotypes	Affective withdrawal, emotional flattening, passivity, indifference, rigidification, stereotypes, mannerisms	Sufficient intellectual and affective stimulation, openness, flexibility, mobility

capacity for the processing of complex information is also in agreement with the observation that excessively blurred identity and status differences in patient-staff relationships appear to have an unfavorable effect on schizophrenics (Beck 1978).

On the other hand in *patients with chronic residual conditions* the greatest danger lies in the understimulation prevailing in old-fashioned and understaffed, rigidly organized hospital departments, nursing homes, or other care facilities. Clearly structured behavioral and sociotherapeutic programs, with opportunities for gradual progression in a network of small half-way institutions, occasionally combined with provoked crisis techniques have been shown to exert the most beneficial effect (Ciompi 1977; Paul et al. 1977; Anthony et al. 1978; Mosher et al. 1980).

By further developing a conceptualization proposed by Mosher (1978), various unfavorable environmental influences can be linked to corresponding behavior disturbances (Table 1, columns 1 and 2). Obviously, exposure to the opposite influences (column 3), whose quality is in striking agreement with the methods and aims of modern environmental and family therapy, should therefore have beneficial effects. Table 1 shows that the presence in the environment of tension, discontinuity, unpredictability refusal, coldness, contradictoriness, irrationality, infantiliation, and stereotyping is bound to aggravate, and even to induce, similiar phenomena in the hypersensitive schizophrenic, while calmness, clarity, simplicity, and trust appear to be particularly favorable. Thus, the attitude (and personality) of the attending staff is of vital importance. Staff members should not be assigned at random to work with these vulnerable patients, as has been hitherto the case, but must be very carefully selected and trained (Mosher et al. 1973) – a claim which, even if unusual, is certainly not exaggerated in the view of the enormous weight and severity of schizophrenia.

Conclusion

The proposed multicausal concept of schizophrenia, integrating genetic, organic, and biochemical factors as well as psychosocial ones, seems to lead to surprisingly coherent therapeutic consequences whose practical relevance and value has already been confirmed to some extent. However, it must be realized that most of the discussed research findings concern only partial aspects of the overall treatment concept that has been tentatively developed in this paper. Research strategies with appropriate tests for a critical investigation of the global efficiency of the various aspects involved remain largely to be developed, as does in many places the required infrastructure. Furthermore, progress is delayed by ideological barriers obstructing the free flow of ideas between representatives of different theories and approaches. Nevertheless, there is one favorable point concerning the proposed methods which must be particularly stressed. The emphasis is not on complicated techniques accessible only to specialists with long years of training (psychoanalysts, family, system and behavior therapists), although particular attention is given precisely to their contributions. On the contrary the therapeutic principles proposed in this paper are very straight forward. Essentially, they correspond to an ancient commonsense wisdom: More than anything else, the "insane" are confused, anxious, hypersensitive, and vulnerable people; therefore, anything contributing to a relaxed, simple, clearly defined environment will have a beneficial effect on the intricate pattern of their thoughts and emotions. Such an approach makes sense not only to the medical specialists but also – and this is far more important in everyday life – to the nursing staff as well as to family members, employers, and lay helpers. Together with the professionals they become able to lay, on these grounds, solid therapeutic foundations without which even the most sophisticated medical treatments will remain suspended in a vacuum, so to speak. Inevitably, the insights and progress achieved during the short therapeutic sessions will continually be invalidated by the negative feedback of experiences from the daily social environment. In fact, a number of theoretical and practical reasons suggest that the polarizing of the entire interdependant, intrapersonal, and interpersonal therapeutic field in one clearly defined direction is the most important prerequisite for a successful therapeutic process. Obviously, this general demand is nothing else but the logical extension of the claim for *a simplified in formation input which appears as the central therapeutic principle in the proposed approach to schizophrenia.*

Summary

On the basis of a synthesis of the recent literature, the usual therapy for schizophrenics is criticized with respect to an often overly one-sided concept of the illness, a lack of clarity and continuity in long-term treatment programs, an unfavorable therapeutic environment, and an inappropriate attitude toward the patients. Schizophrenia is understood as an affliction in which manifold congenital and acquired components lead to a vulnerable premorbid personality with an unclear structure of the internalized reference and coping systems, with disturbed information processing mechanisms, and an increased tendency to psychotic reactions to stress. The long-term development seems to be stronly influenced by psychosocial factors. For this reason in therapy it is essential to provide a maximum of clarity, simplicity, and continuity of all therapeutic measures, including the structure of the therapeutic setting and the communicational attitudes toward the patients. Overstimulation as well as understimulation are to be systematically avoided. In the light of the literature and his own experience the author analyzes the consequences of neglecting these principles, and indicates the possibilities of their practical application.

Bibliography

Anthony WA, Buell GJ, Sharrat S, Althoff ME (1972) The efficacy of psychiatric rehabilitation. Psychol Bull 78:447–456

Anthony WA, Cohen RR, Vitalo R (1978) The measurement of rehabilitation outcome. Schizophr Bull 4:365–383

Bateson G, Jackson DD, Haley J, Weakland JW (1956) Towards a theory of schizophrenia. Behav Sci 1:246–251

Beard JH, Malamud TJ, Rossman E (1978) Psychiatric rehabilitation and long-term rehospitalisation rates: The findings of two research studies. Schizophr Bull 4:622–635

Beck JC (1978) Social influences on the prognosis of schizophrenia. Schizophr Bull 4:86–101

Bellak L (ed) (1979) Psychiatric aspects of minimal brain dysfunction in adults. Grune and Stratton, New York San Francisco London

Bennet D (1978) Social forms of psychiatric treatment. In: Wing JK (ed) Schizophrenia. Toward a new synthesis. Pergamon, London/Grune and Stratton, New York

Birley JL, Brown GW (1970) Crises and life changes preceeding the outset of acute schizophrenia: Clinical aspects. Br J Psychiatry 116:327–333

Bleuler M (1972) Die schizophrenen Geistesstörungen im Lichte langjähriger Kranken- und Familiengeschichten. Thieme, Stuttgart

Bleuler M (1981) Einzelkrankheiten in der Schizophreniegruppe? In: Huber G (ed) Schizophrenie. Stand und Entwicklungstendenzen der Forschung. Schattauer, Stuttgart New York

Broen WE, Storms LH (1967) A theory of response-interference in schizophrenia. In: Maher BA (ed) Progress in experimental personality research. Academic Press, New York London

Brown GW, Birley JTL, Wink JK (1972) The influence of family life on the course of schizophrenic disorders: A replication. Br J Psychiatry 121:241–258

Capstick N (1973) Group homes: Rehabilitation of the long-stay patient in the community. Proc R Soc Med 66:1229–1230

Chapman L (1979) Recent advances in the study of schizophrenic cognition. Schizophr Bull 5: 568–580

Ciompi L (1977) Gedanken zu den therapeutischen Möglichkeiten einer Technik der provozierten Krise. Psychiatr Clin 10:96–101
Ciompi L (1978) Un élément précieux dans un service differencié de réadaptation socio-psychiatrique: L'appartment protégé. Information Psychiatrique 54:5–9
Ciompi L (1980a) Ist die chronische Schizophrenie ein Artefakt? Argumente und Gegenargumente. Fortschr Neurol Psychiatr 48:237–248
Ciompi L (1980b) Catamnestic long-term studies on the course of life of schizophrenics. Schizophr Bull 6:606–618
Ciompi L (1980c) The natural history of schizophrenia in the long term. Br J Psychiatry 136: 413–420
Ciompi L (1982) Affektlogik. Die Struktur der Psyche und ihre Entwicklung. Ein Beitrag zur Schizophrenieforschung. Klett, Stuttgart
Ciompi L, Mueller C (1976) Lebensweg und Alter der Schizophrenen. Eine katamnestische Langzeitstudie bis ins Senium. Springer, Berlin Heidelberg New York
Ciompi L, Ague C, Dauwalder JP (1977) Ein Forschungsprogramm über die Rehabilitation psychisch Kranker. I. Konzept und methodologische Probleme. Nervenarzt 48:12–18
Ciompi L, Dauwalder JP, Ague C (1979) Ein Forschungsprogramm zur Rehabilitation psychisch Kranker. III. Längsschnittuntersuchungen zum Rehabilitationserfolg und zur Prognostik. Nervenarzt 50:366–378
Cotman CW (1978) Neuronal plasticity. Raven, New York
Dohrenwend BP, Egri G (1981) Stressful life events and schizophrenia. Schizophr Bull 7:12–23
Drezdowics-Parizek J (1980) Konstruktion einer Schätzskala zum Sozialverhalten. Lizenziatsarbeit, Universität Bern
Erlenmeyer-Kimling L, Cornblatt B, Friedman D, Marcuse Y, Rutschmann J, Simmens S, Davi S (1982) Neurological, electrophysiological and attentional deviations in children at risk for schizophrenia. In: Henn FA, Nasrallah HA (eds) Schizophrenia as a brain disease. Oxford University Press, New York Toronto, pp 61–98
Freeman H (1978) Pharmacological treatment and managment. In: Wing JK (ed) Schizophrenia. Toward a new synthesis. Academic Press, London/Grune and Stratton, New York, pp 167–187
Gardos G, Cole JD (1976) Maintenace antipsychotic therapy: Is the cure worse than the disease? Am J Psychiatry 133:32–36
Goldberg SC, Schooler NR, Hogarty GE, Roper M (1977) Prediction of relapse in schizophrenic outpatients treated by drug and sociotherapy. Arch Gen Psychiatry 34:171–184
Goldstein WN (1978) Toward an integrated theory of schizophrenia. Schizophr Bull 4:426–434
Gottesman II, Shields J (1976) A critical review of recent adoptation, twin, and family studies on schizophrenia: Behavioral genetics perspectives. Schizophr Bull 2:360–398
Haley J (1959) The family of the schizophrenic: A model system. J Nerv Ment Dis 129:337–375
Hirsch SR, Leff JP (1975) Abnormalities in parents of schizophrenics. Oxford University Press, London
Hogarty GE, Goldberg SC, and the Collaborative Study Group (1973) Drug and sociotherapy in the aftercare of schizophrenic patients: One-year-relapse rates. Arch Gen Psychiatry 28:54–65
Hogarty GE, Goldberg SC, Schooler NR, Ulrich RF, and the Collaborative Study Group (1974) Drug and sociotherapy in the aftercare of schizophrenic patients II. Two year relapse rates. Arch Gen Psychiatry 31:603–608
Huber G, Gross G, Schüttler R (1979) Schizophrenie. Eine Verlaufs- und sozialpsychiatrische Langzeitstudie. Springer, Berlin Heidelberg New York
Imfeld M-Ch (1977) Berufliche Rehabilitation ehemaliger psychiatrischer Patienten. Konstruktion einer Beobachtungsskala für Arbeitsverhalten. Lizenziatsarbeit, Universität Bern
Iversen LL (1978) Biochemical and pharmalogical studies: The Dopamine hypothesis. In: Wing JK (ed) Schizophrenia. Towards a new synthesis. Academic Press, London/Grune and Stratton, New York, pp 89–116
Jacobs S, Myers I (1976) Recent life events and acute schizophrenic psychosis: A controled study. J Nerv Ment Dis 162:75–87
Kallmann FJ (1946) The genetic theory of schizophrenia: An analysis of 691 schizophrenic twin index families. Am J Psychiatry 103:309–322
Katschnig H (1980) Sozialer Stress und psychische Erkrankung. Urban und Schwarzenberg, München Wien Baltimore

Keppler K, Lempp R, Pascheday D, Rebmann HE, Rupps R (1979) Die frühkindliche Anamnese der Schizophrenen. Nervenarzt 50:719–724

Kernberg OF (1980) Internal world and external reality. Object relation theory applied. Aronson, New York London

Kety SS, Rosenthal D, Wender PH, Schulsinger F (1976) Studies based on a total sample of adopted individuals and their relatives: why they were necessary, what they demonstrated and failed to demonstrate. Schizophr Bull 2:413–428

Leff J (1978) Social and psychosocial causes of the acute attack. In: Wing JK (ed) Schizophrenia. Toward a new systhesis. Academic Press, London/Grune and Stratton, New York, pp 139–165

Lempp R (1973) Psychosen im Kindes- und Jugendalter – eine Realitätsbezugsstörung. Huber, Bern Stuttgart Wien

Lidz T, Cornelison AR, Fleck S, Terry D (1957) The intrafamilial environment of schizophrenic patients: II. Marital schism and marital skew. Am J Psychiatry 114:241–248

Matthews SM, Roper MT, Mosher LR, Menn AZ (1979) A non-neuroleptic treatment of schizophrenia: Analysis of the two-year postdischarge risk of relapse. Schizophr Bull 5(2):322–333

McGhie A, Chapman J (1961) Disorders of attention and perception in early schizophrenia. Br J Medi Psychol 34:103–117

Mednick SA (1958) A learning theory approach to research in schizophrenia. Psychological Bull 55:316–327

Mednick SA, Schulsinger F, Teasdale TW, Schulsinger H, Venables PH, Rock DR (1978) Schizophrenia in high-risk children. Sex differences in predisposing factors. In: Serban G (ed) Cognitive defects in the development of mental illness. Brunner & Mazel, New York, pp 169–197

Minuchin S (1974) Families and family therapy. Harvard University Press, Cambridge/Mass

Mirsky AF, Kornetzky C (1964) On the dissimilar effects of drugs on the digit symbol substitution and continuous performance tests. Psychopharmacologia 5:161–177

Mosher LR (1978) The surrogate "family", an alternative to hospitalisation. In: Shershow JC (ed). Schizophrenia: Science and practice. Harvard University Press, Cambridge/Mass, pp 223–239

Mosher LR, Reifman A, Menn A (1973) Characteristics of nonprofessionals serving as primary therapists for acute schizophrenics. Hosp Community Psychiatry 24(6):391–396

Mosher LR, Menn AZ, Matthews S (1975) Soteria. Evaluation of a home-based treatment for schizophrenia. Am J Orthopsychiatry 46(3):455–467

Mosher LR, Keith SJ (1980) Psychosocial treatment: Individual, group, family and community support approaches. Schizophr Bull 6:10–41

Parras A (1979) The mental hospital revisited: a proposal. Schizophr Bull 5:223–226

Paul GL, Lentz RJ (1977) Psychosocial treatment of chronic mental patients. Milieu versus social learning programms. Harvard University Press, Cambridge/Mass, London

Poljakow J (1973) Schizophrenie und Erkenntnistätigkeit. Hippokrates, Stuttgart

Rosenthal D (1969) Problems of sampling and diagnosis in the major twin studies of schizophrenia. Schizophr Bull 1:11–26

Sandall H, Hawley TT, Gordon GC (1975) The St. Louis community homes program: Graduated support for long-term care. Am J Psychiatry 132:617–622

Sartorius N, Jablensky A, Shapiro R (1978) Cross-cultural differences in the short-term prognosis for schizophrenic psychoses. Schizophr Bull 4:102–113

Searles HF (1959) The effort to drive the other person crazy. Br J Medical Psychology 32:1–19

Selvini-Palazzoli M, Boscolo L, Cecchin G, Prata G (1977) Paradoxon und Gegenparadoxon. Ein neues Therapiemodell für die Familie mit schizophrener Störung. Klett, Stuttgart

Shields J (1978) Genetics. In: Wing JK (ed) Schizophrenia. Towards a new synthesis. Academic Press, London/Grune and Stratton, New York

Singer MT, Wynne LC, Toohey ML (1978) Communication disorders and the families of schizophrenics. In: Wynne LC, Cromwell RL, Matthysse S (eds) The nature of schizophrenia. Wiley, New York Chichester Brisbane Toronto

Spadoni AJ, Smith JA (1969) Milieu therapy in schizophrenia. Arch Gen Psychiatry 20:547–551

Spohn HE, Patterson T (1979) Recent studies of psychophysiology in schizophrenia. Schizophr Bull 5:581–610

Stierlin H (1975) Von der Psychoanalyse zur Familientherapie. Klett, Stuttgart

Vaughn C, Leff J (1976a) The measurement of expressed emotion in the families of psychiatric patients. Br J Soc Clin Psychology 15:157–165

Vaughn C, Leff J (1976b) The influence of family and social factors on the course of psychiatric illness. Br J Psychiatry 129:125–137

Venables PH (1978) Cognitive disorder. In: Wing JK (ed) Schizophrenia. Toward a new synthesis. Academic Press, London/Grune and Stratton, New York, pp 117–137

Venables PH, Wing JK (1962) Level of arousel and the subclassification of schizophrenia. Arch Gen Psychiatry 7:114–119

Watzlawick P, Beavin JH, Jackson DD (1967) Pragmatics of human communication. Norton & Co, Inc, New York

Wing JK (ed) (1978) Schizophrenia. Towards a new synthesis. Academic Press, London 1978/ Grune and Stratton, New York

Wing JK, Brown J (1970) Institutionalism and schizophrenia. Cambridge University Press, London

Zerbin-Ruedin E (1979) Genetik endogener Psychosen. Schweiz Arch Neurol Neurochir Psychiatr 125:287–299

Psychotherapy of Schizophrenia in Community Psychiatry

2-Year Follow-up Findings and the Influence of Selective Processes on Psychotherapeutic Treatments

Yrjö, O. Alanen, Viljo Räkköläinen, Juhani Laakso, Riitta Rasimus, and Ritva Järvi

In 1976 we began a project in Turku, Finland, for developing treatment of schizophrenic patients within the framework of the community psychiatric health services of our country (Alanen et al. 1979, 1980, 1982). The project was based on a broad psychotherapeutic treatment approach previously developed in the psychiatric teaching hospital of the University of Turku over several years. It was facilitated by the fact that this teaching hospital is also part of the community psychiatric treatment system of the Mental Health District of the City of Turku (population 165,000), and works in close cooperation with the other treatment units of the district. Ideologically we had two chief goals: that the efforts of our four-member team, although based on an integrated illness model of schizophrenia, should be directed so as to strengthen and to especially develop psychotherapeutic and family-centered treatment activities; and that they should be directed in a way suitable to the community psychiatric framework.

During $1^1/_2$ years we did psychiatric and psychological investigations of 100 successive patients, aged 16–45, entering treatment for the first time for a disorder included in the schizophrenia group at an inpatient or outpatient unit operating in the district. We also interviewed these patients' closest family members in 90 of the 100 cases. These investigations also included establishment in each case of a specific treatment plan within the framework of our general orientation and consistent with available psychiatric services.

A follow-up investigation was performed in each case 2 years after the beginning of treatment by the same team members who again saw both patients and their families. In addition, an independent psychiatric investigator carried out separate psychiatric follow-up investigation of the patient sample. Further data on the patients were collected from various treatment agencies, within or outside the community health service system. The Social Insurance Institution consented to provide information on sickness compensation payments and disability pensions. Five-year follow-up of these patients has begun this year; the results of the new follow-up are not available for this presentation.

Indications for different modes of psychotherapy, as suggested during the initial examinations of our sample, have been described earlier (Alanen et al. 1979). In this paper, we will present data based on the 2-year follow-up examination. The data include information on the extent to which the various types of treatment were realized, on the factors which seemed to have influenced the selection of members and modes, as well as some prognostic findings and observations concerning the effect of different therapeutic modes on the outcome of our patients.

Material

Our sample consisted of 52 men and 48 women. The diagnostic criterion for inclusion in the sample was the presence of distinct, psychotic, schizophrenic-type symptoms reflecting a state of disintegration relative to the previous level of personality functioning. The final diagnostic category was established on the basis of an understanding of the clinical picture of the patient gained over a longer period of time. The ultimate age and diagnostic distribution of the patients are shown in Table 1.

Table 1. Age and diagnostic distribution

Age (years)	Typical schizophrenia	Schizophreniform psychosis	Schizo-affective psychosis	Borderline psychosis	Total
16–25	24	1	3	6	34
26–35	22	5	8	10	45
36–45	10	4	3	4	21
Total	56	10	14	20	100

The group of *typical schizophrenias* was composed of patients who besides a schizophrenic-type thought disorder had some other primary or nuclear symptoms as defined by Bleuler (1911) and Langfeldt (1953). These included an accentuated autism, a hebephrenic affect disorder, a typical schizophrenic auditory hallucinosis, physical delusions and hallucinations (e.g., of electric currents the patient feels passing through himself), massive delusions of influence, catatonic symptoms of severe degree, and depersonalization and derealization experiences in the absence of clouded consciousness.

Among *schizophreniform psychoses* were included brief as well as recurring psychotic states with schizophrenic secondary symptoms – particularly ideas of reference and other paranoid delusions, and including confusional symptoms of a schizophrenic character – but without primary symptoms. *Schizo-affective psychoses* had both schizophreniform and manic or depressive psychotic symptoms. The symptoms revealed by the *borderline psychotic* patients were also schizophreniform and often of a short duration; however, this group also included some patients with more chronic psychotic features. The difference between the borderline psychotic group and the schizophreniform group was determined by the typical borderline personality organization (Kernberg 1967) characteristic of the former but not of the latter. However, this personality structure was not included in our material in the absence of psychotic-level symptoms. The symptomatology of the borderline psychotic group was, as a rule, slight (corresponding appreciably with the criteria of borderline schizophrenia as defined by Spitzer et al. 1979) while that of the schizophreniform group was often stormy even if of short duration.

Implementation of Treatment Activities

In addition to the initial investigation, the members of our team participated in treatment plan meetings concerning patients at various treatment agencies, and they also carried out some actual therapeutic work and therapy supervision. It should be stressed, however, that the responsibility for the treatment of the patients was always carried out by the different units themselves, and that most of the psychotherapeutic work was carried out by mental health workers other than team members.

It is a basic endeavor of our approach that the psychotherapeutic activities should be developed on a broad base, so as to include all professional groups involved in mental health work. Table 2 lists the various professional groups participating in the various treatment modes (individual therapy, family therapy, group therapy) according to the number of patients, the number of therapists in each professional group, and the level of their psychotherapeutic training.

The personnel resources in the Mental Health District of Turku are relatively limited. This is especially true of the central community psychiatric outpatient service center, the Turku Mental Health Office. The personnel capacity of the office counted per population of the district is clearly below the average of the country. This is compensated for by the aftercare treatment visits of discharged patients at the university hospital, as well as by the participation of the private sector in outpatient care. Approximately 20% of the psychotherapies in our material were carried out by private institutions and practitioners.

The breakdown for the different modes of psychotherapy and the numbers of patients during the follow-up period is illustrated in Table 3. The numbers in the first column are those from the initial evaluations.

Table 2. Professional category and training of therapists

Professional category	Number of cases	Number of therapists	Psychotherapeutic training of therapists		
			1	2	3
Psychiatrist	19	12	3	7	2
Other physician	11	7	–	7	–
Psychologist	13	9	5	2	2
Social worker	6	5	–	5	–
Registered nurse specialized in psychiatry	33	11	–	10	1
Registered nurse	1	1	–	1	–
Psychiatric aide (1.5 years of training)	3	3	–	3	–
Total	86	48	8	35	5

1 Some kind of formal psychotherapeutic training program of 2–6 years' duration completed.
2 On-the-job training, long-term therapy supervision, psychotherapeutic special training in progress.
3 No special training.

Table 3. Psychotherapeutic treatment prescription

Mode of treatment	Number of patients	
	Originally indicated	Actually received
Intensive individual therapy	25	33
Infrequent individual therapy	44	23
Conjoint family therapy	16	8
Couples therapy	26	12
Supportive psychotherapeutic contact with family members	36	33
Treatment in a psychotherapeutic community	63	53
Group therapy in an outpatient setting	10	2

Of all the offered modes of treatment, individual and community therapy most closely approached original expectations. As seen in Table 3, intensive individual therapy was received by 33 of our patients – more than suggested in the initial treatment plans – and a more infrequent individual therapy was received by another 23. By intensive individual therapy we here denote a one-to-one therapeutic relationship for at least 6 months with a minimum of one therapy session a week. A minimum duration of 6 months was also taken as a criterion for infrequent individual therapy, with the sessions taking place at least once a month and with the same therapist. Contacts with other outpatient units were excluded in order to eliminate vagueness and uncertainty about their continuity, as well as changes of the caretaking persons.

Joint therapy of the patient and members of his family was carried out in eight cases, and couples therapy, attended by the patient and his or her spouse or partner, in 12. These numbers only amount to a half of that indicated in the beginning of our study. In 33 cases separate supportive therapy was given to some of the patient's relatives or friends, at least for a short period excluding the initial contact. Since in some cases more than one mode of family therapy was used during the follow-up period, the total number of patients who received family-centered treatment in one form or another amounted to 44.

Treatment in a psychotherapeutic community was received by 53 patients. Very brief stays on the ward and other hospitalizations not involving psychotherapeutic process are not included here. More unsatisfactory were the findings concerning group therapy within the outpatient setting, which only two patients in our sample received.

Based on the 2-year follow-up investigation, we could refer to 61 patients in our sample of 100 as "psychotherapy cases." By this we mean patients who had received individual or group therapy ordinarily for a time exceeding 6 months, conjoint family therapy or couples therapy in an ordinary form, and those in long-term intensive treatment in the psychotherapeutic communities of the Turku University Psychiatric Hospital, or a combination of these treatment activities. It must be mentioned that another group of patients, *not* included in these psychotherapy cases, comprised individuals who had received shorter crisis therapy or had been treated for a shorter time in a psychotherapeutic community, and those patients with whom either individual or

Table 4. Extent of neuroleptic drugs administered

Daily dose adjusted to correspond to chlorpromazine	Highest daily dose (number of patients)	Average daily dose during follow-up period[a] (number of patients)
Over 300 mg	46	3
100–300 mg	46	19
Under 100 mg	6	12
Varying doses for more than half of the follow-up period		12
Several brief periods		27
Only one brief period		25
No neuroleptic drugs	2	2

[a] The lines in this column indicate the sequential classification used in statistical calculations.

family therapy had been attempted. In only 20 cases can it be said that no form of psychotherapeutic treatment had even been attempted.

Despite our psychotherapeutic orientation, neuroleptic drug therapy was prescribed for all but two of our patients, though mostly in small or moderate doses as is seen in Table 4. However, only 34 of the 100 patients received drugs continuously during the period of 2 years. A quite deliberate use of medication thus formed part of the treatment of schizophrenic patients in our psychotherapeutically oriented approach.

The Influence of Selective Processes on Psychotherapeutic Treatments

We shall next consider, in the light of certain basic clinical and psychosocial background variables, the influence of the selective processes whereby the patients entered the various categories of psychotherapy actually provided, and certain questions concerning the indications for these therapies.

Intensive individual psychotherapy was not given in the group of schizophreniform psychoses. There were no other statistically significant associations between individual therapies and the various diagnostic subcategories; patients with typical schizophrenia were, however, relatively more common in the group which received infrequent therapy and those with schizoaffective or borderline psychosis in the group which received intensive individual psychotherapy. Patients with long-term ego disintegration received infrequent individual therapy more than the average of the sample, which was of marginal statistical significance. The provision of intensive individual psychotherapy was, in turn, associated at a significant level with the patient's willingness to enter treatment and at a marginally significant level with the patient's insight into his own illness at the time of initial investigation. Its association as well with a slow onset of the disorder also reached a marginally significant level. Cases of typical schizophrenia accounted for approximately half of the group that received intensive individual psychotherapy.

Women received intensive individual psychotherapy somewhat more often than men; the difference was marginally significant. The absence of the divorced and the widowed in the group receiving this mode of therapy was significant. Of the background variables related to social class and education, only the patient's basic education had some association with his presence in this treatment category, and even then at a merely descriptive level.

It is interesting to compare these findings with those concerning the treatment indications determined in the initial study (Alanen et al. 1979). At that time both an above-average level of basic education and an above-average social status were very strongly accentuated among the patients for whom intensive individual psychotherapy was planned. University students were also found to be highly significantly overrepresented. These correlations were no longer found in the case of treatment actually provided, expect for the symptomatic significance of basic education just mentioned. This can probably be considered as evidence of the broad base on which treatment was provided in this instance. The relatively common preconception that intensive individual psychotherapy is suitable only for educated, "enlightened" patients was thus disproved in the course of practical therapeutic work. The fact that the actual provision of this mode of therapy was not distributed among the patients in accordance with the original plan also seems not to have adversely affected the treatment outcome. Only when the patients referred to as psychotherapy cases were studied as a whole did the level of the patient's basic education reach a statistically significant association with the implementation of treatment.

Our experience concerning the implementation and outcome of treatment showed that it is difficult to draw a sharp line between indications for the intensive and the infrequent modes of individual psychotherapy. If there is anything deserving special mention as a distinguishing feature in those patients specifically for whom intensive individual psychotherapy was considered indicated, it is above all their positive attitude toward the treatment, and their insight. On the other hand, considerable development took place, particularly in the patient's attitude toward treatment, during the follow-up period. The process of "ripening" for intensive individual psychotherapy might take place quite gradually, sometimes after prolonged treatment on an infrequent basis or after repeated hospital stays. In the follow-up phase we assessed that almost 80% of our patients would have benefited from an opportunity to explore their problems in the setting of a regular psychotherapeutic relationship.

In connection with this follow-up assessment, the question of greatest interest is probably which patients were regarded at that point as *not* in need of individual therapy. Results indicate these to be married persons in the oldest age group, persons with well-developed occupational identities, and persons with the diagnostic category of schizophreniform psychoses (all at a significant level). A marginally significant association was furthermore found for a relatively low level of basic education, a relatively low social status, a social role other than that of a student, a clinical picture dominated by paranoid solutions, lability in external life, and commitment to hospital by legal measures. When we combine our clinical observations with these statistical correlations, the picture of those patients for whom individual therapies are not indicated emerges as twofold. This group includes, on the one hand, certain married patients in the older groups, for whom couples therapy was considered a more useful mode of treatment than individual therapy. On the other hand, it includes patients – mostly male – whose social background is more unfavorable than usual and whose life has also been labile; it hardly seemed possible to establish a firm individual therapeutic relationship with these patients.

Conjoint family therapy and couples therapy were provided for approximately one-third of the patients for whom such therapy was considered indicated in the follow-up assessment. This low level was particularly so in the case of conjoint family therapy. Tho most important reason for this was the treatment staff. Most of them lacked not only the training but also the attitude and approach required by system-oriented family therapy. Separate support for family members, on the other hand, was provided to a considerably greater extent.

Considering the background variables, the implementation of actual family therapy was quite clearly associated with motivation for such therapy. The willingness of the family members to participate in some kind of family-centered therapy was highly significantly related to its actual implementation, and the patient's own willingness emerged as marginally significant. This was particularly pronounced in couples therapy. The attitude of the spouses toward joint therapy was noticeably more often positive than that of the patients' parents. Couples therapy turned out in our study to be a useful mode of treatment, the possibilities of which were too seldom utilized, in terms of both the number of cases treated and the intensity and duration of therapy.

The majority of cases in which conjoint family therapy of the patient and his parents was chosen included the very severely disturbed patients from family environments characterized by highly pathological binding relationships. The patient's relatively young age and his entanglement with the parents in difficult interrelationships hampering individualization were important indications for this mode of therapy also in the assessments made in the follow-up phase. Although many of the families showed treatment motivation in the initial phase, conjoint family therapy, of all the treatment modes used, involved most resistance on the part both of the patients and their parents and, as already noted, the treatment staff. In our experience conjoint family therapy of the schizophrenic patient and his parents can be undertaken in many cases only after prolonged preparatory work, dealing in an empathic way with the problems of both the patient and his family members. – Since the beginning of this project, we have experienced that an effective training has markedly developed these activities.

As already stated, the treatment which quantitatively followed most closely the indications determined in the initial study was that in a psychotherapeutic community. Of the clinical background variables, this mode of therapy was highly significantly associated with long-term ego disintegration, showing that this type of treatment was received by a large number of the most regressive individuals among our subjects. Of the other clinical variables, the patient's willingness to enter treatment was significantly correlated with this mode of therapy. Of the psychosocial variables, a marginally significant association was found with relatively young age, female sex, and lack of occupational identity, and a descriptive association was found with the social role of a student.

The need for treatment in a psychotherapeutic community was especially recommended on the same grounds in the case of relatively young patients who were psychologically still deeply involved with the childhood family and who showed long-term regression of ego functions. This choice became crucial where family members showed poor empathic capacities at the time of the patient's entrance into treatment. In such a case, the stay in the psychotherapeutic community thus offered an auspicious interval during which it might be possible to establish a successful treatment relationship with both the patient and his family. Finally, patients outside the working community due to unemployment or other reasons were also often considered to need treatment in a psychotherapeutic community.

Treatment Modes and the Initial Psychological Examination

The initial psychological examination of the patients was carried out at the same time as the initial psychiatric interviews, but independently of them and before the initiation of actual therapy. The results support our view that factors associated with the clinical picture did not much affect the selective processes whereby individual patients entered the various modes of therapy. Psychotherapeutic services were provided fairly evenly for patients with varying backgrounds, though greater than average neuroleptic drug therapy was given to those patients in whom fragmentation, difficulties with reality testing, and disturbances in thought processes and in other ego functions were emphasized.

There were, however, certain characteristics assessed by psychological means which explain far better than statistical chance the use of various modes of treatment. Table 5 shows certain essential findings concerning the 20 variables assessed systematically for each patient. The intensity of the psychotherapeutic approach was here determined by using a five-point rating scale, ranging from a total lack of specifically psychothera-

Table 5. Therapies actually provided, in relation to certain psychological background variables, correlations

Variables	Intensity of psychotherapeutic approach	Forms of psychotherapy		
		Intensive individual therapy	Infrequent individual therapy	Therapeutic community
Psychological mindedness	0.32***	0.36***	−0.12	0.04
Capacity for depression	0.22*	0.21*	0.05	−0.06
Chaotic or isolated object images	0.22*	0.14	0.08	0.13
Symbiotic relatedness	−0.21*	−0.22	−0.12	0.00
Development of object representations	0.15(*)	0.19(*)	0.01	0.12
Withdrawal into autism/omnipotency	−0.14(*)	−0.26*	−0.06	−0.16
....				
General intelligence	0.04	0.04	−0.02	−0.10
Self-object differentiation	0.05	0.03	0.02	−0.17

*** $P < 0.001$; ** $P < 0.01$; * $P < 0.05$; (*) $P < 0.1$.

peutic techniques to the most intensive types of individual, family, and psychotherapeutic community treatments.

The patient's ability to explore his problems in a psychologically meaningful manner and his efforts at psychological insight in dealing with the problems – here referred to as "psychological mindedness" – was the most significant of the individual factors. Thus those patients who at the time of the initial study showed interest in psychological exploration and in analyzing how to cope with their difficulties ended up more often than others in the more intensive forms of therapy, and in individual psychotherapy in particular. Those who tried to deny their problems, or approached them in an externalized or nondynamic manner, came into treatment because of other factors; they also generally received neuroleptic drug therapy in higher doses during their treatment ($r = 0.30, P < 0.001$).

The ability to experience depression and express it at an affective level (the capacity for grief work) was also one of the favorable indications for psychotherapeutic treatment. Those patients who actively denied their feelings of depression, who used defenses of the manic type in coping with loss or frustration, who tried mainly to change their environment, or who were easily overwhelmed by inner rage were those most resistant to psychotherapy. In these cases psychotherapy, which may have started on quite an intensive basis, sometimes broke off in the initial phase, and was thus quite short lived.

According to the psychological assessment, the degree of severity of the psychotic disorder, as assessed on the basis of the patient's capacity for self-object differentiation, appeared in itself not to affect the character of the psychotherapies to any great extent. Certain traits reflecting the developmental level of interpersonal relationships and in particular their internalized counterparts (object representations), on the other hand, had higher prognostic value. Generalizing, we can say that the patient's ability to take into account such qualities of object relationships as autonomy, reciprocity, and sense of responsibility was a positive factor clearly contributing from the very outset to his progress in psychotherapy. Those patients whose representational world was characterized by chaotic anxiety or alienation (often in the manner typical of borderline patients) were, however, more likely to have intensive therapeutic relationships than were patients withdrawn into autism, paranoid thinking, or an inner world colored by omnipotent fantasies. Similarly, accentuated symbiotic and passive needs in the object images were associated significantly more often with a modest level of therapy.

Although basic education showed some slight association with the various intensities of treatment, intelligence factors discriminated hardly at all between the treatment intensity groups.

Our results suggest that, of the different modes of treatment, intensive individual psychotherapy created the most involved process of self-selection and made the most demands on the patients' personal characteristics. The group that received infrequent individual therapy was considerably more heterogenous. A differentiating feature typical of the patients treated in a psychotherapeutic community was their need, potential in character, to find an external object substituting for inner structures. In their representational world self-object relationships of the narcissistic type were accentuated more commonly than in other patients.

Prognostic Findings

Treating schizophrenics is work of long duration. This was clearly shown by the fact that, at the time of our 2-year follow-up, the psychotherapeutic treatment of only 17 patients of the 61 psychotherapy cases had ended. The psychotherapy of 44 patients was still in progress. Because of this, the prognostic findings presented in this phase should be regarded as preliminary in nature. Another factor making any comparisons between the effects of different therapeutic modes on prognosis especially difficult has to do with factors influencing the selection of patients, as discussed above. Therefore the real significance of our treatment procedures on the prognosis of our patients must await still later follow-ups.

Our approach to the study of the prognosis was a multidimensional one, and we certainly found confirmation for the observation made by Strauss and Carpenter (Strauss et al. 1974; Carpenter et al. 1977) that the correlation between different prognostic criteria is merely a relative one. We shall first deal with the findings concerning the most traditional of prognostic criteria, i.e., the degree of recovery from psychotic symptoms at the end of the follow-up period. The findings of our two parallel psychiatric follow-up examinations are shown in Table 6.

The findings of our original team and those of the independent investigator are seen in the table side by side. The figures show that patients with psychotic symptoms were found relatively more frequently by the team than by the independent investigator. The independent follow-up investigation was limited to some extent by subject dropout. Out of our original sample of 100 patients, 17 refused to meet the investigator. There patients had died, all by suicide.

There was nevertheless a highly significant correlation between the two sets of findings ($r = 0.66$, $P<0.001$). Thus, to a fairly great extent the same patients were found by the independent investigator to have psychotic symptoms as by the team; she was, however, more cautious in her assessments, or the symptoms were less in evidence during the one interview she had with each patient. In general, the assessments made by the independent researcher as to the patient's prognosis gave a somewhat more favor-

Table 6. Presence of psychotic symptoms at the time of the follow-up (number of patients)

Diagnostic group	Original team					Independent investigator				
	I	II	III	IV	Total	I	II	III	IV	Total
Schizophrenia	28	6	20	2	56	16	9	18	13	56
Schizophreniform psychosis	–	2	8	–	10	–	–	6	4	10
Schizoaffective psychosis	2	1	10	1	14	1	1	11	1	14
Borderline psychosis	5	1	14	–	20	–	4	15	1	20
Total	35	10	52	3	100	17	14	50	19	100

I, Psychotic symptoms; II, Psychotic symptoms suspected, but not actually observed; III, No psychotic symptoms; IV, Not assessed (including the three dead patients).

able picture than did those of our own group; the latter was affected by our more prolonged knowledge of the patients. Thus we can say that the independent follow-up confirmed our own findings, indicating at the same time that our findings were not overly optimistic.

As regards clinical prognosis it was found that the outcome was relatively good. Somewhat over half of our patients were definitely free of psychotic symptoms at the end of the follow-up period, and even in the group of patients with typical schizophrenia the proportion of symptom-free cases was nearly 40%.

The working ability of the patients at the end of the follow-up was normal in 40 and impaired in 24 cases. Thirty-two of the patients were regarded as unable to work. This corresponded well with the fact that 31 patients were receiving disability pension for psychiatric reasons at the end of the follow-up period.

In the light of these figures the social prognosis in our patient sample seems relatively poorer than the clinical prognosis. In our view, this result was affected by unemployment. At the time of entrance into treatment, 22 patients were already unemployed, and during the follow-up period unemployment was experienced by as many as 42 patients, for at least some of the time.

In Table 7, we have selected some prognostic variables for study in their relationship to the implementation of different treatment modes. Of these modes Table 7 separates by group those patients in intensive individual therapy, infrequent individual therapy, psychotherapeutic community, and the patients generally included in the psychotherapy cases. The outcome of patients in each group is always compared with that of all the other patients in the sample. The column indicating the extent of drug therapy is classified sequentially as in Table 4. Positive correlations always indicate a favorable prognosis, and negative correlations an unfavorable prognostic tendency.

The table includes five prognostic variables, two of which are duplicated on the independent follow-up investigation. Besides the absence or presence of psychotic symptoms, two psychodynamic and two psychosocial variables are evaluated. The psychodynamic variables have the greatest significance in measuring the effects of

Table 7. Therapies actually provided, in relation to prognostic variables: correlations

Prognostic variable	Intensive individual therapy $N = 33$	Infrequent individual therapy $N = 23$	Therapeutic community $N = 53$	Psychotherapy case $N = 61$	Extent of drug therapy (See Table 4)
Psychotic symptoms	0.15	0.05	−0.03	0.18*	−0.07
Psychotic symptoms[a]	0.21*	0.04	0.09	0.20*	−0.17*
Independence from family	0.11	0.05	−0.06	0.09	−0.17*
Independence from family[a]	0.29**	−0.05	0.08	0.10	−0.25**
Nature of interpersonal relationships	0.21*	−0.12	0.04	0.12	−0.19*
Retention/loss of the hold	0.29**	−0.15	0.11	0.16	−0.26**
Able to work	0.20*	−0.08	0.00	0.18*	−0.33***

[a] Assessment made by the independent investigator.
*** $P < 0.001$; ** $P < 0.01$; * $P < 0.05$; (*) $P < 0.1$.

therapy because they are based on assessments of the patient's development during the follow-up period. The first of the two psychosocial variables indicates whether the patients in the end-phase of the follow-up period have retained or lost their hold on the interpersonal and social needs inherent in the life of an adult person. The second psychosocial variables indicates the degree of working ability of the patients.

We can clearly see a positive correlation between intensive individual therapy and the psychodynamic and psychosocial variables, as well as with clinical prognostic variables. The difference, when compared with infrequent individual therapy, is conspicuous, even when the initially somewhat greater severity of the clinical disorder of those patients who received the infrequent therapy is taken into account.

The status "psychotherapy case" is also positively correlated with the prognostic variables, though not at a quite statistically significant level. The extent of drug therapy, on the contrary, is negatively correlated with the prognostic variables and in most cases at a significant level. The negative correlation is more pronounced in the case of psychosocial than clinical prognosis. This kind of comparison, however, does not clarify the effects of the drug treatment since the amount of drugs used was greatest in the most severely disturbed patients. Still, no statistically significant associations were found between the extent of drug therapy and the various diagnostic subcategories, and the patients with initial long-term ego disintegration were highly significantly overrepresented both among the psychotherapy cases and among the patients who received the largest amount of drugs.

It may also be noted that treatment in a psychotherapeutic community, which also involved a selection of patients with disorders of above-average severity, consistently had more positive and fewer negative correlations with prognosis than did the drug therapy variable. The same was also true of the ordinary modes of family therapy which, however, were left out of our table because of the small number of cases involved.

It may be noted that a third clinical prognostic variable (not included in Table 7), the decline or increase in the amount of nuclear symptoms of schizophrenia during the follow-up period, was found to have very clearly positive correlations to treatment in a psychotherapeutic community as well as in conjoint family therapy, but no correlation with the amount of drug treatment. The changes indicated by this prognostic variable were greatest in the data referring to the most disturbed patients (cf. Alanen et al. 1982).

The view that factors other than those dependent on the patient's clinical picture also have important prognostic consequences was most markedly supported by the findings regarding our patients' retention or loss of a hold on the needs and goals of an adult person. A total of 62 patients were found to have retained this hold and 35 to have lost it. The correlation of this prognostic variable with the patient's diagnostic subgroup and original clinical picture was statistically nonsignificant. On the other hand, correlation with employment or unemployment at the time of the initial psychiatric investigation, as well as with a well-developed occupational identity at the time of the onset of the treatment, was statistically highly significant.

Discussion

Our study is apparently the first attempt at a systematic survey of integrated treatment with an emphasis on psychotherapy, our patient sample uncompassing all newly admitted patients with a disorder included in the schizophrenia group in a given area. Perhaps the most important of our findings is that a psychotherapeutic treatment orientation within a community psychiatric framework is not only possible but yields useful results.

Our prognostic findings, despite their preliminary nature, clearly point to a favorable effect of psychotherapeutic modes of treatment. In this respect, our findings resemble more closely those reported by Karon and VandenBos (1972) and Ugelstad (1978) than those put forward by May (1968) and Grinspoon et al. (1972), according to whom drug therapy entailed a better prognosis for schizophrenic patients than psychotherapy. As we earlier pointed out (Alanen et al. 1980), a rigidly method-oriented approach typical of May's study, for example, cannot give an adequate picture of the possibilities of psychotherapeutic treatment modes in the group of schizophrenias. This is due to the fact that the diagnostic and psychodynamic heterogeneity of these patients calls for a more diversified psychotherapeutic management. We realised that the psychotherapeutic approach should be individually planned in each case, taking into consideration the patient as well as his most significant interpersonal relationships. In the course of our study, we developed the concept of need-adequacy (case-specific appropriateness) in the treatment of schizophrenic psychoses, dealt with more closely in other papers (Räkköläinen et al. 1981; Alanen et al. 1982b).

Of the various psychotherapeutic modes of treatment, treatment in a psychotherapeutic community on the one hand and individual psychotherapy on the other were provided most adequately in relation to need. Especially the results obtained with more intensive forms of individual therapy speak in favor of incorporating such therapy, to a greater extent than at present, into the activities of the community health care systems.

In the area of family therapy our achievements remained modest, both in regard to numbers and results, because of less developed training and supervision opportunities. However, a family-oriented approach practiced during the initial investigation seemed to notably support treatment of many patients, and some actual family therapies led to promising results. Our personal feelings is that further development of this treatment sector is of particular importance. We consider the role of group therapy in the treatment of new psychotic patients to be less important, compared to individual and family therapy; it too, however should be offered to a greater extent than was done in this study.

We found that the selective processes influencing the actual psychotherapeutic treatment had less to do with the patient's diagnostic category than with some other characteristics. Even though the patient's social status played a lesser role, because of the wide-ranging participation of various professional groups in the various treatment activities his willingness to enter treatment and his psychological mindedness remained significant selective factors. The absence of the divorced and the widowed among our psychotherapy cases was highly significant, the overrepresentation of women as compared with men only marginally so. According to the psychological investigation, we treated more patients who were relatively mature, cooperative, and object-oriented than ones lacking these qualities. Hence the challenge: How to include in treatment more of those whose unfavorable psychological and interpersonal characteristics make them appear evasive and difficult patients yet who are nonetheless very much in need of care? Extending our work with families should help here among other things.

Our treatment project in the Mental Health District of the City of Turku was helped by the inclusion of the resources of a university teaching hospital. Our findings show that an integrated, psychotherapeutically oriented treatment for schizophrenic patients in a community psychiatric setting can not yet be provided in such a way as to satisfy all potential needs, but in any case on a relatively large scale and with encouraging results. The question remains, however, whether such a project can also be realised elsewhere, and without being supported by a psychotherapeutically oriented teaching center.

As far as the quantitity of resources is concerned, this question can be answered in the affirmative. As mentioned earlier, the manpower resources of the community psychiatric outpatient care are no greater in Turku than elsewhere in the country; rather, the opposite is the case. Likewise, the number of hospital personnel per bed available remains within the average. Even in the university hospital – with the exception of the physicians holding a university position – it is not higher than the average for the central mental hospitals in Finland.

The personnel capacity of the Turku Mental Health Office, counted per population of the district was 1.2 per 10,000, and the average for the country was then 2.2 per 10,000. However, the number of psychotherapeutic treatments carried out by the personnel of the Office amounted only to a third of all the outpatient treatments in our patient sample. The number of treatments carried out by the personnel of the university hospital, in the context of aftercare visits of discharged patients, came to the same number, and a third part of the treatments, again of the same quantitative level, was carried out by other institutions and private practitioners. The goal in terms of personnel resources for outpatient care in community psychiatry, as determined by the Central Medical Board of Finland, is 4.2 persons per 10,000 inhabitants. If only this number can be reached in the future, the quantitative factor would not form an insurmountable obstacle to realizing psychotherapeutically oriented treatment activities even more extensive than ours. Before that happens – and also later – good cooperation with the private sector is needed.

More critical than this quantitative factor are the qualitative ones. These fall into two categories: the development of the needed theoretical orientation, and the training of caretaking personnel and further development of their therapeutic skills.

The model developed by us for the treatment of schizophrenic patients reflects a consistent theoretical base. It is characterized, first, by a basic psychotherapeutic attitude toward the patient and his disorder within an integrated illness model of schizophrenia (Räkköläinen et al. 1981; Alanen et al. 1982b). Secondly, it assumes that the genesis and current state of the patient's disorder and the nature of his interpersonal relationships are mutually interdependent. Thirdly, it values the patient as a member of the community who should achieve psychosocial and occupational rehabilitation.

In terms of training, an essential objective is the organization of a broad-based system of on-the-job training and therapy supervision for the caretaking personnel. The data concerning psychotherapeutic training of the therapists (cf. Table 2) show that the great majority of them had no formal completed psychotherapeutic training but had acquired their psychotherapeutic skills through on-the-job training and long-term psychotherapy supervision. Our 2-year follow-up results seemed to indicate that there was no noticeable difference between the results obtained by these therapists – many of them registered nurses specialized in psychiatry – and by those who had received formal psychotherapeutic training. According to our experience, empathic staff members who have plenty of experience in dealing with schizophrenic persons often have acquired the necessary qualifications for developing into good therapists for these persons. Continuous therapy supervision, however, seems to be an absolute condition for this to happen.

In developing our own treatment orientation, a crucial role was played by supervisors who had received specialized psychotherapeutic training in psychoanalytically oriented individual therapy, as well as in family therapy. Where such persons are not locally available within the treatment team, efforts should be made to recruit them in some other way to run regular seminars and provide supervisory sessions. In our experience, many of the therapists lacking formal training in psychotherapy may with time even become quite capable of providing supervision for others. In the 1980s a multiprofessional program of psychotherapeutic training including both individual and family therapy as well as group therapy, geared to field work should be developed in Finland for the psychiatric personnel employed within the community health care system.

The views put forth above are also relevant to the organization of an integrated treatment system with continuous cooperation between the outpatient and inpatient settings. In Turku, the community psychiatric service system is still too hospital-centered as reflected in the fact that the treatment of as many as 74 of our 100 study patients was initiated in the hospital, and that of an additional five by day hospital care, while that of only 21 patients was initiated in an outpatient setting. The participation of the hospital personnel in outpatient treatment through continuous aftercare of discharged patients was vital to the accomplishment of treatment. In the future, we hope that the share of the outpatient center will grow so that more patients may be treated outside the hospital from the outset, and transitory hospitalizations may be more easily handled within the hospital setting. We are at present further developing our day hospital activities.

Clear leadership is necessary in this kind of work in order to make possible the most efficient and sensible use of resources. At the same time, the organization of the treatment community should be flexible and due consideration should be given to the members' own initiatives and spontaneous choices both as regards the patients with whom they want to work and in the arrangement of their supervision. Those in a high administrative position should primarily prevent unrealistic decisions and expectations and take an active responsibility in the management of the evasive and difficult patients referred to above. Without the security provided by the institution and leadership, and without the support of the broader working community, the work will not succeed.

References

Alanen YO, Räkköläinen V, Rasimus R, Laakso J (1979) Indications for different forms of psychotherapy with new schizophrenic patients in community psychiatry. In: Müller C (ed) Psychotherapy of schizophrenia. Excerpta Medica, Amsterdam Oxford, pp 185–202

Alanen YO, Räkköläinen J, Laakso J, Rasimus R (1980) Problems inherent in the study of psychotherapy of psychoses: Conclusions from a community psychiatric action research study. In: Strauss JS et al. (eds) Psychotherapy of schizophrenia. Plenum, New York, pp 115–129

Alanen YO, Räkköläinen V, Rasimus R, Laakso J, Järvi R (1982) Developing the treatment of schizophrenia in a community-psychiatric setting. A psychotherapeutic and family-centered approach. Psychiatr Fennica 1982, pp 101–120

Alanen YO, Räkköläinen V, Laakso J (1982b) Krankheitsmodelle bei der Schizophrenie und die Bedürfnisangemessenheit der Behandlung. Nervenarzt 53:150–153

Bleuler E (1911) Dementia Praecox oder die Gruppe der Schizophrenien. Deuticke, Leipzig

Carpenter WT, McGlashan TH, Strauss JS (1977) The treatment of acute schizophrenia without drugs: An investigation of some current assumptions. Am J Psychiatry 134:14–20

Grinspoon L, Ewalt JR, Shader R (1972) Schizophrenia: Pharmacotherapy and psychotherapy. Williams & Wilkins, Baltimore

Karon BP, Van den Bos GR (1972) The consequences of psychotherapy for schizophrenic patients. Psychotherapy: Theory, Research and Practice 9:111–119

Kernberg O (1967) Borderline personality organization. J Am Psychoanal Assoc 15:641–685

Langfeldt G (1953) Some points regarding the symptomatology and diagnosis of schizophrenia. Acta Psychiatr Scand [Suppl] 80:7–26

May PRA (1968) Treatment of schizophrenia. Science House, New York

Räkköläinen V, Laakso J, Alanen Y, Rasimus R (1981) Need-adequate treatment of schizophrenic psychosis. A paper presented in Oslo, unpublished

Spitzer RL, Endicott J, Gibbon M (1979) Crossing the border into borderline personality and borderline schizophrenia. The development of criteria. Arch Gen Psychiatry 36:17–24

Strauss JS, Carpenter WT (1974) The prediction of outcome in schizophrenia. II. Relationships between predictor and outcome variables: A report from the WHO international pilot study of schizophrenia. Arch Gen Psychiatry 31:37–42

Ugelstad E (1978) Chronic psychotic patients in psychiatric hospitals – new treatment experiences (in Norwegian). Universitetsforlaget, Oslo

The Open Hospital and the Concept of Limits[1]

Daniel P. Schwartz

An understanding of the dimensions of what we call "action," not simply as a "discharge" phenomena, an all-or-nothing occurrence, but an understanding which is coordinate with current psychoanalytic knowledge, is yet to be evolved in our science. One dimension required of such an understanding would be a definition of the concept of "limits" in action terms. This paper attempts part of such a definition.

Our modes of thought deal more centrally with concepts of state rather than process. Hospitals *are*, rather than *do*. They are places of warmth or terror, places of healing or decay. Conceptions of patients too – schizophrenic patients more than most – are often discussed in state, not process terms. He is said to be ill, regressed, has a memory, is deluded, is recovering, even "existing." Yet all of us find this less than satisfying and search for a language that relates state to process, as did Freud (1914), centrally in exploring transference; Strachey (1934) in explicating interpretation; Sullivan (1962) in investigating the self and interpersonal processes; Lidz and Fleck (1965) in their studies of the family and its dynamism; and Erikson (1959) primarily in his clarification of the place of the historical past and future rootedness in the processes of evolution of an individual's identity.

How might we try to understand hospitals and their patients in process terms? What do they do – or attempt to do – with each other? Hospitals – psychiatric hospitals, that is – do take action. The extent of the range of that action is often called the "limit" of that action. And reciprocally, though ambiguously enough, that limit of the hospital's action often marks out a boundary and determines the extent of the range of action – the limit that is available and possible for the patient, upon whom the hospital's action limit impinges. The hospital puts a patient who is assaulting others into seclusion and thereby defines its own actions, its limits, and reciprocally limits and marks out the range of possible behaviors of such a violent patient. Many, but by no means all, such definitions of extent or range – such behavioral boundaries – have the quality of a restriction, a stop, a "no," a "delay," to them.

Psychiatrists, psychoanalysts, and psychologists as a group are opposed to limits. Indeed, we specifically search out and oppose those destructive constraints an individual puts unconsciously on himself. We measure the individual human costs of destructive societal constraints, such as sexist and racist discrimination, as well. It is, therefore,

1 The author has freely used the helpful conceptual clarification of Dr. Martin Cooperman and Dr. Ess A. White, Jr., as well as clinical material generously provided by Drs. Martin Cooperman, Richard Q. Ford, Ann C. Greif, and Jill D. Montgomery, all of the Austen Riggs Center staff. They are not, however, in any way responsible for the faults in the paper or its arguments.

with some discordant surprise that we find in psychotherapeutic hospital work that we act in a limiting fashion toward our patients, impose constraints, and often this appears to be *helpful.*

A young schizophrenic man recently admitted to a hospital locked ward becomes, as he talks with his therapist and patient-staff groups on the ward, progressively more disorganized. His thinking appears looser, he becomes more abusive in his behavior. Addressing this verbally seems to excite him further, and as he progressively becomes more assaultive, tears the ward furniture apart; the therapist arranges that he be put against his will in a seclusion room. Upon seeing the patient in the seclusion area, then, the therapist finds the patient has become suddenly quite calm and better organized. The patient states that somehow he had thought the therapist and/or the ward staff expected him to be either crazy or incompetent, as his mother had, it seemed to him, when she used to run down the path in front of his bicycle to remove all stones or obstacles that he might encounter as he rode his bike when he was younger.

There is abundant evidence that the felt and actual absence of clear limits in a situation is one of the conditions which with adequate stress can precipitate severe psychological problems. In some patients psychotic disorganization can arise, for example, upon their coming suddenly from a restrictive puritanical home environment into the dormitory atmosphere of apparent free sexual expression on today's college campus, or upon promotion to a position which appears to give unlimited license to aggression. (Perhaps Freud's Herr Doctor Schreber belongs here.)

Finding, then, that we do act in hospitals toward our patients and that some of those actions define boundaries, and these limits constrain the possibilities of behavior of our patients on occasion helpfully, how can one describe the useful functions of those limits? They appear to be of service in three somewhat different situations: (a) that of aiding the literal survival of the patient, (b) that of aiding the patient's intrapsychic state of regression or disorganization, and (c) that of playing an important part in growth and learning.

Survival includes those painfully obvious examples where having imposed a limit which placed someone upon a locked ward against his will he tells you in time: "I felt all the people in the world were tyring to tell me that they wished me dead and it was therefore my moral obligation to try and kill myself." Such patients often say that they appreciate your having prevented that by having put them against their will in a locked hospital. Or, having committed a young person to a closed hospital to avoid probable death when he was found standing mute without food and shirtless in below zero winter cold on the street, that patient says later, as he describes his behavior to a therapist, that he was trying to modulate some awesome rage, some loathsome sexuality, and the only option which he felt was available was to stop all human functions – eating, protective clothing, need for warmth, etc.

Intrapsychic organizational states are modified on occasion by limit-setting processes. The simplest of those involves confrontation techniques to limit denial and splitting behaviors. A schizophrenic girl, denying her feelings of grief and betrayal by her therapist's absence, initially is filled with self-loathing and persecutory ideas. She cries in another doctor's presence for her dead father and explains to him that she is afraid that her absent therapist is probably going to die as well. She indirectly asks her mother to intervene and remove her from the hospital. The denial and suicidal regression can be modified only when that behavior can be limited, *constrained* within her therapist's office and she heeds the demand that it be discussed with her therapist. Regressive psychotic states seen in acute hospitals often appear to lyse when the current task *must* be directly addressed and the regressive withdrawal limited.

Growth and learning, too, are complexly served by actions involving limits. In particular, with schizophrenic patients whose capacities for intrapsychic object constancy are so centrally troubled, and so centrally important in their recovery, there is considerable evidence that internalization processes and limits are related. The early work of Wexler (1952), Cameron (1961), and Hoedemaker (1955) all suggest that it is in the process of defining a limit – of saying no – that the schizophrenic patient is able to evolve an internal image of his therapist.

The question, of course, is how, in very different hospital settings, does this definitively evolve. There are amongst hospitals of psychotherapeutic emphasis, that is, where electroconvulsive therapy is not used, and antipsychotic medication is used to facilitate psychotherapeutic treatments, two quite different categories: those hospitals which are mostly concerned with antiregressive measures, and those which are interested in the facilitation of growth. Acute, short-term treatment hospitals are best described as consistently opposed to regression. In terms of our perspective of action, they use forceful limits to insure survival and rapidly alter the patient's intrapsychic state in an antiregressive fashion. They use locked doors, restrictions, group pressure, here-and-now focus, family therapy, confrontation and often punitive and authoritative direction, prescribe behavioral routines, focus upon external tasks, and search persistently for previously established adaptive family equilibrium. Limits are involved in prescribing focus, sanctions, behaviors, avoidance of intimacy and introspection, and directive leadership activities. And one can see how useful all these limits are. They do focus on the precipitating events and forces; they do foster task-directed attention, affective response, clarity of required action; they do limit the time sequences, the withdrawal; they do compel the systematic behaviors previously and adaptively operative to be reassembled. These limits facilitate the ego's delay functions, locate the ego's attention function, use the superego in the service of clear task definition, and modulate arousal of the instinctual life by the hospital and treatment team.

Psychotherapeutic hospitals also include those whose major commitment is toward the facilitation of the patient's growth. Those hospitals' interest is not simply in symptomatic recovery of the schizophrenic patient – though that is difficult enough – but also in providing an environment in which the patient can find a way to evolve a capacity for a viable life through participation in the hospital's milieu and psychotherapeutic procedures. This involves, like all growth, long periods of time, and such hospitals are called long-term hospitals. Such institutions are colloquially characterized as closed or open depending on whether they have locked wards, that is, depending on the character of their limits.

Closed psychotherapeutic hospitals are characterized by their limiting activity and indeed are empowered by our society to do so, for they attempt by such limits to insure, first, the survival of the patient and of the society of others. Their limiting actions, including that of accepting involuntary admissions, may be so routinized as to escape notice. They write orders on each patient, restrict space, define clothing, confine to a locked ward, grant step-wise privileges, require attendance at group meetings, assign individual therapy, assign the therapist and family treatment, prescribe activities, regulate contact with families, friends, jobs, and outside community affairs. All who have and do work with such institutions hear patients explain again and again the relevance and value of such limiting activities, limiting actions. Personal and societal survival dictates the presence in a society of such institutional processes and their limit-setting capacities. Patients in locked hospitals say, after they have been stopped from killing themselves, that they were evil and deserved only death, that they felt their parents or spouses needed them to die, and they were compelled to cooperate with this slowly or rapidly by taking suicidal steps. Limits which separate patient from family are commonly necessary. A young person intent upon suicide required being placed in a seclusion room lest he hang himself, yet he was repetitively sent razor blades by his parents unwittingly inviting him to kill himself in the face of the family treatment dealing verbally with these matters. Survival of the treatment process and the patient are often inseparable in these matters, though in our discussion of open hospitals, it should become clear how wisely and usefully they can be separated.

In closed hospitals it is often the case that the patient, after a period of engagement in his therapy, appears to be involved in a host of destructive acts involving various degrees of displacement toward the therapist and hospital. These behaviors often are accompanied by regressive disorganization. Only after the therapist takes a limiting action – says you can't do that with or to me in my office; I will see you on the ward until you have better means to express what you are trying to say – does the patient, seen on the ward, rapidly organize and then tell the therapist that he was afraid, perhaps correctly afraid, that he was about to hit or hurt the therapist. The therapist's introducing a limit, a behavior, reciprocally limits and helps the patient's own delay functions, modulating their range and forcefulness. This appears as well to allow a more organized, less regressed, intrapsychic organizational state to develop. And it is noteworthy that it is often the case that the limit is imposed *before* it is possible to fully articulate the nature of the conflict. It is often only after the limit is imposed that the patient can say: "I was afraid I would kill you." It is as if the conflict needs to be solved first before it can be addressed.

A limit which appropriately *focuses* upon a task often has a particularly organizing effect. For example, the therapist and the patient's focus on dependency processes and the limit this focus put upon grandiose and distracting expectations may be markedly organizing.

In closed psychotherapeutic hospitals, growth occurs in many dimensions. One of those appears to be those internalizations which involve a limit. This has been described in various settings by Wexler, Cameron, and Hoedemaker as noted previously.

One of the most profound of limiting behaviors in hospitals is that involving what in psychoanalysis is correctly called "termination" and was one of the first parameters introduced by Freud in the analytic situation (Freud 1955). We in psychotherapeutic hospitals are all too often occupied by the externals of this limit; that is, hospital discharge. Indeed, this is one thing we do to patients, this imposition of a limit; we discharge them. All too often in our work with patients who have been previously hospitalized our prejudices interfere with our analytic inquiry about such matters. We would not accept at face value a patient saying that he left home a long time ago and that the only thing he can think about is that he hated living at home. We often do accept, incorrectly I believe, at face value patients who say I was hospitalized at "X" and that was a place I was so glad to escape from.

Having noted many ways in which limits – particularly restrictive, punitive, freedom-denying actions limiting patients' behavior – are useful, let me clearly state the cautionary note. Limits are often, possibly most often, used in the service of the hospital's, the society's, or the therapist's destructive sadism. Power motives pervade their use and the opportunities for the use of locked wards to neglect, promote nonrelatedness, indulge obsessive needs of staff for control, avoid the high cost of good care, good treatment, recovery, and growth all hide under the psychology of limits.

Locked wards, seclusion rooms, electroconvulsive therapy, and high dose antipsychotic medication are used most often to warehouse patients, and to avoid providing the personnel necessary and the treatment programs required to aid in modern medical, societal, and therapeutic responsibility for the mentally ill. Often, and sadly, they are used to remove patients and their troubles from their families, from their communities, and from their environments in ways which bar any hope for recovery.

Token economies and adversive conditioning all too easily employ limits to dehumanize whatever useful effect may be intended, and indeed they have under careful management. Too often such conditioning degenerates into sadistic torture, including the use of "paddling," and worse on occasion. Noting the value of limits, implicitly and incorrectly, risks giving license to such dangerous or destructive practices. Commonly enough, it must be noted, a closed hospital's limit-setting capacities to lock up, to separate from community, to restrict behavior, however therapeutically intended, are used by the patient's pathological processes in the service not of growth but of destruction, not of organization but of regression.

At the other end of the spectrum is the type of growth-facilitating psychotherapeutic hospital called properly an open hospital. Austen Riggs Center is one of those open hospitals. It is the one which I know best, and I want to note that my description of it starts with limits, but in this case signally with what it *does not do*. It receives only voluntary admissions of patients who are at least young adults, who intend to be there for an appreciable period of time, and who can afford the costs of such care. These characteristics of young adulthood involve a family-patient interaction which will allow a patient to be somewhat removed from his family. That is a part of the process of separating.

The open hospital does not admit patients who need crisis intervention. It has no locked wards, no locked doors, no seclusion rooms, no fences. There are no orders written on our patients; no system of privileges exists. Patients are free to come and go as they please; most have private rooms. Regular attendance is not required at the various community meetings which are forms of group therapy. The patients can request a change of therapist within the hospital staff and often consult with the Director of Psychotherapy in regard to such a change. The hospital is on the main street of the small town of Stockbridge, Massachusetts, and indeed our Austen Riggs Theatre is an ensemble company in which both patients and other citizens of our local community compete for roles through auditions and jointly participate in staging productions. Patients hold jobs in town, drink at the local inn, and attend colleges in the neighborhood. While we have physicians and internists in constant attendance upon the premises, for more serious medical care our patients consult with the individual experts at a local community hospital. We use antipsychotic medications, only with the cooperation of the patient, as an adjunct to psychotherapy. We do not prescribe activites and until recently we did not have a social worker on the staff. So we don't detain, we don't regulate activities, we don't stop visitors, we don't stop visiting home, we expect the patient to tell us when he is going to be away so that we don't worry unnecessarily, but we don't expect them to ask our permission.

My point is not to be an advocate of this kind of psychotherapeutic hospital environment, but simply to note how important it is that one cannot describe such a hospital and how it acts upon patients without using as the central point the concept of limits. This is an open hospital for patients whose age, capacities, responsiveness, and situations are all engaged in the process of separating from their families. This hospital is an open hospital which is best described by its limits – the range of behaviors it does *not* do. Indeed, the tension between the limit defined as the hospital's range of behavior and the reciprocally defined limit of the behavior of the patient creates and locates possibilities for useful discussion between the patient and staff. Such discussions of reciprocal limits take place where the potential for change and growth is often the clearest. As I was writing this paper, one of our schizophrenic patients stopped me on the way to the store, and after inquiring after my welfare, said he thought I should be aware of the difficulties covered by some of the hospital's limitations. He meant by that that one of our nurses wouldn't marry him, nor would his therapist invite him home to dinner.

This open hospital, the Austen Riggs Center, cannot be simply described by what we don't do, but, of course, by what we do do as well. We do provide many things, not the least of which is intensive, individual psychotherapy of four or more hours each week with an experienced therapist, a very special activities program using sculptors, poets, and theatre directors as teachers, the presence and focus of nurse-clinicians, community programs, and much more. But in much the same spirit that Glover evidenced when he described psychoanalysis as the articulation of the basic rule of free association and the study of the patient's various attempts to avoid or distort that rule, so here I wish to call attention to that which most characterizes an open hospital; that is, the limits, the range, and extent of behaviors which it doesn't do. These are clearly related to what it "can't" and "shouldn't" do as well. The creative and central tension between that system and the patient, between the staff and the patient, is part of where the patient might grow.

Perhaps most noticeably and helpfully these limits function in an open hospital in their relation to survival. A typical situation might involve a "cutter," a patient who slashes her wrists. To the uninitiated visitor at our daily hospital morning staff conference, which includes all therapists, nurses, administrators, and activities personnel, the report of such a patient's wrist cutting incident may indeed seem bizarre. The nurse, describing the highlights of the previous 24 hours' activities, says among other things: "Millie has come back from her job as an usher in the local music festival and cut her wrists." The nurse, having come upon her and checked, sees that the patient's life is not in danger, applies first aid, tries to talk with the patient to understand what is going on, calls the psychiatrist on call who evaluates that the wound is not dangerous, who agrees with the recommendation that the patient go to the local general hospital and have the emergency room physician see if sutures are advisable. Often a patient then is taken to such an emergency room by another patient, though occasionally by our own nurses. Contact is made with the local emergency room physician, the cut is sutured, and the patient returns to the hospital, called locally the "Inn," and sleeps through the night.

The morning report continues with other incidents of patients. Various patients attended a canoe trip, Billy has isolated himself in his room, and the competition between the anorexic patients who are in a seeming gorge-and-vomit contest is reported. Upon completion of the report, questions and comments are asked for, and Millie's therapist tries to convey a bit of what she understands the patient may be dealing with in therapy. Some of the other nurses add that the patient was hysterically thrashing about at the time of the cutting and that the mother was hysterically overwrought upon hearing of this incident, feeling that the patient's beauty was being destroyed, and other staff share information on this and other matters. The conference moves on. No one locks the patient up, no one takes her over, no one on the staff behaves hysterically in a concerned manner, or indeed appears terribly in great distress. There is no change in the treatment plan. And this reasonable unresponsiveness, this view that it is the patient's treatment, the patient's risk, the patient's wound (not the hospital's), the patient's responsibility, appears to be helpful. One has the impression that, more easily than in a closed hospital, it is clear to patients that it is their wrist, their risk, and their treatment that is at stake.

Observing such events is made all the more clear by those patients who have transferred to open Riggs from closed hospitals. One such typical patient worked intensively and closely with a young therapist and an art therapist at a closed hospital. Upon getting into a heated transference at that hospital, she cut her wrists and the therapist and art therapist were suddenly taken off the case, the patient's therapy was limited to once-a-week reality-oriented work, after which she, the patient, made a shambles of her hospitalization and of the hospital as best she could. Upon cutting her wrists at Riggs she had sutured herself up before presenting herself for staff attention. Her therapy was not interrupted. It is my conviction from watching many such events that part of the trouble in each such event is that a closed hospital could not define their limits in such a closed setting by nonresponding. They have to act by virtue of their ordinarily protective task. And one might add that at the Austen Riggs Center often we have just the reverse kind of difficulty. We have to not act in the face of what might very well be better for the patient – if we had acted – even if this meant interrupting the treatment and sending the patient elsewhere.

Other patients in our open setting faced with this increasing involvement in an intensive psychotherapy and hospital community climb mountains at considerable risk and engage in solitary, long distance hikes and find in these activities, and in their freedom to leave, to miss a therapy hour or a community meeting, their freedom to be where no one can see them, relief from their persecutory anxieties. Such mountain climbing trips are not without risk; indeed, the risk of which often only their therapists know involves their literal survival. It seems not a chance phenomena that it was in this very open setting some years back that Erikson, studying the problem of identity, choice, and negative identity, pointed out that many growing young people have to know that they have the *real* choice of throwing their life away – of not surviving – if the choice of actively living and working is to become owned by such a person with any valued meaning. Perhaps Albert Camus (1955) said the same thing in his discussion of the myth of Sisyphus.

Not infrequently in the course of those regressions and disorganizations which threaten all schizophrenic patients upon engagement in exploratory psychotherapy, the patient attempts to alter that inner state, that sense of trapped and fiercesome intimacy by requiring or requesting a change of therapist. Indeed, after consultation with our Director of Psychotherapy, when that is a persistent request, such a change is made. That is, we have applied the limit that we *do not* compel the choice of therapist or the continuity of the treatment. And reciprocally the choice and the responsibility is the patient's. Such changes of therapist often, but not always, work out, and one wonders whether one of the forces which facilitate that, is not the superior skill of the second therapist, but rather the clarity of the limit – "it's your choice, your treatment."

Clarity of focus of action is often valuable to our patients in this setting. One such patient had regularly removed all of her clothing in seclusion areas of her previous hospitalization where she thought she was a male lion whose task it was to fornicate with all other patients who were female lions. She reported to her therapist the contrast in her feeling here in this *open* Riggs setting. In her room that previous night she had, while half dressed, been listening to her stereo at high volume. A male aide on duty had entered her room after knocking and requested that she turn the stereo volume down. She felt quite guilty, she said, since he saw her half clothed and she wondered whether her blasting stereo had really not been an unwitting invitation to intrusion by this aide. What a contrast there was, she thought, in her feeling. She had been, as far as she could recall, totally lacking in self-consciousness about her nudity in the other hospital seclusion area in front of men and women there. Most of it, she supposed, was that she felt herself to be in charge in our open setting here. While in the locked seclusion area in the other hospital, it was as if she belonged to them, was their responsibility.

Growth, in any event, is multifaceted, and difficult to describe but one has the impression that limit is involved here, too, and in our open hospital the limit is imposed by what one does not do.

A young schizophrenic man has had persistent delusions that his mouth is ugly and deformed and can only be repaired by extensive reconstructive surgery. Unmodified by medication, family therapy, other attempts at outpatient psychotherapy, and inpatient psychotherapy in a closed hospital, he gradually puts his delusions and medications aside in the course of intensive psychotherapy in our open hospital. During the process of this therapy, oral rage emerges, dominates the field more directly, but is never felt in the presence of the therapist. The patient finds he cannot stand the sound of eating and talking, "mouth noises," while in the dining room, and he runs screaming from the dining room at the sound of other people's chatter while eating. He volunteers to cook a meal for a group of patients and finds himself enraged, wishing to throw all of the food on the ground, to tear the food apart, tear the patients themselves apart like pieces of barbequed chicken, limb from limb. He stays in his room and avoids his therapy, in a rage that his therapist doesn't come to seek him out. He calls his parents and reports his therapist as negligent because he, the patient, is not going to his therapy. His therapist, after a time, does visit him in his room, and they walk back to the office together. "You are to blame," the patient says, "you're not looking after me, you don't know what's happening, you're not helping me, you're not talking to the nurses about me. I'm not getting any better." The therapist notes that the patient is very angry at him, and in the process of responding acknowledges his (the therapist's) knowledge from the nurses, in fact, about what the patient has been doing, what the patient has been saying to other people in his ward behavior and during avoided therapy hours. The therapist says to the patient: "You are the one who is avoiding me, not coming to your hours, not talking to me, and I gather you must feel like you're torturing me with that, reporting me to your parents, documenting my failure as a therapist, while you miss your hours – not me." "I know," says the patient after a thoughtful moment. "I feel as if you were devouring me. It is as if you ate up bits of information each time you see me and I talk to you. The more I talk to you, the more I enjoy being with you, the more it is as if I were a fish on a string, and you're reeling me in and going to eat me up, and I'll disappear." "You do disappear," said the therapist, "by not coming to your hours." The hour ends.

The limit here is not coercing attendance upon the hour. And it is no accident that the example makes it possible to confuse who is doing what to whom. For between these attached invested people – patient and therapist – there is partial fusion, and the limit – that is, the therapist in this open hospital does not regularly coerce attendance upon him – allows, demands the reciprocal limit of the patient's responsibility to choose to attend or not attend and is a part of the critical juncture. It is the limit which marks out a boundary – a newly evolved separateness between those people – out of the fusion. And yet it begins to partake of an internalization. For it seems to me that it is as the patient says, it is I who am afraid of being devoured and want to devour, it is not my therapist eating me up in the hours. He begins the demarcation of a boundary between them which contains as part of its definition the image of the other who is not oneself, not devoured, not devouring, and still there. The relation of this to previous psychoanalytic work in my supposition is obvious. The work of Pious (1961) on the organization of an image of the therapist is central. The related work of the child analysts upon the formation of object constancies, e.g., by Solnit (1979), is invaluable. And discussions of the process of internalization are, I believe, reciprocally related to that process partially described by Loewald (1960) as an element in the therapist's formation of a "mutative interpretation." That is the process by which a partial identification of the therapist with the patient is formed unconsciously and as an aspect of that identification is resolved it is possible for the therapist to formulate and communicate to the patient the interpretation. What one is adding here in its reciprocal form is that the patient for that "resolution" requires the evolution not only of the attachment, the fusion and projection, but *then* the limit, which occurs in action defining the extent of a range of behaviors ("It is you who devours"). A boundary then is established, a beginning separateness which is a crucial part of the internalization by the patient of the *image* of the other.

There is much more to be said of limits and open hospitals, of course. It is the case that such hospitals are not without rules, both crude and subtle sanctions. Of interest to me is that Mosher (1978) reports of Soteria House, another very different open hospital, rules and constraints which we at Riggs repetitively also *must* arrive at as well – no violence, no incest, obey the laws of the land, and some regulation of the visitors into the house.

Perhaps most interesting in this is the fashion in which every institution must define its limits relative to its societal tasks. A closed hospital empowered by society to limit by restriction must define its limits differently from an open hospital, which defines its task as that of maintaining the dignity and locus of choice within the patient himself, and therefore must try to limit by "not doing." In Erikson's terms, the patient's ego, in order not to be inactivated, must fashion out of its societal tasks some variant of organization which involves a centrality of integration of constitutional givens, idiosyncratic libidinal needs, favored capacities, significant identifications, effective defenses, successful sublimations, and consistent roles (Erikson 1959). Perhaps in addition one must integrate the limits, the evolved boundaries of action. In that evolving centrality of which Erikson (1981) speaks so cogently, in the sense of continuity, that evolution of active choice and boundary process which such an "I" evolves, the psychology of limits of action constitutes an important element.

References

Cameron N (1961) Introjection, reprojection, and hallucinations in the interaction between schizophrenic patient and therapist. Int J Psychoanal 1961:42

Camus A (1955) The myth of Sisyphus. Hamish Hamilton, London

Erikson E (1959) In: Klein GS (ed) Identity and the life cycle. Psychological issues, vol 1, no 1, monog 1. International Universities Press, New York

Erikson E (1981) The Galilean sayings and the sense of "I." The Yale Review, vol 70:3

Freud S (1914) Remembering, repeating and working-through. 1918 standard edn, vol 12, pp 145–156. Hogarth Press, London, 1958

Freud S (1918) From the history of an infantile neurosis. 1918 standard edn, vol 17, p 10–11. Hogarth, London, 1955

Hoedemaker ED (1955) The therapeutic process in the treatment of schizophrenia. J Am Psychoanal Assoc 3:89–109

Lidz T, Fleck S, Cornelison A (1965) Schizophrenia and the family. International Universities Press, New York

Loewald H (1960) On the therapeutic action of psycho-analysis. Int J Psychoanal 41:16–33

Mosher L, Menn A (1978) The surrogate "familiy," an alternative to hospitalization, chap 10. In: Shershow SC (ed) Schizophrenia, science and practice. Harvard University Press, Cambridge

Pious W (1961) A hypothesis about the nature of schizophrenic behavior. In: Burton A (ed) Psychotherapy of the psychoses. Basic Books, New York

Solnit A (1979) Some applications of the theory of object constancy in childhood. Given at a joint meeting of the Western New England and Boston Psychoanalytic Societies, Stockbridge, Massachusetts, October 20, 1979. Submitted for publication as "developmental perspectives on the self and object constancy"

Strachey J (1934) The nature of the therapeutic action of psycho-analysis. Int J Psychoanal 15: 127–159

Sullivan H (1962) Schizophrenia as a human process. Norton, New York

Wexler M (1952) The structural problem in schizophrenia. In: Brody E, Redlich FC (eds) Psychotherapy with schizophrenics. International Universities Press, New York

Scientific Evidence and System Change: The Soteria Experience

Loren R. Mosher[1] and Alma Z. Menn[2]

Introduction

The Soteria project is now more than 10 years old. Since 1972 (Soteria House opened in May 1971) more than 25 scientific papers have been published about various aspects of it. In 1974 a replication of the original study was initiated by opening a second facility called Emanon ("no name" spelled backwards). The project has received a million dollars of National Institutes of Mental Health (NIMH) research support. Despite what would appear to be the record of a "winner" or a "survivor," at least, it is likely that the psychological model of care the project developed, implemented, evaluated, and showed to be effective will not go beyond a one-time demonstration. Emanon closed in January 1981 due to our inability to find local resources to support its continuation as a clinical facility. Its research support was not continued; despite an approved NIMH grant request, it was not a high priority project. Soteria House itself may survive for a year or so because of an ongoing Community Mental Health Center (CMHC) staffing grant. Its research support has ended. The county in which Soteria is located allocates about $20 million per year for publicly funded mental treatment. Soteria House has never received any of this money. The reasons given are that it is a research facility and too small to be a significant addition to the country's services.

The major focus of this report is to try and analyze why Soteria is unacceptable to public and private treatment funding sources, despite scientific evidence that it represents a cost-effective form of treatment for some segment of persons who would otherwise be psychiatrically hospitalized. So readers can evaluate the quality of the scientific evidence for themselves, it is necessary to present the projects's background, research design, and results thus far.

Background

Difficulties the authors encountered with the treatment of psychosis in hospital settings provided a major impetus for the establishment of Soteria, a home where schizophrenics who would otherwise have been hospitalized live through their psychosis with a non-

1 Uniformed Services University of the Health Sciences 4301 Jones Bridge Rd., Bethesda, Md. 20814.

2 Institute for Psychosocial Interaction 555 Middlefield Rd., Palo Alto, Ca. 94301.

professional staff. To wit, hospitals – even well-staffed "progressive" ones – invariably have institutional characteristics which create barriers to establishing the types of relationships which could maximally facilitate the process of recovery from psychosis. The "barrier" characteristics to which we refer (present to varying degrees in different settings) are the following.

Theoretical Model

Although a variety of other models may be mixed in, or explicitly avowed, most psychiatric wards function primarily within a medical model: Doctors have final authority and decision-making powers; medications are accorded primary therapeutic value and used extensively; the person is seen as having a disease, with attendant disability and dysfunction which is to be "treated" and "cured"; and labeling and its consequences, objectification and stigmatization, are almost inevitable.

In contrast, at Soteria (from the Greek, salvation or deliverance) the primary focus is on growth, development, and learning. The staff are to "be with" the patients, or residents as we call them, to facilitate these processes insofar as they can. They share decision-making powers and responsibility with residents. They are not there either to treat or cure the residents. Neuroleptic medications are infrequently used. Although we have no quarrel with the demonstrated heuristic value of the medical model, we do believe its application to psychiatric disorders can have unfortunate (and unintended) consequences for individual patients. We are not proposing an alternative model, however, because we know of none that satisfactorily explains what we label "schizophrenia." We *do* propose an alternative attitude or stance: Basically, we advocate a phenomenologic approach to schizophrenia, i.e., an attempt to understand and share the psychotic person's experience without judging, labeling, derogating, or invalidating it.

Size

Most psychiatric hospital wards have at least 20 patients. Thus, the staff/patient group is apt to be 40–60 persons.

For severely disorganized persons, however, a social reference group of no more than 12–15 persons is especially important. We believe a group of this size, when combined with a homelike atmosphere, maximizes the possibility of the disorganized person's getting to know and trust a new environment and to find a surrogate family in it; at the same time, it minimizes the labeling and stigmatization process. This number is, interestingly, about the maximum number able to live under one roof as an extended family or commune. Most clinicians also believe 12 is about the upper limit for group therapy. Finally, experimental psychology's small task groups have been shown to function most effectively with not more than 12 members. Thus, rather than a 20-bed ward, Soteria is a home that sleeps 8–10 comfortably, with 6 beds occupied by residents and 2 by staff.

Social Structure

This aspect interacts closely with size: To function effectively, every organization, large or small, needs structure. In general, the larger the organization the greater the structure. Unfortunately, more elaborated structures have consequences which impinge negatively on persons undergoing psychotic disorganization: inflexibility, reliance on authority, institutionalization of roles, and decision-making power residing in the hierarchy – outside client's control. Inevitably, those at the bottom of the hierarchy feel powerless, irresponsible, and dependent. Because of this, at Soteria we are attempting to be as unstructured as is commensurate with adequate function. Structure which develops to meet functional needs is dissolved if the need is not a continuing one. There is no institutionalized method of dealing with a particular occurrence. For example, overt aggressive acts are dealt with in a variety of ways including physical control, depending on a myriad of contextual variables.

Medication

We live in an overmedicated, too frequently drug-dependent culture. Our ambivalence about drugs is resolved by creating two categories of drugs: good ones (e.g., alcohol), and bad ones (e.g., LSD). Psychiatry's attitude is no different from that of the wider social context; we are looking for the magical answer from a pill. The antipsychotic drugs have provided psychiatry with real substance for their magical cure fantasy with regard to schizophrenia. As is the case with most such exaggerated expectations, the fantasy is better than the reality. After 2 decades, it is now clear that the phenothiazines do not *cure* schizophrenia. It is also clear that they have serious, sometimes irreversible toxicities (Crane 1973), that recovery may be impaired by them in at least some schizophrenics (Goldstein 1970; Rappaport et al. 1978), and that they have little effect on long-term psychosocial adjustment (Niskanen and Achte 1972). This is not to deny their extraordinary helpfulness in reducing and controlling symptoms, shortening hospital stays, and revitalizing interest in schizophrenia. One aim of the Soteria project is to seek a viable, informed alternative to the overuse of, and excessive reliance on, these drugs – often to the exclusion of psychosocial measures. We use them infrequently and when prescribed, they are kept primarily under the individual resident's (patient's) control. That is, the resident is asked to monitor his response to the drug carefully, to give us feedback so we can adjust dosage, and after a trial period of 2 weeks he is given a major voice in determining whether or not the drug will be continued.

Soteria is a reaction to criticisms of existing facilities in each of the four areas mentioned above. However, much of what is involved in the program is based on the positive contributions of a variety of other researchers, clinicians, and theorists. In fact, we have come to recognize that no individual element of the Soteria program is new; it is their combination in one setting we believe to be unique.

To identify some of Soteria's roots: the era of moral treatment in America (Bockhoven 1963); the tradition of intensive interpersonal intervention in schizophrenia (Sullivan 1962; Fromm-Reichmann 1948); therapists who have described growth from psychosis (Menninger 1959; Perry 1962); the group of psychiatric heretics (Laing 1967;

Szasz 1961); and descriptions of the development of psychiatric disorder in respone to life crisis (Brown and Birley 1968).

Research Design

Sample Selection

All subjects are obtained from a screening facility that is part of the CMHC complex containing our control wards. Approximately 600 new patients are seen there per month, of whom about 250 are hospitalized. Anyone meeting the following basic criteria is a potential study candidate:

1. Clearly schizophrenic
2. Deemed in need of hospitalization
3. No more than one previous hospitalization for 2 weeks or less with a diagnosis of schizophrenia
4. Age 16–30 (either sex)
5. Unmarried, separated, widowed, or divorced

The selection criteria are designed to provide us with a relatively homogeneous sample of individuals diagnosed schizophrenic, but a group at risk for prolonged hospitalization or chronic disability. Early onset and being unmarried have both been shown to be predictive of need for chronic care (Strauss et al. 1977).

Treatment Assignment

Subjects meeting study selection criteria are identified without knowledge of the group to which they will ultimately be assigned. Study requirements are explained, and informed consent is obtained from the patient and his family, or significant other, if available. As only six residents can be accommodated in the experimental setting, intake is limited by bed availability. Therefore, consenting subjects are admitted to the experimental program if a bed is available. If no experimental bed is available, eligible consenting subjects are admitted to the comparison treatment group. Basically, this procedure results in treatment group assignment on a consecutively admitted, space-available basis. It should be emphasized that our experimental and control subjects are remarkably similar on demographic and baseline psychiatric symptomatology variables.

Research Assessment

The measures below are a partial list of those completed at baseline (admission to the study) and at followup (6, 12, and 24 months postadmission). All assessments are conducted by an independent research team that has no direct treatment responsibilities in either setting.

Baseline Assessment

Diagnosis. As per DSM-II (American Psychiatric Association 1968). For a subject to be included in the study, three independent diagnoses of schizophrenia must be in agreement.

Diagnostic Symptoms. A checklist of seven symptoms. Four of seven symptoms are required for inclusion in the study (Cole et al. 1964).

Certainty of Diagnosis. A seven-point scale (Mosher et al. 1971).

Mode of Onset. Assesses acute/insidious onset types (Vaillant 1964).

Paranoid/Nonparanoid Status. A short scale for rating paranoid schizophrenia (Venables and O'Conner 1959).

Inpatient Multidimensional Psychiatric Scale. A widely used symptom rating scale producing scores on ten psychotic syndromes (Lorr et al. 1963).

Global Severity. An overall measure of psychopathology.

Brief Social History Form. A detailed description of a patient's and family's psychiatric and social history (Boothe et al. 1972).

Follow-up Assessment

Patient Progess Report. For each 6-month interval, information on the subject's medication history, use of other treatment, living arrangements (including any hospital readmissions), work status, social contacts, global severity, and improvement is obtained.

Clinical Settings

Experimental

Soteria is a 1915-vintage, 12-room house located on a busy street in a "transitional" neighborhood of a San Francisco Bay Area city. Bordering Soteria on one side is a nursing home and on the other, a two-family home. The neighborhood has a mixture of small businesses, medical facilities (a general hospital is one block away), single-family homes, and small apartments (usually homes that have been remodeled for this purpose). It is a designated poverty area inhabited by a mixture of colllege students, lower-class families, and ex-state hospital patients. Some 15%–20% of residents in the area are Mexican-American and there is a sprinkling of blacks.

Due primarily to licensing laws, the house can accommodate only six residents at one time, although as many as ten persons can sleep there comfortably. There are six paid nonprofessional staff plus the project director and a one-fourth time project psychiatrist. One or two new residents are admitted each month. In general, two of our specially trained nonprofessional staff, a man and a woman, are on duty at any one time. In addition, there are usually one or more volunteers present, especially in the evening. Most staff work 36- to 48-h shifts to provide themselves the opportunity to relate to "spaced-out" (their term) residents continuously over a relatively long period of time. Staff and residents share responsibility for household maintenance, meal preparation, and cleanup. Persons who are not "together" are not expected to do an equal share of the work. Over the long term, staff do more than their share and will step in to assume responsibility if a resident cannot do a task to which he has agreed. The project director acts as friend, counselor, supervisor, and object for displaced angry feelings by staff. The part-time project psychiatrist supervises the staff and is seen as a stable, reassuring presence (in addition to his formal medicolegal responsibilities).

Although staff vary somewhat in how they see their roles, they generally view what psychiatry labels a "schizophrenic reaction" as an altered state of consciousness in an individual who is experiencing a crisis in living. Simply put, the altered state involves personality fragmentation, with the loss of a sense of self.

Few clinicians would disagree with a description of the evolution of psychosis as a process of fragmentation and disintegration. But, at Soteria House, the disruptive psychotic experience is also believed to have unique potential for reintegration and reconstitution if it is not prematurely aborted or forced into some psychologically straitjacketing compromise. Such a view of schizophrenia implies a number of therapeutic attitudes. All facets of the psychotic experience are taken by Soteria House staff members as "real." They view the experiental and behavioral attitudes associated with the psychosis – the clinical symptoms, including irrationality, terror, and mystical experiences – as extremes of basic human qualities. Because "irrational" behavior and mystical beliefs are regarded as valid and as capable of being understood, Soteria staff try to provide an atmosphere that will facilitate integration of the psychosis into the continuity of the individual's life. Thus, psychotic persons are not to be considered "diseased," nor are they to be related to in a depersonalized way, for to do so would invalidate the experience. When the fragmentation process is seen as valid and as having potential for psychological growth, the individual experiencing the schizophrenic reaction can be tolerated, lived with, related to, and validated, but not "treated" or used to fulfill staff needs. Limits are set if the person is clearly a danger to himself, others or the program as a whole – not merely because others are unable to tolerate his madness. Phenothiazines are ordinarily not used for 6 weeks. If the resident shows no change at that time and is either paranoid or has an insidious onset, chlorpromazine (300 mg/day or more) is given.

A word about the background for our use of specially trained nonprofessionals as primary staff (see also Mosher et al. 1973). We believe that relatively untrained, psychologically unsophisticated persons can assume a phenomenological stance vis-à-vis psychosis more easily than highly trained persons (e.g., MDs or PhDs) because they have learned no theory of schizophrenia, whether psychodynamic, organic, or a combination of both. Because they lack the preconceived ideas of professionals, our nonprofessional staff members have the freedom to be themselves, to follow their visceral responses, and to be a "person" with the psychotic individual. Highly trained mental health professionals tend to lose this freedom in facor of a more cognitive, theory-based, learned response that may invalidate a patient's experience of himself if the professional's theory-based behavior is not congruent with the patient's felt needs. Professionals may also use their theoretical knowledge defensively when confronted, in an unstructured setting, with anxiety-provoking behaviors of psychotic persons. This pattern of response is not so readily available to our unsophisticated nonprofessional therapists; nor is it reinforced by a professional degree with its accompanying status and power.

CMHC Comparison Ward

The Community Mental Health Center's inpatient service consists of two locked wards of 30 beds each. About 250 patients are admitted (including readmissions) per month. It is a well-staffed (1.5/1 staff/patient ratio) active treatment facility oriented towards crisis intervention, employing high doses of neuroleptics, rapid evaluation, and placement in other parts of the county's treatment network as its immediate goal. All of the control patients reported here received phenothiazines during their inpatient stays. Only one was discharged off drugs.

The CMHC staff is generally well trained, experienced, and enthusiastic; they see themselves as doing a good job. Patients are assigned to one of five treatment teams on each ward which meet daily to decide treatment plans. Patients are assigned a therapist who provides 30 min of psychotherapy daily and takes a major role in treatment planning. The therapist may be a technician, community worker, or any of the other treatment specialists. There are 90 min per day of occupational therapy and a daily community meeting led by any member of the treatment team. A crisis group meets for 90 min 5 times per week (all patients); a couples group, 2 h per week (married patients and spouses); a psychodrama group, 2 h per week (all patients who are able); a women's group, 2 h per week; and a survival group (for readmitted patients) 90 min 3 times per week.

Because the Center inpatient service takes patients from all over the county (it is the only facility with a 24-h-a-day psychiatric emergency service and locked wards), most patients are referred back to one of four regional centers nearest their homes for outpatient care. This care may include partial hospitalization (day or night care); individual, family, or group therapy; and medication followup. The county also has an extensive board and care system and eight halfway houses for adolescents and adults.

Results

Two-year outcome data from this group of subjects have been reported in detail elsewhere (Mosher and Menn 1978; Matthews et al. 1979). Briefly summarized, the significant results are:

Table 1. Demographic data at admission

Variable	Experimental group	Control group
Age		
N	37	42
Mean ± SD	21.1 ± 3.3	22.5 ± 4.1
Range	15–28 years	16–31 years
Sex		
N	37	42
Male	19(51%)	26(62%)
Female	18(49%)	16(38%)
Social class[a]		
N	33	27
Mean ± SD	3.1 ± 1.1	3 ± 1.1
Range	1 to 5	1 to 5
Education		
N	37	36
College graduate	2(5%)	4(11%)
Some college	19(51%)	20(56%)
High school graduate or some high school	16(43%)	12(33%)

[a] Based on the Hollingshead-Redlich Index of Social Class for father.

Admission Characteristics. Subjects in the two programs are remarkably similar on most demographic and admission psychiatric variables (Tables 1, 2). However, the CMHC sample is significantly older by about 2 years ($P \leqslant 0.05$) than the Soteria sample, and the CMHC sample stayed a significantly shorter duration of time in the hospital ($P \leqslant 0.001$) during their original stay (a difference expected because of the treatment orientation in each facility).

Milieu Assessment. Because of our conception of the Soteria program as a recovery-facilitating social environment, systematic study and comparison of the two milieus are particularly important. We have used Moos' WAS and COPES scales for this purpose (Moos 1974). The between-program differences, we find, have been remarkable in their magnitude and stability over 10 years. As may be seen in Fig. 1, the Soteria environment is perceived as significantly different from the CMHC milieu on nine of ten subscales of the Moos instrument. They are seen similarly on only the order and organization variable. This pattern has remained stable (with minor fluctuations) for the project's 10-year life (Fig. 2, 3). Thus, we may conclude that the two environments are, in fact, very different with Soteria milieu conforming closely to our predictions (Wendt et al. 1983).

Readmissions. Utilizing the lifetable method (Klerman et al. 1974; Fleiss et al. 1976) to study community survivorship, Soteria patients had a better chance (by about 20%) than CMHC patients of having never been rehospitalized over the 2-year follow-up interval. At 12 months postdischarge the cumulative probability of having not been

Table 2. Psychiatric assessments at admission

Variable	Experimental group	Control group
Diagnostic symptoms (maximum, 7)		
N	37	32
Mean ± SD	5.2 ± 1.3	5.3 ± 0.7
Thought disorder	95%	74%
Hallucinations	87%	57%
Delusions	68%	62%
All three	60%	41%
Certainty of diagnosis[a]		
N	37	33
Mean ± SD	6.2 ± 0.8	6.3 ± 0.8
Range	4 to 7	5 to 7
Mode of onset[b]		
N	35	34
Mean ± SD	2.4 ± 1.2	2.7 ± 0.9
Acute	49%	59%
Insidious	51%	41%
Paranoid-nonparanoid status[c]		
N	37	33
Mean ± SD	11.9 ± 5.2	11.6 ± 5.4
Paranoid	41%	34%
Nonparanoid	59%	66%

[a] Maximum rating 7, indicating definitely schizophrenic.
[b] Maximum score 4: 1 or 2 indicates insidious, 3 or 4 acute.
[c] Maximum score 25: 13 or more indicates paranoid.

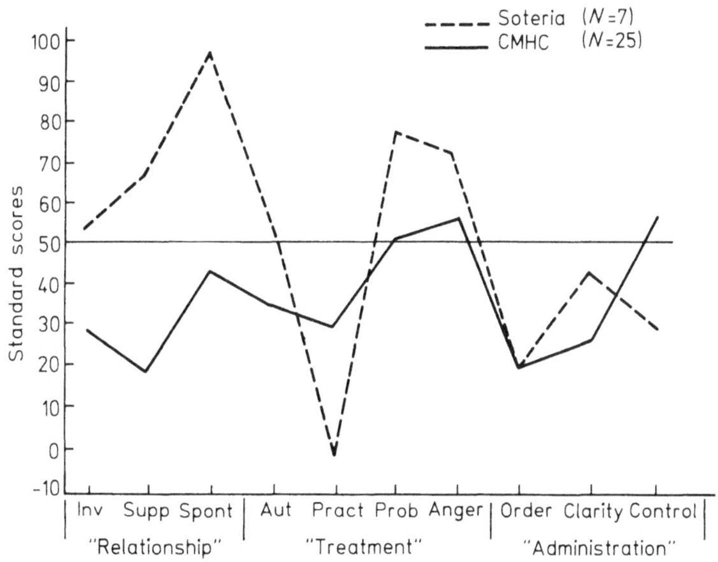

Fig. 1. Comparison of Soteria and CMHC staff WAS "real" testing: Based on staff norms for 160 wards

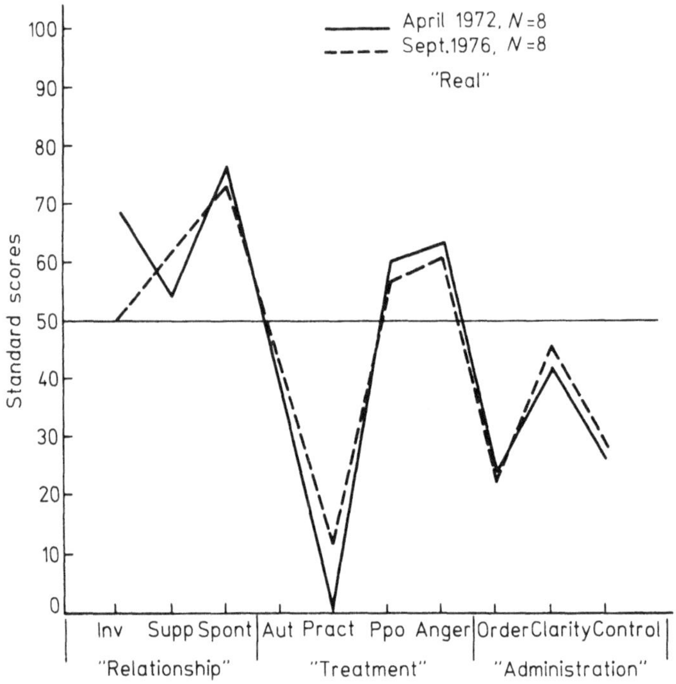

Fig. 2. COPES change over time: Soteria staff

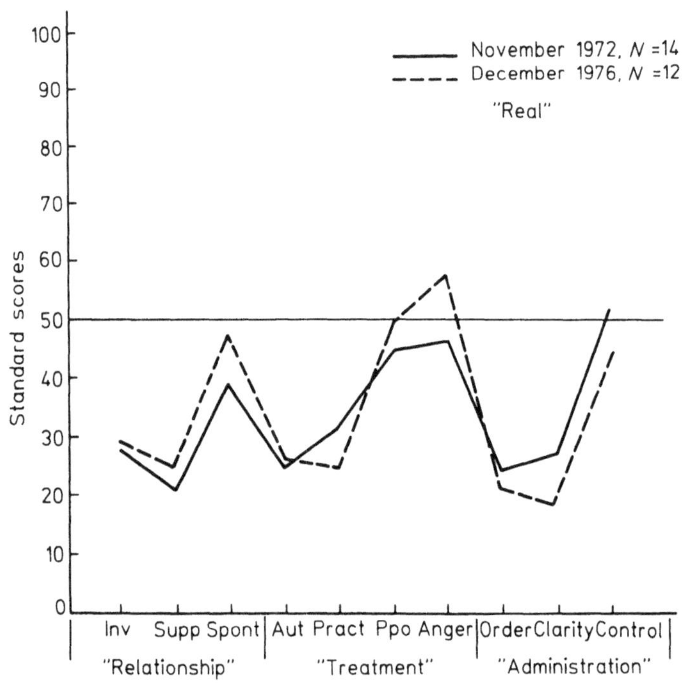

Fig. 3. WAS change over time: Valley staff

rehospitalized significantly favors ($P \leqslant 0.05$) Soteria subjects. These differences occurred despite the fact that 50% of the CMHC sample was maintained on neuroleptics up to the point of readmission or until 24 months postdischarge, whereas only 19% of the Soteria sample received postdischarge neuroleptic drug treatment, with half of the 19% maintained continuously on neuroleptics.

Community Psychosocial Adjustment. At 2 years postadmission, Soteria-treated subjects were working at significantly higher occupational levels and were more often living independently or with peers.

Cost. Despite the large differences in lengths of stay during the initial admissions (about 1 vs 5 months), the cost of the first 6 months of care for both groups is about $4000.

System Change

Based on what we have presented in the Research Design and Results sections of this report, it is fair to say that the Soteria project has presented evidence that suggests that newly diagnosed schizophrenic patients can be treated as well – or better – at no greater cost in a nonhospital community setting as in hospital. Our results are consistent with those of others who have studied nonhospital alternative treatments, e.g., Fairweather et al. 1969; Pasamanick 1967; Stein and Test 1976; Langsley et al. 1968; Polak and Kirby 1976. Have these presentations of scientific evidence resulted in a shift away from the use of hospitals to use of alternative methods of care in the United States? Basically, the answer is no.

The evidence has not persuaded psychiatry that nonhospital alternatives are a useful ingredient in the therapeutic smorgasbord. Why, in the era of so-called scientific psychiatry, have these types of facilities and clinical care paradigms not been widely implemented? The answer(s) to this question is both complex and elusive. The most facile answer is that the studies were either insufficiently rigorous, did not provide convincing evidence, or were one-time, unreplicable products of the investigators' enthusiasm and dedication. As one of these enthusiastic investigators, I must ask how many comparative outcome studies of variations in hospital treatment are there? Despite the vast numbers of patients psychiatrically hospitalized each year (more than a million in the United States), there are very few controlled outcome studies of systematically varied inpatient care (Glick et al. 1974; Herz et al. 1971; Caffey et al. 1972). While the evidence supportive of the use of alternatives may not be incontrovertible, there would appear to be more hard data relative to their usefulness than there is for in-hospital treatment.

If the evidence presented is in itself *acceptable,* why is the next step – its application to clinical care settings – not? I would posit that the implementation of alternatives is unacceptable because they represent a threat to in-hospital psychiatry's turf. What are the elements of the Soteria program (these are true to a greater or lesser extent for most alternatives) that are perceived as threats to hospital psychiatry?

In brief, the elements of the Soteria program most relevant to this discussion are:

1. The facility is not a hospital and its program is not run by doctors or nurses by delegation. However, it admits only clients who would have otherwise been hospitalized.
2. Neuroleptics, the standard treatment for schizophrenia, are used as infrequently as possible, preferably not at all.
3. Primary treatment responsibility, power, and authority are vested in the nonprofessional staff.

What are the means by which traditional hospital psychiatry has defended itself against this rather radical attempt to demedicalize psychosis? We will describe four that we believe to be most used to maintain the status quo.

Lack of Third-party Payers

Foremost, and most effective, there are no third-party payers in the United States willing to underwrite this form of care. The United States does not have a national health insurance system. Those who can afford it pay for their health care by the purchase of insurance from private carriers like Blue Cross and Blue Shield and others. The government pays for health care for those who cannot afford private insurance through its Medicaid and Medicare programs. Whether privately or governmentally supported this form of payment is referred to as "third-party" (i.e., not paid directly by the patient). Without reimbursement from these sources Soteria and other programs like it cannot survive. Through complex negotiations and good luck, we were able to obtain a staffing grant from a local CMHC to partly support the Soteria staff. Although Federal CMHC regulations allow it, this use of staffing grant money to support alternatives is unusual. The facility does not qualify for Medicare or Medicaid and our attempts to change the relevant regulations have been unsuccessful so far. The responses of the private insurance carriers to our requests to be included as a reimbursable service at least on a trial basis were interesting. The typical third-party payer response is:

a) "It's not a hospital and therefore is not providing a reimbursable medical service".
b) "It's still experimental and has not provided sufficient data about cost-effectiveness to warrant consideration for inclusion."
c) "We might consider it on a 1- or 2-year experimental basis if you are willing to meet JCAH[3] hospital staffing standards." Two-day hospitals had previously been supported in this way. Because those standards require extensive MD and RN coverage, the program would become much more expensive that it is and its nonmedical basic philosophic tenets violated – hence a catch-22 situation.
d) "We are already paying for too many psychiatry hospital beds; covering alternatives would only expand bed capacity futher and hence increase our (insurer) costs. If you (i.e., the Soteria project) would close six existing hospital beds we might consider it."

---

3 Joint Commission on Accreditation of Hospitals (JCAH) is a national organization which sets staffing and record-keeping standards for medical facilities in the United States.

I do not mean to imply that psychiatry actively moved to prevent third-party payment for alternatives; rather only that it has not joined in to actively seek it.

This situation is an example of bureaucratization in the insurance industry. In the case of Blue Cross/Blue Shield it is also an example of a professional group controlling its funding source.

The ultimate viability of alternatives in the therapeutic market place resides with funding sources. The degree of interest these fiscal intermediaries will have in paying for innovations in care is strongly influenced by the prevailing zeitgeist. In the last decade or so there has been a substantial shift in psychiatry's zeitgeist – away from a socioenvironmental one to a more medical biologic point of view. Thus, there is little pressure to pay for a basically nonmedical treatment. What are other relevant manifestations of the biomedical zeitgeist? It would appear that psychiatry is doing what it believes it must to continue to qualify for third-party payment, i.e., sticking with hospital-based wards.

The Medicalization of Community Psychiatry

It is ironic that the now nearly 20-year-old community psychiatry movement in the United States has moved the mental health system back into closer juxtaposition with the somatic health system. That is, the relative isolation of mental health before the 1960s – as manifested in the state hospital systems – was broken down with the advent of community psychiatry with its emphasis on inpatient care on wards in general medical hospitals. The growth of such wards was also given impetus by psychiatric coverage in various health insurance programs. For the most part, payment for inpatient care in general hospitals has been the only consistently available mental health benefit. These two factors account in large part for growth of these wards and the increasing numbers of patients treated in them. For example, between 1967 and 1971, the numbers of schizophrenic patients treated on such wards nearly doubled – from 90,000 to 170,000 (Taube 1969, 1973).

This process of bringing "mental illness" back into the mainstream of medicine was given further impetus by a flurry of developments in medical technology. That is, a whole array of new sophisticated techniques became available for use in the search for the "schizococcus" and other specific etiologies of mental illness. Application of these techniques to "mental illness" has provided us with a deluge of new information but has as yet failed to discover specific etiologic factors in psychosis. In addition, in a characteristically American fashion, a new generation of technology-oriented biological psychiatrists has risen preferentially to positions of influence and power in many medical school departments of psychiatry.

Neuroleptics: The answer at last; or wishes transformed to myths

Another important factor in the progressive medicalization of madness has been the introduction and widespread use of neuroleptic drugs – clearly efficacious treatments for psychosis. Because drugs can only be prescribed by MDs, so long as drugs are viewed as "the answer" to mental illess, doctors' power and control of the treatment system are inevitable and will increase.

Because pills are given to individuals, they maintain medicine's traditional focus on *a* person as "sick." This can prevent the doctor and the system over which he presides from looking at the family and wider social contextual factors that might have exerted important influences on the development of psychosis – and might also therefore be amenable to intervention. Thus, medications can narrow conceptual sights and unnecessarily limit treatment possibilities.

The drugs have also produced at least one widely held myth (at least in the United States) that they are responsible for the massive deinstitutionalization that began in the early 1960s and crescendoed after 1967. This is a gross overinterpretation of their power. Deinstitutionalization began in earnest when federal Medicare dollars become available to states. Ergo, elderly patients were moved from hospitals to nursing homes – and their cost shifted from state to federal dollars. In Europe, for example, where an economic incentive does not exist, deinstitutionalization has been slower and more modest in scope.

The Waning Influence of Psychoanalysis

I believe it is fair to say that the 50s and early 60s were the heyday of psychoanalytic influence on more traditional psychiatry. Psychoanalysts and analytic theories were widely used for both descriptive and etiologic purposes. For a number of years it was almost de rigueur for residents in the best known training programs to enter analytic training.

In the late 60s and through the 70s their influence has been much diluted by waves of findings from the new technologists and technology. The appeal of analytic constructs, so pervasive in the 50s and 60c, has been replaced by more reliable, identifiable, and quantifiable neurotransmitters, endorphins, etc. The sometimes poetic, slightly gossamer, often convoluted, and difficult-to-grasp analytic variables have been replaced by ones with known and reproducible norms, means, and standard deviations. Whether these high tech findings have made a substantial contribution to clinical practice remains a moot point.

This evolution is complex in its derivation but nevertheless psychoanalysis as a discipline does not seem to be as interested in psychosis as it was during its halcyon days. The neuroleptics, development of rapid turnover wards in general hospitals, and community psychiatry each contributed to what I perceive as a withdrawal of psychoanalysis' cathexis of psychosis. In a sense, exploration of the uncharted territories of psychosis seems to have been given up in favor of a return to the original turf of analysis – the outpatient treatment of neurosis. This brief discussion is obviously oversimplified, biased, and subject to many exceptions. However, it does give one person's perception – with little vested interest in the process – of a facet of recent history.

References

Bockhoven J (1963) Moral treatment in American psychiatry. Spring Publishing Co, New York

Boothe H, Schooler N, Goldberg S (1972) Brief social history for studies in schizophrenia: an announcement of a new data collection instrument. Psychopharmacol Bull 8:23–44

Brown GW, Birley JLT (1968) Crisis and life changes and the onset of schizophrenia. J Health Soc Behav 9:203–214

Caffey EM, Galbrecht CR, Klett CJ (1972) Brief hospitalization and aftercare in the treatment of schizophrenia. Arch Gen Psychiatry 24:81–86

Cole J, Klerman G, Goldberg S (1964) Effectiveness of phenothiazine treatment in acute schizophrenics. Arch Gen Psychiatry 10:246–261

Crane G (1973) Clinical psychopharmacology in its 20th year. Science 181:124–128

Fairweather G, Sanders D, Cressler D, Maynard H (1969) Community life for the mentally ill: An alternative to institutional care. Adline Publishing Co, Chicago

Fleiss J, Dunner L, Stallone P, Fiever R (1976) The life table: a method for analyzing longitudinal studies. Arch Gen Psychiatry 33:107–112

Fromm-Reichman F (1948) Notes on the development of treatment of schizophrenia by psychoanalytic psychotherapy. Psychiatry 11:263–273

Glick I, Hargreaves WA, Goldfield MD (1974) Short vs. long hospitalization: a controlled prospective study. Arch Gen Psychiatry 30:363–369

Goldstein M (1970) Premorbid adjustment, paranoid status, and patterns of response to phenothiazine in acute schizophrenia. Schizophr Bull 3:24–37

Herz MI, Endicott J, Spitzer R, Mesnikoff A (1971) Day vs. inpatient hospitalization. Am J Psychiatry 127(10):107–118

Klerman G, DiMascio A, Weissman M, Prusoff B, Paykel ES (1974) Treatment of depression by drugs and psychotherapy. Am J Psychiatry 131:186–191

Laing R (1967) The politics of experience. Ballantine Books, New York

Langsley DG, Kaplan DM, Pittman FS, Machotka P, Flomenhaft K, DeYoung CD (1968) The treatment of families in crisis. Grune and Stratton, New York

Lorr M, Klett C, McNair D (1963) Syndromes of psychosis. Macmillan, New York

Matthews SM, Roper MT, Mosher LR, Menn AZ (1979) A non-neuroleptic treatment for schizophrenia: analysis of the two-year postdischarge risk of relapse. Schizophr Bull 5(2):322–333

Menninger K (1959) Psychiatrist's world. In: Hall B (ed) The selected papers of Karl Menninger. Viking Press, New York

Moos RH (1974) Evaluating treatment environments: A social ecological approach. John Wiley and Sons, New York

Mosher L, Pollin W, Stabenau J (1971) Identical twins discordant for schizophrenia: neurologic findings. Arch Gen Psychiatry 24:422–430

Mosher L, Reifman A, Menn A (1973) Characteristics of nonprofessionals serving as primary therapists for acute schizophrenics. Hosp Community Psychiatry 24:391–395

Mosher LR, Menn A (1978) Community residential treatment for schizophrenia: two-year followup data. Hosp Community Psychiatry 29:715–723

Niskanen P, Achte K (1972) The course and prognosis of schizophrenic psychoses in Helsinki: A comparative study of first admissions in 1950. Monogr No. 2 from the Psychiatric Clinic of the Helsinki University Central Hospital

Pasamanick B, Scarpitti FD, Dinitz S (1967) Schizophrenics in the community. Appleton-Century-Crofts, New York

Perry J (1962) Reconstitutive process in the psychopathology of the self. Ann N Y Acad Sci 96: 853–876

Polak PR, Kirby MW (1976) A model to replace psychiatric hospitals. J Nerv Ment Dis 162: 13–22

Rappaport M, Hopkins HK, Hall K, Belleza T, Silverman J (1978) Are there schizophrenics for whom drugs may be unnecessary or contraindicated? Int Pharmaco-psychiatry 13:100–111

Stein LI, Test MA (1976) Training in community living: One year evaluation. Am J Psychiatry 133:917–918

Strauss JS, Kokes RF, Klorman R, Sacksteder JL (1977) Premorbid adjustment in schizophrenia: concepts, measures, and implications. Part I. The concept of premorbid adjustment. Schizophr Bull 3(2):182–185

Sullivan H (1962) Schizophrenia as a human process. W. W. Norton and Co., New York

Szasz T (1961) The myth of mental illness: Foundations of a theory of personal conduct. Hoeber-Harper, New York

Taube C (1973) Length of stay of discharges from general hospital psychiatric inpatient units, United States 1970–1971. Statistical Note 70. Biometry Branch, NIMH

Taube C (1969) General hospital inpatient psychiatric services 1967. Survey and reports section, Biometry Branch, Office of Program Planning and Evaluation, NIMH

Vaillant G (1964) Prospective prediction of schizophrenic remission. Arch Gen Psychiatry 11: 509–515

Venables P, O'Connor N (1959) A short scale for rating paranoid schizophrenia. J Mental Sci 105: 815–818

Wendt J, Mosher LR, Matthews S, Menn A (1983) A comparison of two treatment environments for schizophrenia. In: Gunderson JG, Will OA Jr, Mosher LR (eds) The principles and practices of milieu therapy. Jason Aronson, Inc, New York, pp 17–33

Community Work and Participation in the New Italian Psychiatric Legislation

Paolo Tranchina and Paolo Serra[1]

Introduction

With this chapter we have the opportunity to continue the discussion which we started 6 years ago at the 5th Symposium on Psychotherapy of Schizophrenia in Oslo (Arezzo Group 1975). Many things have happened since then.

First, we must remember the premature death of Professor Franco Basaglia who, with his practical and theoretical work, opened up the road to a new type of psychiatric practice based on the rejection of institutional violence, on a review of the social mandate given to psychiatrists, and on research into social participation and the collective response to suffering.

In 1978 a new psychiatric legislation, which reflected the ideas of alternative work being carried out in recent years, was enacted in Italy. Before examining the concrete aspects of the new law it is necessary to go back and sum up schematically the distinguishing elements of Democratic Psychiatry.

Fundamental Aspects of the Alternative Italian Experience

The practical work which has been carried out, beginning in the 1960s at the psychiatric hospital of Gorizia and then in other places such as Trieste, Arezzo, Ferrara,

---

1 Paolo Tranchina, analytical psychologist, specialized in 1971 at the C. G. Jung Institute in Zurich, has worked as an analyst in Milan and afterwards at psychiatric hospitals in Arezzo and Florence. He currently works as a full time psychologist at local health unit No. 9, in Prato (Florence). Since 1972 he has directed, together with Professor Agostino Pirella, the "Fogli di Informazione," the bimonthly magazine of the alternative psychiatric movement in Italy. In 1978 he published the book *Norma e antinorma* (Feltrinelli, Milan), which deals with the connection between psychoanalysis and alternative psychiatry.
Paolo Serra, M.D., specialized in psychiatry in 1975 at the university of Rome. He worked at the mental hospital in Gorizia in 1972. From 1973 to 1977 he worked in the Arezzo Psychiatric Hospital and since 1978 he has been head of the psychiatric hospital services of the Casentino valley (province of Arezzo). Since 1981 he has also been director of part of the psychiatric hospital of Arezzo.

and Perugia, and is now in the process of development also in big cities such as Turin and Genoa,[2] has the following basic features:

1. It began in public mental hospitals by taking over the responsibility for all types of psychiatric suffering. It was not simply a case of pilot studies using chosen staff, selected patients, and privileged economic and institutional conditions. Starting work in public mental hospitals favored the expansion of the alternative experience (Basaglia 1968; Pirella 1975).

2. The democratic workers did not limit themselves to technical work which was more highly qualified than traditional psychiatry, but tried continually to create ties with all administrative, political, social, trade union, popular, and citizen bodies, to place the fight for the renewal of psychiatry in the center of the greater fight for health reform.

3. The struggle against institutional segregation has mobilized to a great extent all the country's communications media, taking psychiatry out of its traditional isolation and continually trying to tie it to the national political and social context, to work organizations, and to the processes of exploitation (Basaglia 1971).

4. The actual destruction of the mental hospital and the search for territorial alternatives was not only a technical fact, but went hand in hand with a collective examination of the processes of social rejection typical of our society, and of all types of contradictions whether economic, social, historical, or domestic, which manifest themselves as psychological problems in concrete individuals. This study has also stripped the therapeutic pretense from the mental hospital, revealing the latter's true repressive function along with that of all other total institutions (Basaglia 1974).

The Practical Work of Opening Up the Mental Hospital

The practical work, initially inspired by the experience of M. Jones, took the following form:

1. Progressive opening up of all departments and elimination of the highest levels of violence: physical isolation, electroshock, and the abuse of drugs.

2. Frequent use of departmental and general meetings as a tool for reopening dialogue and allowing contradictions to emerge into the open (Ferrara and Tranchina 1980). This therapeutic tool went hand in hand with other personal meetings to increase understanding and communication.

2 Franco Basaglia at the time of his death had the responsibility for all the mental health services of the province of Rome and the whole Lazio region. At present Agostino Pirella is the director of the mental health services of the Piedmont region. Antonio Slavich directs the mental hospital at Genoa and Sergio Piro is director of a mental hospital in Naples.

3. Constant questioning of the institutional hierarchy and increasing psychiatric nurses' responsibility by going beyond their exclusive role of control and observation.[3]

4. Progressive reconstruction of the personality, history, and social role of the patients by continually breaking down physical and psychological barriers between the inside and the outside of the hospital; examination of the general processes which caused the isolation and disturbance of each individual patient, and research into economic and occupational alternatives to the old forms of ergotherapy.

The processes of collective rehabilitation for long-term patients and nonrepressive treatment for short-term cases have permitted the reevaluation of the subjectivity of patients through an encounter which is open to exchange, research into alternatives, and to the discovery of the common basis of suffering beyond all diagnostic labels and standard therapeutic treatment.

The continuous exchange between hospital and community has been essential and has permitted, as soon as the discharges of long-term patients increased, the transfer of the intervention center from the hospital to the community, using structures like family houses, outpatient services, social centers, and so on, and a massive use of home treatment (Berger 1979; Haugsgjerd, Engelstad 1977; Jantzen 1980).

The New Law

The essential aspects of the new law are:

1. Progressive elimination of psychiatric hospitals. The law in fact states: "It is in any case forbidden to build new psychiatric hospitals and to utilize those already existing as specialized psychiatric divisions of general hospitals."

2. Only the patients who have been already admitted are allowed to be readmitted, and this, with varying time limits for each region, up to December 1981.

3. With regard to compulsory admissions, it is obligatory to use exclusively special services "for diagnosis and treatment" in the general hospital up to a maximum of 15 beds. Three circumstances are indispensable for carrying out a compulsory treatment: (a) "That there exist psychic alterations such that urgent therapeutic interventions are required," (b) that these interventions "are not accepted by the patient," (c) "that there may not exist conditions and circumstances that would permit the adoption of immediate and adequate mental health measures outside the hospital." Even in these cases the admission is temporary, the patient does not lose his civil rights, he can communicate with whom ever he wishes, and he enjoys wide democratic guarantees.

---

3 As Maccacaro observed: "... the definition of mental illness ... is only an opinion of deviance related to a referent whose definition changes continuously as the verifier changes." (Maccacaro 1978)

4. Finally, the law gives favor to community interventions and states: "The interventions of prevention, cure, and rehabilitation relative to mental illness are put into effect as a rule by the community services and by those facilities not located in the hospital."

Commentary on the Law

The progressive elimination of the psychiatric hospital, recognized as a nontherapeutic and alienating place, is one of the most unique aspects of the new law. The fundamental institution of isolation is broken down in this way, with a clean cut for the short-term patients and limitations for long-term patients. The use of the general hospital as a last resort for compulsory treatment means of course using medication to treat the most serious psychic suffering, but it is also a fundamental step in freeing psychiatry from its isolation as compared with medicine in general. The stigma associated with psychiatric suffering is in this way notably diminished.

The law has eliminated the concept of danger in the use of compulsory treatment; at one time the patient was declared "dangerous to himself and/or to others or a public scandal." The notion of danger has been replaced by an assessment which together with the seriousness of the illness considers also the absence of necessary community alternatives. Compulsory treatment, therefore, is not carried out using only parameters connected to the seriousness of the illness and to the ontological definition of the same illness, but also makes precise reference to the scarce community organization in the patient's treatment (Amministrazione Provinciale di Arezzo 1977). Compulsory treatment is no longer used exclusively for the defense of society against its deviant members, but as the awareness of the scarcity of the community answers to psychic problems increases, it involves more respect for the individual and less stigmatization. The center of treatment has moved from the hospital to the community. This aspect indicates the recognition of the right of the patient to be cured, normally, within the environment in which his contradictions evolved and thus indicates the necessity of mobilizing all available social resources to counter his suffering. Participation and collective solutions, which can create solidarity and help through enhanced awareness of the common aspects of suffering, are part of a trend which opposes the logic of segregation and of research on the sacrificial lamb.

The Enforcement of the Law

Like any socially advanced law, this one too is enforced with varying resistance. The delays, polemics, and objections are many. In some towns the new law is often transgressed or minimally applied with a massive use of drugs and almost no community work. In the experience inspired by Franco Basaglia's work, however, the law offers the possibilities of alternative treatment and permits starting new points of examination of the essence of mental diseases and the course these take within the framework of community treatment and the involvement of nontechnical forces (Simons 1980).

In the first year of enforcement there was a decrease of about 17% of the population of the psychiatric hospitals in Italy; this population has fallen from 52,305 inmates to 43,526. Compulsory admissions have decreased by 63%, declining from 33,287 to 12,244. This trend, which is continuing, shows the progressive erosion of the old mental institutions and demonstrates how many of the compulsory admissions carried out in the past were completely arbitrary.

One can also note relevant differences between the north and the south of Italy. This confirms how strongly socioeconomic conditions influence the general health organization.

The delays in creating intermediate structures are very serious and widespread and are due to several facts: (a) opposition on the part of traditional psychiatry, generally established in general hospitals, towards community work; (b) bureaucratic inefficiencies of the new administrative organization; (c) government and spending cuts which, in respect to health and other social services, heavily influence the treatment of the less privileged classes.

From this general view, indispensable to an understanding of the parameters within which our present work is operative, we will now move on to some considerations more directly connected to the problem of participation.

New Significant Facts

Examining our direct experience over these years of enforcement of the new law, the following significant facts emerge:

1. In new cases we practically never resort to hospitalization and crises seem to manifest themselves with lesser significance.
2. The major problems are with patients who have had many admissions to psychiatric hospitals, for whom it is often difficult not to use general hospitals.
3. In every case in which nonprofessionals together with psychiatric staff offer the patient their solidarity and help we note a remarkable decrease in the intensity of symptoms.

Home Treatment of Crises

The possibility of avoiding hospitalization of new cases through intensified relations with the patient, his relatives, and the environment means that it is possible to follow particularly problematic and acute situations at home, on condition that sufficiently elastic services and the necessary community connections with general practitioners, political forces, and the public exist. Obviously this requires great responsibility, reliability, and a rejection of the traditional codes of working hours, as well as a deep knowledge of the community and the ability to mobilize various forces and to invent solutions case by case.

We believe that a change can be observed in the seriousness of the symptoms through which the most dramatic crises are manifested, whether they be treated at home or in hospitals. It seems that immediate treatment, coupled with the certainty that hospitalization is an exception, modifies the way patients express their psychotic experience.

The understanding of suffering in the environment in which it is manifested allows us to ascertain and try to modify a series of variants which absolutely cannot be identified in separate situations, such as searching for immediate solutions to the principal contradictions. On this subject we would like to relate a case which, we believe, shows interesting features.

R. C. is a 27-year-old worker, an only child, who lives with his parents in a small village in the Casentino valley in the province of Arezzo. One Sunday his parents telephoned the psychiatric hospital and asked for immediate admission for their son. After a period of several months of only spasmodic communication, he began to feel he was being followed when driving, being observed when sleeping, and was bothered by voices and noises. A few days before his parents' telephone call to us, he had become aggressive towards them to the point of threatening his father with a hatchet, because he believed that his father knew his persecutor but would not tell him who this persecutor was. After various interviews with the parents, who refused to enter the house, one of us went to visit the son, who had shut himself in the house and gave no signs of life. The doctor called him repeatedly by name and when R. partially opened the door, holding a hatchet, the doctor identified himself as a physician on duty called by his parents, who were worried about his health. Before entering the house the doctor declared his intention was only to talk, that he was alone, and that R. had nothing to fear. Once inside the house the doctor asked R. to put down his hatchet because a hatchet invokes fear, and when one is afraid it is more difficult to communicate. After this they began to discuss R. 's persecution. R. accurately described his experiences and declared that his persecution was objectively true. The doctor then questioned his fears, and proposed the hypothesis that they were figments of his imagination. At this point R. said: "If these things are not real I belong in a mental institution." The doctor replied that in Casentino no one belonged in a mental home any longer and that no one could be admitted, due to the new law, not even if one wanted to be. The problem was to understand what was causing his suffering. The hypothesis of illness undermined R. 's certainty about his persecution. The possibility of being ill without automatic psychiatric isolation appeared as a less terrifying alternative to persecution, as if the patient believed: "I prefer to be ill, if this does not include the risk of ending up in a psychiatric hospital, rather than being sane but in mortal peril caused by this persecution." The dialogue continued on these lines and the parents' return to the home was discussed.

After house calls twice a day over a period of 2 weeks, R. continued the treatment in the doctor's office. Three days after the first session, the patient agreed to take haloperidol 2 mg twice daily.

During the sessions it became possible to understand the dynamics of his persecution. R. lived in cultural proverty, as expressed by his phrase: "I work every day and go to the ballrooms on Sunday." This way of life had become intolerable after an unfortunate platonic love affair with a girl about whom R. had endless fantasies, encouraged by his parents' haste for an unrealistically early marriage.

The symptoms progressively disappeared and the patient now permits himself experiences outside his normal surroundings. He continues to visit the psychiatrist's office occasionally and he recently said: "Crises are important, because without them one cannot change his own way of life."

This case permits us to understand the new relationship between the service and the client without the threatening interference of the psychiatric hospital. It seems to us that the absence of an alien space, totally isolated from normality, reacts as a powerful reassuring factor significantly favoring dialectical exchange and the thrust of treatment. This absence seems to us to permit, even during acute crises, an experience of lesser alienation; the specter of social exclusion at a maximal level, present and feared in the past, no longer lurks on the scene. We also note enhanced adherence to the reality principle as related to psychotic experience, precisely because in reality each crisis has an outcome involving less exclusion and stigma. The continuity of the environment allows us to evalute the positive aspects present, without previous alienation of the threatened identity of the patient; this favors the preservation of higher levels of self-esteem. It was exactly on these levels of self-esteem that the mental institution gouged wounds beyond healing, because it represented a total fracture of the patient's relationship with everyday life. The absence of the psychiatric hospital therefore eliminates not only its real damage, but also its symbolic destructiveness in the patient's crisis.

In the past the mental institution has socially represented punishment, violence, irrationality, and injustice. Now the possible reactions to these threats have diminished. The psychotic experience thus becomes more and more suffering to be understood by the patient together with the professional and other people, instead of a deviance to be punished by separation from the community.

Former Inmates in General Hospitals

Avoiding the readmission of patients who have previously been hospitalized in mental institutions is frequently more difficult. In fact we have seen that when admitted for the first time to a general hospital patients often demand psychiatric repression, or they behave as though they were in a mental institution, but usually, during successive stays in hospitals, they modify their behavior. Some patients gave us the impression they wanted to test the new law to reassure themselves and to see whether they would really not end up in a mental institution. We believe that these patients wanted to check the new limits of repression. We have, however, noted that patients more willingly accepted admission to a general than to a mental hospital. The use of an already familiar structure creates less alienation as they are treated in a place frequented by everybody with any kind of disease. Furthermore the contact with patients not suffering from psychiatric illness permits them to remain anchored more easily to reality.

We do not wish to defend with these remarks the medical approach to mental illness, but only to underline the less negative aspect of medical treatment as compared with psychiatric institutionalization. On the other hand experiments such as the Arezzo one demonstrate that it is possible to treat any type of patient without separation of psychiatric departments from general hospitals. For every admission, there must be found a free room, or a bed, in a ward of the general hospital. Psychiatric assistance must be organized with varying intensity according to the individual case. Obviously this type of work implies profound cooperation with the doctors and nurses of the general hospital, with whom it is vital to discuss the case before admission. The use of drugs must be discussed as well, and meetings must be organized to discuss the irrational aspects of fear and stigma.

The experience gained in past work involving the opening up of the psychiatric hospital has enabled us to detect the repressive institutional processes also present in general hospitals. We see in particular rigid division of work and roles, nonresponsibility of nurses, authoritarian planning of a patient life-style, and all the other things which make of an ill person an object to look after instead of the subject of a healing process.

The Problem of Social Participation

To us community work means involving the greatest possible number of nonprofessionals in the suffering of the patient. We believe, in fact, that the psychotic patient needs a profound understanding of his interior processes. At the same time, he must have the possibility of extended contact in everyday life.

These interpersonal relationships seem to us indispensable in combatting the patient's deep sense of loneliness and his difficulties in coping with others. The availability of friends, young people, and community groups acts as a potent stabilization factor. We have seen, for example, that temporary overnight stays with groups of friends or in other nonpsychiatric community situations, when the family situation becomes intolerable, allows us to avoid admitting the patient to a general hospital.

Obviously the first step is the involvement of relatives who, feeling themselves supported by the service, show lesser degree of anxiety and fear. This also allows us to mitigate the explosive valences and to understand together with the patient and his relatives how the relationship among themselves has developed, which are the hardest aspects to tolerate, and so on.

Sometimes there is no family to rely upon and thus the discovery of other groups becomes the only alternative to hospitalization. Such a case is related below:

M. M. is a 30-year-old man, orphaned of both parents, with many prior institutionalizations and a 1-year internment in a hospital for the criminally insane for the rape of an adolescent. Upon his release, after a long stay in the general hospital due to the unavailability of other choices, we were able to find him a place to live: a small nonpsychiatric community led by a progressive priest. M. had always worked sporadically for some months before suddenly abandoning his job with an intense crisis during which he either became completely stupified or lived for weeks on end with the feeling of being persecuted. Since M. has been living in the community he has greatly improved in spite of two crises. We elaborated his fears and his habit of experiencing his job as a type of vengeance, a growing internal rage about which he felt guilty. We worked over a long period on his aggression toward the adolescent and the feelings of guilt which tortured him for having been in a criminal asylum. He always feared that his past might be discovered by his workmates.

Recently M. allowed himself for the first time in his life to be ill from work for a day and to report to his employer without excessive fear. He took 15 days of holiday alone, by the sea, and resigned from work – communicating his resignation to his employer – instead of abandoning his job in a crisis as in the past. Naturally the introspective work with us, twice a week, was fundamental, but without the presence of the community, with the members of which we often verify our work and occasionally spend an evening, he would not be at his present stage of recovery. This also because, like many of our patients, he has so little influence that his relationship with us is not enough for significant improvement.

Our coinvolvement in the field involves a network between the local institutions and significant situations for the patients. This means having contacts with, among others, general practitioners, employers, trade unions, old age homes, administrators, and the courts to promote solutions which we could never achieve on our own. This means also modifying ways of thinking and rejecting attitudes consolidated over the years, finding practical situations of socialization, work, free time, holidays, and, at the limit, to acting on the change of demand and the public's culture modifying them and, therefore, the organization of the services and their logic of excessive specialization.

What we are trying to do therefore is to direct our attention – until now focused solely on patients and their families – toward a general view which includes processes of collective reflection about hazardous situations, damage, and suffering which are common to all.

Conclusions

The majority of our work is actually carried out in the patient's own home, or in buildings independent of hospitals, such as offices, or community centers. Within the interpersonal relationships we construct with the clients, once the initial difficulties have been overcome, the clients react to our friendly and open manner usually by confiding in us. They often wish to know about us the things we know about them. During the interviews we do not refuse to talk about life's general aspects or politics. We go into personal problems accepting the different levels at which the patient is disposed to face them. When the relationship deepens, we try to pass from public problems to private ones, and vice versa, with scientific curiosity, searching together for new relations rather than referring to standard model theories. The step from personal to political problems is a work of ideological socialization which attempts to tie the particular to the general. On the other hand the step from the political to the personal moves towards an insight which is not cut off from the outside world. Either way the steps seem to us useful for a wider understanding of individual experiences. In fact if what is personal, the inner world, is – taken on its own – felt to be different, deviant, ill, its connection to the general, to the political, permits us to refer it to others, to what is somehow felt to be reassuring and normal.

The work we carry out is to cross and cross this bridge, to understand and experience it with the greatest possible number of variations, in its own history and in everyone's history, to strengthen it until it breaks less frequently or not at all. When the patients feel that their bridge is strengthened they suddenly abandon the relationship for a few months or years and then return, at times, with the air of an expert who has heard a creak or a malfunction, and who feels the need to understand what it is and to do something about it. These withdrawals are not escapes or negative resistances. It seems they are the expression of the need for autonomous experiences through which the patients try to prove themselves in life by loosening a relationship that can be immediately rejoined in case of need. The intensity, quality, and length of a relationship are therefore established little by little in a setting which is open to the needs of the patient, instead of being closed within the borders of a technique. At times the relationship may be upheld by a nurse or a social worker and it may take place in the most unlikely places depending on the circumstances. The collective verifications within the psychiatric service is the unifying moment in the differing modes of approach. Contradictions and problems rematerialize in reflection and mature understanding through past experiences and present practical work. We thus practice a continuous collective dialectic between theory and practice.

The tendency is to work with an approach as little technical as possible, with the least possible formality, but closer to the way of life and needs of the patient. We know that these are not the major tendencies in our country. The use of general hospitals has created in many cases small mental institutions imbedded like foreign bodies in the needs of the community. Hospitalization, which for us is an exception, is the norm in many situations. Often what we call "community priority" is completely unknown.

The problem is that many aspects of coinvolvement and participation are carried out in moments of ideological, political, and economic crisis, by which not only psychiatric reform, but health care reform itself, is seriously threatened. The battle therefore remains in progress, and even if bureaucratic delays, reactionary political pressures, and the medical bodies, oriented towards profit and private professional interests, should lead to a modification of the law, we think that there is a definite end to psychiatric hospitals and that psychiatry in Italy will never again be what it was in the past.

In fact, as Sergio Piro confirmed in his article to commemorate the first anniversary of the death of Franco Basaglia: "It is perhaps possible, if political conditions exist to permit it, for a reform to be temporarily retracted, subdued, or devalued. However, it is not possible for an epistemological fracture to be healed, for an outworn or insufficient system of reference to be reestablished, or for a body resting on bases which are clearly false and misleading to reconstruct itself on new and solid foundations" (Piro 1981).

It was precisely the consideration of the practical difficulties and the anticipated resistance that made the change from mental institutions to psychiatric services in general hospital an indispensable step. If, even now, at a national level, the problems are so difficult, let us ponder upon the intolerable situation which would have arisen if we had directly proposed solutions such as crisis centers and social centers. We realize that there are serious risks in reestablishing a medical approach to the treatment of psychic diseases. It seems to us, however, that the brief periods of hospitalization, the search for community structures, and the increase of community work offer to the dedicated professional the possibility to limit as much as possible the use of general hospitals and also to work for the dismissal of long-term patients.[4] On the other hand our presence in a general hospital, by continuous interventions through psychiatric advice in the various medical and surgical departments, allows us to act on a preventive level.

In our opinion it will only be possible to overcome the priority of the hospital and the isolation of therapeutic activity if the problem of health becomes a collective movement involving the entire population. This is necessary to fight against the exclusive attention to the symptoms only at a technical level. This is happening today in medicine, as it happened in old style psychiatry. These sciences, notwithstanding their differences, have always been closely allied in maintaining their domination over a sick body or mind, studying its processes, searching for remedies while keeping it strictly separated from social and economic contradictions. In our work we try, on the contrary, to reconstruct these connections, to open this bridge made of participation.

Participation means trying to understand together why people develop cancer of the bladder or depression, understanding that illness and suffering are not exceptions unconnected with the normal way of life, but results of a globality of aspects which need investigation. Too readily the exceptions become monsters to be stigmatized or insignificant cases to be forgotten. To whose advantage is it that they remain so?

It is therefore necessary to seek the collective roots of suffering and at the same time to connect them to the individual's unrepeatable variables, trying to reinforce the processes of solidarity, help, socialization, and collective struggles to change existing social reality. Only by following this course, we believe, can we obtain real prevention and reach a higher truth. The alternative is to try only to cure in a more efficient way, content with our own technical, professional role, in a world whose productive processes and social, political, and economic contradictions produce ever increasing suffering, illness, and death.[5]

References

Amministrazione Provinciale di Arezzo (1977) I tetti rossi. Mazzotta, Milan

Arezzo Group (1975) Schizophrenia and psychotherapy in the light of class struggle and democratic psychiatry. In: Jørstad J, Ugelstad E Schizophrenia '75. Universitetsforlaget, Oslo, pp 159–172

Basaglia F (1968) L'istituzione negata. Einaudi, Turin

4 At Naples, for example, a commission was formed to decide how many of the 100,000 homes which have to be built for the earthquake victims should be used for the rehabilitation into society of long-term patients who still live in mental hospitals.

5 We wish to thank Dr. Norman Elrod for his correction of the English translation of our paper.

Basaglia F (1971) La maggioranza deviante. Einaudi, Turin
Basaglia F (1974) Crimini di pace. Einaudi, Turin
Berger P (1979) Neue Psychiatrie, Erfahrungen aus Italien und Deutschland. Psychiatrie Verlag, Rehburg Loccum
Ferrara M, Tranchina P (1980) Theory, praxis, utopia in the general assembly of the mental hospital of Arezzo. In: Fogli di Informazione No. 70. Editrice Centro di documentazione, Pistoia
Haugsgjerd S, Engelstad F (1977) Seks samtaler om psykiatri. Pax Forlag, Oslo
Jantzen W (1980) Arbeit und Arbeitslosigkeit als pädagogisches und therapeutisches Problem. Pahl-Rugenstein, Cologne
Maccacaro GA (1978) Notes for a research on epidemiology of psychiatric institutions as a social disease. In: Fogli di Informazione No. 50. Editrice Centro di Documentazione, Pistoia
Pirella A (1975) Sozialisation der Ausgeschlossenen, Praxis einer neuen Psychiatrie. Rowohlt, Hamburg
Piro S (1981) He has not destroyed only the mental hospital. In: L'Unità 29th August
Simons T (1980) Absage an die Anstalt, Campus Verlag, Frankfurt New York

III. Individual Psychotherapy

Introduction

The First International Symposia on the Psychotherapy of Schizophrenia, held in the Swiss towns of Lausanne and Brestenberg some 25 years ago, focused largely on individual therapy. In fact, psychotherapy of schizophrenic patients was then almost synomymous with individual therapy. Things have since changed. Individual therapy figures in this volume only as one among several therapeutic modalities, and in the following review article by Gunderson it receives about the same coverage as milieu therapy and family therapy. (Group therapy was omitted because it was the subject of several other recent reviews.) In Gunderson's as well as Cancro's contribution to this section, drawing on the authors' wide-ranging knowledge of the field, we can discern some reasons for this relative decline of individual therapy within the gamut of psychosocial interventions. For example, we can no longer dismiss the many comparative studies which question the value and feasibility of individual, particularly psychoanalytically oriented therapy for the masses of schizophrenic patients in psychiatric institutions. We are reminded that patients who see their therapist for 1 h a day or so have an additional 23 h of contact with other hospital personnel and fellow patients who may reinforce or counteract whatever therapeutic gains they derived from their individual sessions.

And we have to take into account further the experiences of family researchers and family therapists, partly reported in other sections, which suggest that even in cases where direct contacts between the patient and his family have ceased, powerful, albeit invisible, family bonds (or systems forces) may continue to influence heavily a schizophrenic patient's symptomatology and life course.

And yet, despite the growing importance of the milieu, the group, and particularly the family, a powerful argument can still be made for the legitimacy, if not primacy, of individual therapy for certain selected schizophrenic patients. Benedetti's work is a case in point. He describes movingly, and illustrates with impressive pictures drawn by the patient herself, a therapeutic journey that led the patient from deep despair and confusion to growth and recovery. This journey gives evidence of what the author has called a "therapeutic symmetry" or "therapeutic symbiosis" in which therapist and patient share in one "psychometabolism," as it were, out of which then a stepwise mutual individuation of the partners can develop.

Also other findings, as cited by Gunderson, appear to confirm the value of a close therapeutic relationship for certain, maybe many, nonchronic schizophrenics whereas chronic patients seem in general to benefit, initially at least, more from structuring interventions than from such an intense relationship.

Matussek directs our attention to one, perhaps the, central feature of a successful individual therapy with schizophrenics: the facilitation of a positive transference relationship. It requires, among other things, a patient, accepting, noncritical, and nonintrusive attitude on the part of the therapist, apparently not unlike the attitude which Kohut recommends for analytic work with fragile narcissistic individuals.

The final chapter by Frosch et al. examines some basic differences in the attitudes and approaches of individual therapists of schizophrenics, thereby further elucidating the preconditions, feasibility, and risks of an individual therapy with these patients.

Helm Stierlin

Clinical Considerations from Empirical Research[1]

John G. Gunderson and Alexander Carroll

This chapter derives some clinical implications from empirical efforts to study psychosocial treatment of schizophrenic patients. Since the earlier review written in 1975 (Gunderson 1976), many other efforts to review the growing literature on psychosocial treatment of schizophrenia have been completed (West and Flynn 1976; Schooler 1978; Gunderson 1977, 1979; Mosher and Gunderson 1979; Mosher and Keith 1979, 1980; May and Simpson 1980; Klein 1980). There have even emerged reviews on how to evaluate this body of research (Mosher 1972; May 1974; May and VanPatten 1974; Carpenter et al. 1981). Ours will be a more selective review aimed at identifying and formulating issues of practical clinical importance. Where relevant, we have cited previously described (Gunderson 1978) general therapeutic processes which seem to be operative in effective treatments. Thus, this review reflects more of a synthetic effort to combine results and will give little attention to the critical tasks of describing and evaluating the designs and methodology of the various individual studies. Group therapy will not be reviewed because of the extensiveness with which this area has been recently reviewed by others and because we felt little could be added to what they have said.

Institutional Treatment

During the past decade, four studies have evaluated the relative merits of brief hospitalization versus longer-term hospitalization (Table 1). Most of these studies (Caffey et al. 1971; Mattes et al. 1977a, b, 1979; Glick and Hargreaves 1979) found more clinical improvement by the time of discharge in those who had the longer-term stays. Nevertheless, these differences were very quickly lost after discharge allowing the general conclusion that, because short-term hospitalization is less expensive and in some instances may offer advantages (Herz et al. 1975, 1976, 1977, 1979), it is a preferable form of treatment. The major exception to this generalization comes with respect to nonchronic schizophrenics (Glick and Hargreaves 1979; Mattes et al. 1979). For this group alone, there appeared to be some modest advantages from the longer-term hospitalization which were evident in the follow-up evaluations of posthospital function.

---

1 This study supported in part by NIMH Grant # 25246-07. The special contributions of Arlene Frank, Ph.D. are gratefully acknowledged.

Table 1. Long-term (ST) vs short-term (ST) hospitalization

Study	Diagnoses	Hospital Setting	LT	ST	Results
Caffey et al. (1971)	Schiz	14 VA Hspt'ls many wards	a) $N = 67$ 75 d b) $N = 66$ 83 d + aftercare grp.	$N = 68$ 29 d + aftercare grp.	St grp better at 3 wks, but no difference in follow-ups at 6 mo. and 1 yr.
Herz et al. (1975)	Multiple dx – pts. with families	CMHC different wards	$N = 63$ 50 d	a) $N = 61$ 10 d hosp + day care b) $N = 51$ 9 d hosp'n	Grps equal at 1–3 months, ST grp resumed work earlier and less family burden
Glick et al. (1974–1977)	Schiz non-chronic	Univ. Hspt'l 1 ward	$N = 70$ 90–120 d	$N = 71$ 21–28 d	ST grp better at 1 mo. LT grp better at 1 yr. and 2 yr – esp good premorbid females
Mattes et al. (1977a, b, 1979)	Mixed psychoses	Pvt. Hspt'l different wards	$N = ?$ 179 d	$N = ?$ 89 d	LT grp rated as less ill by relatives. Grps generally equal. No diffs seen for small Sz sample alone (N = approx. 23)

Another series of studies has shown that patients randomly assigned to day hospital care did as well, if not better, than those who were assigned to full hospitalization (Wilder et al. 1966; Washburn et al. 1976; Herz et al. 1978). Here also, there is some suggestion that schizophrenic patients may be the exception insofar as full hospitalization might have some advantages for them which do not apply to other diagnostic groups (Michaux et al. 1973). More recently, a major study involving ten day treatment centers in Veterans Administration hospitals has been reported by Linn et al. (1979). This study focused exclusively on schizophrenic patients randomly assigned either to day treatment or to an aftercare consisting largely of drug management. Linn found advantages for the patients who received the day hospital treatment compared to those receiving drugs alone over a 2-year period in terms of relapse, social function, and attitudinal changes. Of more interest was that this study demonstrated differences in the effectiveness amongst the ten day treatment centers. As with the inpatient studies, more effective day treatment centers had less rapid turnover, i.e., longer stays.

Taken together, these studies indicate that schizophrenic patients may profit more from longer-term residential stays with gradual unpressured transition into the community. Two possible reasons for this are the following:

1. Longer-term treatment programs are useful primarily to facilitate engagement of schizophrenic individuals with aftercare programs which then exert their enduring positive therapeutic effects on social function and community tenure. This has been suggested by a number of investigators (Glick and Hargreaves 1979; Mattes et al. 1979; May and Tuma 1981; Alanen et al. 1981) and will be discussed further in a later section of this paper.
2. Well-designed inpatient or day treatment milieus contain therapeutic activities which are beneficial to schizophrenic individuals and which grow in their effectiveness with more prolonged exposure. In this respect, effective short-term wards seem to require milieu characteristics (e.g., high control, low expression of feeling, low support) which are different than and probably incompatible with the characteristics of effective long-term wards (Ellsworth et al. 1972; Moos et al. 1973) and which may render them less suitable for schizophrenic patients. The next section will examine the available evidence with respect to this explanation, i.e., that positive therapeutic processes can exist within milieus which make them effective for schizophrenic patients.

In summary, these studies of institutional treatment underscore the schizophrenic patient's need for stable, gradually tapering, long-term supports. In this regard, Kellam (1981) has convincingly described the importance of maintaining continuity of treatment location, programs, and staff during the transition into greater community life.

Milieu Treatment

The most impressive evidence for the value of psychosocial treatments in the 1970s has come from a series of studies evaluating milieu treatment. These studies have measured the milieus' effectiveness as an addition to or instead of drugs or therapy which had convincingly established its effectiveness in the prior decade. This literature indicates that optimal milieus are active and intensive, but beyond that differ in what characterizes milieus which are best for chronic and for nonchronic patients. Fairweather et al. (1960) initially described this by showing how chronic patients responded poorly to the intensive milieu which seemed to be preferable for many nonchronic patients. From a different vantage point, Heim et al. (1976) described two patterns of participation by schizophrenic patients within active therapeutic communities – one group who could join and use the group processes, and others who were excluded by virtue of their passivity and withdrawal and needed a more homogeneous environment.

Nonchronic Patients

A series of studies with nonchronic schizophrenic patients summarized in previous reviews (Gunderson 1975; Mosher and Gunderson 1979; Mosher and Keith 1979; Gunderson 1980) has indicated that 3–6 months of intensive milieu treatment is as good as or even better than drug treatment for comparable nonchronic patients. This is true whether the drugs are given in different, but nonintensive milieus (Carpenter et al. 1977), or within a different but equally intensive milieu, (Mosher and Menn 1976, 1978), or even when the drugs are given within the same intensive milieu (Carpenter et al. 1977; Rappaport et al. 1978). The advantages for the milieu-treated patients who did not received drugs over their drug-treated counterparts were uniformly evident in social functioning, and more surprisingly, in recidivism 1 year (Mosher and Menn 1976) to 3 years (Rappaport et al. 1978) after discharge.

Although each of these studies has serious methodologic limitations, by their cumulative weight they establish a therapeutic potential for intensive milieus with nonchronic schizophrenics which equals or surpasses that of drugs. One wonders whether more profound advantages might have been observed if these milieu programs had provided concurrent drug therapy – especially in the early phase of treatment. Moreover, since the milieu programs in these outcome studies seem in some respects similar (i.e., active, well staffed, employing principles of therapeutic communities) to the milieu programs offered at those hospitals (Langley Porter and Hillside) where longer-term treatment appeared to benefit schizophrenic patients, the question naturally arises whether further benefits might have been found if the patients had stayed longer.

The results of these outcome studies can be joined with the results of those studies that correlate milieu process variables with community tenure (see reviews by Ellsworth 1981, and Liberman 1981) as a basis from which to derive the following characteristics which milieus designed to optimally affect nonchronic schizophrenics should include:

1. Distribution of power and decision-making authority (Ellsworth et al. 1972)
2. The use of peers with an emphasis on establishing new and corrective relationships
3. A high sense of involvement attained through frequent staff/patient and patient/patient interactions (Kellam et al. 1967; Linn 1970) and a tight sense of community
4. An enthusiastic and hopeful attitude, extending to a view of psychosis as a time-limited experience from which learning can take place
5. A high staffing ratio and small 6–8 bed units with a minimum length of stay of 3 months

These milieu characteristics emphasize the therapeutic benefits of involvement, i.e., they are accepting, highly interpersonal, and utilize some therapeutic community principles.

The Chronic Patient

With respect to the chronic patient, one finds a remarkably clear and persuasive delineation of those milieu principles which are best suited for their treatment in the work by Paul and Lentz (1977). Paul's study compared two different forms of intensive milieu program – in the absence of drugs – to drug-treated patients who remained in a custodial ward. In a 3-year follow-up, it was found that patients treated in the active milieu programs showed significantly more discharges, less recidivism, and better symptom remissions than the group who remained in a custodial setting. Of special interest is the comparison between the two forms of intensive treatment – one of which embodied the principles of the therapeutic community (including characteristics similar to those recommended above for nonchronic schizophrenics). The other was a social learning program based on the principles of behavior modification through rewards and punishments à la Ayllon and Azrin (1963). In this comparison, the social learning program had substantial advantages over the therapeutic community program in terms of release to the community, but also within the hospital program itself with regard to more dramatic reduction of psychopathology and in managing severely aggressive behaviors. Dangerous and aggressive behavior constituted the most obvious failure of the therapeutic community compared to the social learning procedures. Aside from the impressive claims for the benefits of the social learning program,[2] the careful baseline matching of staff, patients, and amount of therapeutic activity makes it possible to infer from the differences in outcome something about the optimal milieu processes for chronic patients, i.e., differences in outcome can be inferred to be a function of the specified milieu interventions.

The most obvious beneficial characteristic of the social learning program is structure. Clarity of roles, expectations, consequences, leadership, and responsibilities appear helpful to the chronic patients – and useful to the staff as well in dealing with angry behavioral disruptions. The application of structure was flexibly sensitive to individual differences such that the degree and type of environmental stimulation or demand was sustained at a tolerable and useful level for each patient.

A variety of studies suggests that a highly structured, control-oriented environment of this type is also advantageous for nonchronic patients during the acute phase of hospitalization (Caffey et al. 1971; Mosher and Menn 1976; Glick and Hargreaves 1979) but, as described already, gives way to the advantages of more stimulating, demanding, interactional processes. The chronic patient seems less able to tolerate environments with high interpersonal demands or unpredictability without regression to disruptive

2 Paul states that the social learning program could rehabilitate the most severely debilitated chronic patients to a point of institutional release into board and care facilities by 26–30 weeks and that, if continued for 2–3 years in a less intensive but still operative social learning aftercare program, a significant number of chronic patients could achieve stable independent functioning.

behaviors. Linn's study (Linn et al. 1979) of day treatment for chronic schizophrenic patients seems to require a similar conclusion. Of the ten day treatment centers that were studied, six were found to be clearly preferable in terms of lowering relapse rates, reducing symptoms, and changing attitudes. What characterized these six effective day treatment milieu programs – in addition to slower turnover rates – was less active group and family intervention programs. The only form of specific therapy which appeared to positively correlate with effectiveness was occupational therapy. The authors summarized their study by advocating a sustained, nonthreatening environment where the demands are clear and practical. The promising work by Liberman et al. (1980) which utilizes specific social learning techniques appears to be consistent with these reports.

These studies of milieu treatments for chronic patients highlight the role of sustained structure as a critical process ingredient. They do not appear to support Fairweather's (1960) conclusion that too much intensity of intervention is toxic to chronic patients. Rather, as both Paul (1977) and Liberman (1981) have pointed out, it is the form or type of intervention that determines the effects. Concurrent with the positive emphasis placed on providing a structured, clear, and predictable environment is a deemphasis on an approach which asks the chronic patient to examine his motives, the historical antecedents to his condition, or requires emotional involvement. While there is a forceful emphasis on improving the amount of social interaction, these interactions frequently have a structured task focus and the emotional content of such interactions is deemphasized. Finally, these studies suggest that the second major characteristic of effective milieus for chronic patients is that they allow continuity of structured programs beyond the inpatient period. In this respect, the work by Paul continues in the tradition of Fairweather's lodges (Fairweather et al. 1969) in developing carefully planned environments which address the chronic patient's passivity and attempts to make his grossly maladaptive symptomatic behaviors more alien.

Individual Therapy

Of the controlled studies on individual psychotherapy for schizophrenic persons, the evidence supporting its value (Rogers et al. 1967; Karon and O'Grady 1969) has been limited and nonpersuasive (see reviews by Feinsilver and Gunderson 1972; Dyrud and Holzman 1975; Gunderson 1979; Heinrichs and Carpenter 1981). Evidence of at least occasional dramatic success can be found in the literature in the form of case reports. However, the question of whether these patients were truly schizophrenic has recently been raised (North and Cadoret 1980). More persuasive evidence is found in the reports on groups of patients treated at various centers with a tradition of intensive psychoanalytic psychotherapy – Massachusetts Mental Health Center (Vaillant et al. 1964), Yale Psychiatric Institute (Rubenstein 1972), Michael Reese Hospital (Kayton 1975), Karen Horney Clinic (Rubins 1976), McLean Hospital (Gunderson and Gomes-Schwartz 1980), and most recently, the Turku Mental Health Care District (Alanen et al. 1981). Such reports are not convincing of the widespread value of individual psychotherapy for schizophrenic patients, but they do underscore the need to recognize more about what can make individual psychotherapy at least occasionally therapeutic.

Some generalizations can be made from examination of nearly all the reported successes with this method:

1. Its advantages become evident after patients have been seen for a year and a half or more.
2. It is provided within a supportive psychosocial context.
3. It involves at least twice weekly and generally more frequent meetings.
4. Psychoanalytically oriented explorations require close supervision or an experienced, personally analyzed therapist.

May et al. (1981) have recently reported more definitive follow-up information from their study which indicates that the patients who received individual psychotherapy during their initial hospitalization appeared to do worse in the 3–5 year period following that initial hospitalization than patients who receive a variety of other treatments. This had initially been reported with respect to recidivism (May and Tuma 1976), but more surprisingly and more convincingly, it has now been shown to be true with respect to social function and interpersonal relations. In another recent report from Hogarty's important study on supportive psychotherapy in aftercare programs Goldberg et al. (1977) point out that this form of therapy actually increased relapse among patients assigned to it who were initially quite symptomatic whereas it appeared to have benefits which emerged after a year and a half for the remaining patients who were initially essentially asymptomatic. From this well-controlled study comes the best available evidence that long-term, supportive therapy can benefit some significant subsample of schizophrenic patients, but it also offers the sobering conclusion that it may be contraindicated until schizophrenic patients are essentially asymptomatic. Because of the nonintensive supportive nature of this psychotherapy, it cannot be equated with the claims made for or against the efficacy of the exploratory psychotherapy used in the successfully treated cases cited above.

Together, the May and the Hogarty studies suggest that for the more acute phases of disturbance, that is, during the phase of hospitalization or for symptomatic outpatients, individual therapy may increase relapse or otherwise increase symptomatic exacerbations by the demand implicit in these therapies for greater responsible participation or examination of issues which may be intolerable. In this regard, as noted earlier, both Glick (1979) and Mattes (1979) attributed the benefits for nonchronic schizophrenics who received longer-term inpatient treatment to the fact that such patients were more likely to become engaged in an aftercare program of individual therapy. We recently examined this hypothesis on the patients assigned to individual therapy on a variety of wards as part of a collaborative outcome study (Stanton, Knapp). Willful discontinuance of psychotherapy was very highly correlated with short hospitalizations, but for patients who remained in therapy beyond 6 months there was no relationship between length of hospitalization and duration of continuance in psychotherapy after discharge. This suggests that short-term hospitalization may cause some patients to discontinue individual therapy after discharge, but that longer hospitalization offers little assurance of continuation in individual therapy. On the other hand, the longer a patient is in psychotherapy, the more likely he is to continue in it.

Thus, there is evidence that one function of hospitalization is to support and encourage the development of an attachment to an individual therapist which is more likely to enable patients to accrue the potential positive benefits of this form of treatment which can only occur if it is continued long term. Here, however, it must be emphasized that there remains no strong evidence that long-term, individual therapy necessarily benefits schizophrenic patients more than comparable patients who do not receive it. Nevertheless, a broad variety of studies, including some already alluded to, support the idea that for some schizophrenic patients, there are advantages for those who continue in long-term treatment (Hogarty et al. 1974; Rubins et al. 1976; Gunderson and Gomes-Schwartz 1970; Alanen et al. 1981; Beck et al. 1981). It is presumably because of this evidence that May ends up recommending an important role for individual psychotherapy in the aftercare of schizophrenic patients despite the discouraging long-term negative effects he found in his follow-up study.

Important questions emerging from this consensus are: (1) For what fraction of schizophrenic patients is an individual psychotherapy indicated? (2) What characterizes the subgroup for whom it will be appropriate? (3) What factors determine whether a patient continues in therapy or not? In our collaborative outcome study, approximately 50% of the patients assigned near admission to individual therapy discontinued it within 6 months. An additional 50% of those who remained in psychotherapy beyond 6 months discontinued it before 2 years. The attrition rate in the first 2 years of therapy did not depend on which of the two forms of individual therapy the patient was assigned nor did it depend to a very large extent upon which of the collaborating hospitals and on what ward these assignments took place. Our results show that when selection of patients for individual psychotherapy is not made on the basis of a clinical judgment of suitability, only about one in four nonchronic schizophrenic patients can be expected to continue in individual psychotherapy for 2 years, i.e., into the time period where its benefits might be expected to become evident. Rogers et al. (1967) found that less than half of the inpatients who were assigned individual therapists actually became engaged in therapy even though attending sessions was supported by the therapist's proximity and the encouragement of nursing staff. O'Brien et al. (1972) found that 40% of the schizophrenic patients assigned to supportive individual psychotherapy at the time of discharge continued for 2 years and that the attrition rates tapered over time. In Alanen's study in which selection for therapy was based on a clinical judgment, over 50% of his schizophrenic sample was assigned to an individual psychotherapy (33% received an intensive form of psychotherapy, while another 22% received supportive psychotherapy). Of that number, how many continued into long-term therapy has not been reported.

A preliminary picture of those patients who are most likely to be suitable candidates for long-term individual therapy is emerging from some recent studies. This picture includes the following characteristics: males who are poorly functioning (Beck et al. 1981), being largely asymptomatic (Goldberg et al. 1977), and being aware of having serious psychiatric problems and having some capacity for adaptive regression (Stanton et al. 1979). With one exception – having low denial of illness – none of these qualities are those which experienced therapists consider to be important for selecting their patients (Gunderson and Hirschfield 1975).

In sum, the conclusion that schizophrenic persons who continue in long-term individual psychotherapy will be better off than comparable patients who do not can be reasonably inferred from numerous reports, but this conclusion is still not firmly established. Recent evidence suggests that between one-fourth and one-half of nonchronic patients are likely to be able to engage in such treatment.

Family Therapy

After a wave of enthusiasm for the benefits of ongoing or intensive therapy for families with schizophrenic members, there has been a shift towards more sober claims and more limited therapeutic strategies (Mosher 1976; Leff 1979). The need for family support and the use of time-limited family interventions at critical points has become more frequently recommended (Wynne 1979). In this context, a series of British investigations (Brown et al. 1962, 1972; Scott 1974; Vaughn and Leff 1976) and one from the United States (Hogarty et al. 1979) have demonstrated that the family context is an extremely important determinant of relapse. These studies have raised the question as to whether family interventions could significantly alter families in ways which could diminish relapse rates. A series of studies (Table 2) has now been undertaken which evaluate this question.

Goldstein and collaborators (1975, 1978, 1980, 1981) have studied brief (six session) family therapy, with drugs as an aftercare strategy. At 6 weeks, when therapy ended, the patients in the family therapy sample were significantly less symptomatic and had fewer relapses; by 6 months the benefits of family therapy were a trend which didn't quite reach statistical significance, and by 3 years there were no longer any discernable benefits for those who had received the family therapy. These results echo Langsley's (Langsley et al. 1969) earlier study by showing that crisis-oriented family interventions can be effective but don't lead to enduring benefits.

Another series of studies, still in progress, has attempted to provide longer-term family interventions specifically designed to decrease the overinvolved or critical interactions (high expressed emotion [EE]) within families which has been shown to increase relapse. Preliminary reports from both Leff et al. (1981) and Falloon et al. (1981a, b) show that family interventions can markedly shift high EE relatives to low scores and that there is a correspondingly significant decrease in relapse rates during the 9 months after discharge. Another preliminary report (Snyder and Liberman 1981) confirms that a family intervention similar to Falloon's can be used on inpatients to greatly reduce EE. These studies have not yet shown whether the benefits of these family interventions endure beyond the period in which the treatment is being given.

Having demonstrated such promise, it becomes increasingly important to learn about the family interventions used in these studies. The common clinical characteristics of these familiy interventions which Anderson (1980) has aptly named psychoeducational can be summarized as follows:

1. Short-term family interventions have short-term positive effects.

2. Conjoint therapies have focused topics, directive leadership, and do not depend or lean upon the authority or experience of the therapist – transference work is not included.

3. The parents or other significant relatives are met with apart from the designated patient. These meetings include the following agenda items:

Table 2. Studies of family therapy

Study	Samples	Rx Comparison	Amount Rx	Outcome Measures
Goldstein et al. (1975, 1978, 1980, 1981)	104 discharged non-chronic patients	Fam. Rx vs No Fam. Rx	$1^1/2$ hrs. x 6 wks.	psychopathology and relapse at 6 wks, 6 mos. and 3 yrs.
Leff et al. (1979, 1981)	24 remitted pts with high EE families	Relatives grps + prn fam and cpls Rx vs Routine clinic care	Biweekly grps for indef duration	EE, psychopathology and relapse at 2 yrs[a]
Falloon et al. (1981a, b)	40 discharged pts with high EE families	Fam. Rx vs Supportive Indiv. Rx	40 sessions tapered over 2 yrs	EE, psychopathology and relapse at 9 months[a]
Snyder and Liberman (1981)	28 inpatients with high EE families	Fam. Rx vs No Fam. Rx[b]	2 hrs x 9 wks	EE and relapse at 9 mos[a,b]

[a] Preliminary reports, not all of the sample have completed follow-up evaluations.
[b] Because of differences in milieu treatment between those given Fam. Rx and others and non-random assignment to Fam. Rx, it is not possible to attribute results as due to the Fam. Rx.

a) Relatives are informed about what is known about the etiology and treatment of schizophrenia with obvious emphasis on the long-term handicaps and the need for drug compliance.

b) Relatives are openly discouraged from being angry toward or critical of the schizophrenic family member.

c) Relatives are asked to identify everyday stressful situations related to living with the schizophrenic person and to develop alternative coping responses.

d) Relatives are encouraged to discuss their family situations with relatives from other families with schizophrenic members.

4. Illness producing or sustaining patterns of family relationships are not identified as such. The concept of schizophrenia as one manifestation of a larger family disorder is not accepted.

5. A flexible and pragmatic approach is taken with regard to the composition, scheduling, and location of meetings involving all or parts of families.

There is an obvious discrepancy between what characterizes the psychoeducational approach employed effectively in these research projects and those which are recommended by well-known advocates of family therapy (e.g., Palazzoli et al. 1978; Haley 1979). Stierlin recently divided the approaches of experienced family therapists into three types: (1) to open up dialogue about major conflicts, secrets, and myths within a family; (2) to ally with certain family members and use this alliance as a lever to shift patterns of control and power; and (3) to directly address and disrupt the most central distortions in the families' orientation (Stierlin 1982). In contrast, the psychoeducational approach clearly discourages family members from confronting patients with their disturbing behaviors – however maladaptive. Such behaviors are considered symptomatic of illness. Leff (1979) has noted in his relatives' groups how "the low EE relatives show a tolerant, even collusive, attitude toward the patient's symptoms and retain a remarkable ability to make light of the most fraught situations. There is no hint of blaming or criticizing the patient." He closes this description by expressing optimism that high EE relaltives can respond to treatment so as to eventually emulate such collusive tolerance.

There is still uncertainty as to how often and when family therapy is indicated. Vaughn and Leff (1976) estimate that about 50% of schizophrenic patients with available families will be in the high EE category. By examining their samples for treatment responders, both Goldstein and Leff have suggested that some low EE families also respond positively – thereby suggesting a more widespread use for psychoeducational family therapy. Obviously when samples are not selected on the basis of having an available family, the number of instances where family therapy of any kind will be indicated are greatly reduced. Alanen et al. (1981) have found that on the basis of clinical judgment conjoint family therapy was provided to only 8 of a series of 108 patients whereas supportive contacts with family members were utilized 33 times. At McLean, we found that ongoing conjoint family therapy for more than 3 months duration was considered clinically indicated for 8 of 50 nonchronic schizophrenic patients. Sporadic, prn, or crisis-oriented interventions were usual. In four of the eight family therapies, it was initiated by the patients' therapists after they had concluded it was essential for the individual work to be productive. The family therapies in the Alanen and McLean series have been of the kinds described by Stierlin whose effectiveness has not been evaluated. There are suggestions throughout this literature that the patients for whom family interventions are provided are a poor prognosis group.

No doubt the current wave of studies on psychoeducational family therapy will provide a welcome stimulus to both the expanded use of family therapy and to a reassessment and shift of techniques for interventions. There is much more that needs to be learned about the relative benefits and indications for the various forms of family treatment that traditionally have been employed.

Discussion

These empirical studies call for some unexpected and difficult revisions in thinking about treatment of schizophrenia. One common assumption is that good quality psychosocial treatments are so expensive that they must regardless of their benefits, be restricted in practice to only the well-to-do. A series of studies has now shown that effective psychosocial treatments cost no more than minimal treatment (because of reduced hospitalizations) and are far less expensive than ineffective psychosocial treatments (Karon and Vandenbos 1975; Paul and Lentz 1977; Mosher and Menn 1978; Linn et al. 1979). In addition, the milieu programs used in Mosher's and Paul's studies modestly improved the likelihood of subsequent employment for some patients. This means that the cost benefits are potentially far greater in the long run.

A more profound conception which is challenged by these studies concerns the mechanisms by which change occurs in treatment. The traditional psychodynamic approach has been to modify an individual's inner life and expect this will bring subsequent changes in his symptoms and relationships to his environment – an "inside-out" strategy. This approach is based on the hope of altering the individual's personality to allow him to more successfully adapt to the endless vicissitudes of circumstance. Insight-oriented individual therapy is the purest example of this approach and may explain why, as noted earlier, measurable behavior change can be expected to occur only after long-term treatment. Gains from this approach are measured by the degree to which they produce enduring changes which go beyond the exposure to the therapeutic intervention. Of the studies reviewed here, the milieu studies with nonchronic patients come closest to emphasizing this strategy by attempting to make the schizophrenic person's inner life understandable and acceptable.

In contrast to this approach, most of these recent studies have been directed at providing a social context for schizophrenic individuals which make symptomatic relapses less likely and only secondarily have considered that such favorable environmental conditions might bring about internal changes. So much has this been the trend that Klein (1980) has legitimately questionsed whether these studies can be considered to evaluate the treatment of schizophrenia per se – or rather just its social consequences. Although such studies obviously take seriously the Sullivanian tradition in which the schizophrenic's pathology is located in the interpersonal world, the goals of such treatments (to prevent relapse) sound similar to those previously ascribed to drugs and frequently criticized by those with psychosocial orientations. Schooler (1980) has pointed out the irony that psychotherapists view relapse after termination of their therapy as evidence of failure, whereas pharmacotherapists view relapse after the termination of drug treatment as evidence of the drug's efficacy.

The principles for this "outside-in" strategy are most clearly found in Paul's milieu program for chronic patients, but they are also found in studies with nonchronic patients receiving other forms of therapy – family therapy most particularly. Although the results from these studies are impressive, it has long been thought that gains made from supportive and directive techniques will remain highly context dependent; i.e., the question has been whether such learning experiences could be enduringly internalized. In this regard, a variety of studies where schizophrenic patients made gains within the treatment context have shown rapid reversals after termination (Goldstein 1981; Lindberg 1981) or discharge (Caffey et al. 1971; Herz et al. 1975; Linn et al. 1979).

Paul's work has shown that social learning experiences based on behavior modification techniques were occasionally internalized to the extent that independent function was achieved after the treatment program was discontinued. This suggests that internal change did occur secondary to behavioral improvement. In line with this, it has been noted that the family interventions which reduce EE may do more than decrease symptomatic relapses – they may allow improvements to occur (Falloon 1981). The changed home environment may allow schizophrenic persons to experiment with new and more adaptive forms of self-expression. Such signals of successful "outside-in" changes seem to reflect dynamic or psychological growth. Such results are consistent with recent reports of patients treated in short-term therapy who achieved symptomatic improvement without dynamic changes, but who – without further treatment – acquired dynamic changes when evaluated at a later follow-up (Malan 1980). In any event, these suggestions of internal change as a direct or indirect result of treatments directed primarily at manipulating the social context of symptomatic behaviors requires an expansion of traditional views of change.

These studies also offer a fresh perspective on the overall processes within treatments which facilitate change in schizophrenic persons. Many of the studies we've reviewed (Linn, Paul, Goldberg, Leff, Falloon) show that the overt psychopathology of schizophrenic individuals is ameliorated by being within treatment programs that are stable, emotionally undemanding, and involve structured tasks. As a result, some reviews of these studies have concluded that schizophrenic patients need deintensified stimulation (West and Flynn 1976; Goldberg et al. 1977; Anderson et al. 1980; May et al. 1981). Studies by Silverman et al. (1975) have found that hospitalized schizophrenic patients will respond to subliminal stimulation of their symbiotic wishes by diminished ward behavior pathology and thought disorder. Moreover, subliminal stimulation of themes of aggression or object loss increase cognitive and behavioral symptoms (Litwack et al. 1979). These results are consistent with the explanation that relatively stressless, need-gratifying environments simulate symbiosis in ways which cause remissions in psychotic symptoms. It is also consistent with the unfortunate frequency with which such gains are disrupted (i.e., by introducing loss of this symbiotic attachment) at the time of discharge – especially when aftercare programs are discontinuous. If a state of homeostatic symbiosis is responsible for decreasing symptomatic relapse, this could help explain why added benefits can occur from longer-term treatment programs but are lost upon discharge; why decreases in EE may diminish relapses; and why discontinuities in treatment as disparate as behavioral modification and individual therapy may result in relapses. If the mechanism of action whereby treatments prevent relapse is via gratification of the illusion of a symbiotic attachment, the obvious question is whether and under what conditions a schizophrenic person can give up a symbiotic attachment once it is established.

Searles (1966), who helped formulate symbiosis as part of the psychology of treating schizophrenia, believes that growth out of symbiosis depends upon corrective emotional experiences. Such growth requires considerable therapeutic activitiy – in his case, interpretations – within the context of symbiotic attachment. Silverman (1975) also found that the potentially harmful effects he anticipated from gratifying symbiotic fantasies could be offset by concurrent focused tasks which assisted differentiation. This model can be applied to institutional programs wherein the patient's symbiotic wishes may be gratified but within which active milieu processes may gradually facilitate the giving up of the attachment. As we have seen, the critical processes within the milieu programs which are best for nonchronic patients are different than those for chronic patients. For nonchronic patients in addition to insight, these programs heavily emphasized interpersonal involvement. Paul's treatment of chronic patients led some to achieve independent functioning – obviously without benefits of interpretation but also without reliance on involvement. His work would emphasize the benefits of the affectively bland, interpersonally neutral, but relentless intrusion of progressive expectations as the critical process variables. The psychoeducational approach similarly would emphasize a highly active but detached – "nothing personal" – problem-oriented approach based on clear identification of tasks, roles, behavioral responses, and consequences. The effectiveness of these treatments is consistent with a variety of clinical observations whereby even very sick patients can respond with dramatically improved function when they don't perceive the requirement to do this as some form of personal – and therefore cruel or arbitrary – demand. It is consistent with such clinical observations as how very sick patients can respond with periods of much better function to crises, or when they have jobs which are satisfactory, or, why they can survive discharge from short-term wards better than when discharged after short-term stays from long-term wards.

Thus, while it may be critical in order to prevent relapses for any treatment's success that it provide an environment – whether it is an institution or an individual – that allows the schizophrenic individual to believe he is symbiotically attached, this should only be considered the first step. The more difficult task is to provide the types of interactions with that environment which will allow that attachment to be relinquished. The evidence supports the idea that there are a variety of ways of doing this and they need to be tailored to the patient's particular form of schizophrenia.

Summary

In summary, a number of general clinical qualities emerge from this review:

1. Treatment of schizophrenia is a long-term process which requires support and continuity whether the goals are simply to diminish relapses or to promote independent functions.

2. Two strategies of treatment – arranging a special environment to decrease toxic stresses, or trying to rearrange the person's inner life – both seem to be effective and are capable of leading to subsequent changes in the other sphere.

3. Chronic patients are most likely to benefit from highly structured, clearly prescriptive, and impersonal therapeutic strategies.

4. Nonchronic patients are most likely to benefit from strategies involving the formation of durable new relationships, and those which involve the patient in the process of becoming more aware of himself.

5. Psychosocial treatments are very expensive where ineffective but can quickly pay for themselves when they are well conceived and effectively delivered.

6. Much more needs to be learned about the subgroups for whom the various therapeutic methods and strategies are best suited and about the proper sequencing of these methods.

References

Alanen YO, Rakkolainen V, Rasimus R, Laakso J, Jarvi R (1981) Developing the treatment of schizophrenia in a community-psychiatric setting: a psychotherapeutic and family-centered approach. Unpublished manuscript

Anderson CM, Hogarty GE, Reiss DJ (1980) Family treatment of adult schizophrenic patients: a psycho-educational approach. Schizophr Bull 6:491–505

Ayllon T, Azrin NH (1963) The measurement and reinforcement of behavior of psychotics. J Exp Anal Behav 8:357–383

Beck JC, Golden S, Arnold F (1981) An empirical investigation of psychotherapy with schizophrenic patients. Schizophr Bull 7:241–247

Brown GW, Monck EM, Carstairs GM, Wing JK (1962) The influence of family life on the course of schizophrenic illness. Br J Prev Soc Med 16:55–68

Brown GW, Birley JLT, Wing JK (1972) Influence of family on the course of schizophrenic disorders: a replication. Br J Psychiatry 121:241–258

Caffey EM, Galbrecht CR, Klett JC, Point P (1971) Brief hospitalization and aftercare in the treatment of schizophrenia. Arch Gen Psychiatry 24:81–86

Carpenter WT Jr., McGlashan TH, Strauss JS (1977) The treatment of acute schizophrenia without drugs: an investigation of some current assumptions. Am J Psychiatry 134:14–20

Carpenter WT Jr., Heinrichs DW, Hanlon TE (1981) Methodologic standards for treatment outcome research in schizophrenia. Am J Psychiatry 138:465–471

Dyrud JE, Holzman PS (1975) Evaluation of psychotherapy. In: Gunderson JG, Mosher LR (eds) Psychotherapy of Schizophrenia. Aronson, New York, pp 269–280

Ellsworth RB (1983) Characteristics of effective treatment settings: a research review. In: Gunderson JG, Will OA Jr., Mosher LR (eds) Principles and practice of milieu therapy. Aronson, New York

Ellsworth RB, Dickman HR, Maroney RJ (1972) Characteristics of productive and unproductive unit systems in V.A. psychiatric hospitals. Hosp Community Psychiatriy 23:261–271

Endicott J, Cohen J, Nee J, Fleiss JL, Herz MI (1979) Brief vs. standard hospitalization. Arch Gen Psychiatry 36:706–712

Fairweather GW, Simon R, Gebhard ME, Weingarten E, Holland JL, Sanders R, Stone GB, Reahl GE (1960) Relative effectiveness of psychotherapeutic programs. Psychological Monographs 74: no 492

Falloon IRH, Boyd JL, McGill CW, Strang JS, Moss HB (1981) Family management training in the community care of schizophrenia. Unpublished manuscript

Falloon IRH, Liberman RP, Lillie FM, Vaughn CE (1981) Family therapy of schizophrenics with high risk of relapse. Family Process 20:211–221

Feinsilver DB, Gunderson JG (1972) Psychotherapy of schizophrenia: is it indicated? A review of the relevant literature. Schizophr Bull 6:11–23

Glick ID, Hargreaves WA (1979) Psychiatric hospital treatment for the 1980's: a controlled study of short vs. long hospitalization. Lexington Press, Lexington

Goldberg SC, Schooler NR, Hogarty GE, Roper M (1977) Prediction of relapse in schizophrenic outpatients treated by drug and sociotherapy. Arch Gen Psychiatry 34:171–184

Goldstein MJ (1980) Family therapy during the aftercare treatment of acute schizophrenia. In: Strauss JS, Bowers M, Downey TW, Fleck S, Jackson S, Levine I (eds) The psychotherapy of schizophrenia. Plenum Medical, New York

Goldstein MJ, Kopeikin HS (1981) Short and long term effects on a program combining drug and family therapy. Unpublished manuscript

Goldstein MJ, Rodnick EH, Evans JR, May PRA (1975) Long acting phenothiazines and social therapy in community treatment of acute schizophrenics. Psychopharmacol Bull 11:37–38

Goldstein JJ, Rodnick EH, Evans JR, May PRA, Steinberg MR (1978) Drug and family therapy in the aftercare of acute schizophrenics. Arch Gen Psychiatry 35:1169–1177

Gunderson JG (1976) Recent research on psychosocial treatments of schizophrenia. In: Jorstad J, Ugelstad E (ed) Schizophrenia 75. Lie, Norway

Gunderson JG (1977) Drugs and psychosocial treatment of schizophrenia revisited. J Continuing Educ Psychiatry, December 25:40

Gunderson JG (1978) Defining the therapeutic processes in psychiatric milieus. Psychiatry 41: 327–335

Gunderson JG (1979) Individual psychotherapy. In: Bellak L (ed) Disorders of the schizophrenic syndrome. Basic, New York

Gunderson JG (1980) A reevaluation of milieu therapy for nonchronic schizophrenic patients. Schizophr Bull 6:64–69

Gunderson JG, Hirschfeld R (1975) Factors influencing the selection of patients for individual psychotherapy. In: Gunderson JG, Mosher LR (eds) Psychotherapy of schizophrenia. Aronson, New York

Gunderson JG, Gomes-Schwartz B (1980) The quality of outcome from psychotherapy of schizophrenia. In: Strauss JS, Bowers M, Downey TW, Fleck J, Jackson S, Levine I (eds) The psychotherapy of schizophrenia. Plenum Medical, New York

Haley J (1979) Leaving home – a study of disturbed young people. McGraw-Hill, New York

Heim E, Johnsen E, Lilienfeld C, Stauffacher H, Wirz P (1976) Application of the principles of the therapeutic community with the participation of schizophrenics. In: Jørstad J, Ugelstad E (eds) Schizophrenia 75. Oslo, Norway

Heinrichs DW, Carpenter WT (to be published) The efficacy of individual psychotherapy: A perspective and review emphasizing controlled outcome studies. American Handbook of Psychiatry

Herz MI, Endicott J, Spitzer RL (1971) Day vs inpatient hospitalization: a controlled study. Am J Psychiatry 127:1371–1381

Herz MI, Endicott J, Spitzer RL (1975) Brief hospitalization of patients with families: initial results. Am J Psychiatry 132:413–418

Herz MI, Endicott J, Spitzer RL (1976) Brief versus standard hospitalization: the families. Am J Psychiatry 133:795–801

Herz MI, Endicott J, Spitzer RL (1977) Brief hospitalization: a two-year follow-up. Am J Psychiatry 134:502–507

Herz MI, Endicott J, Gibbon M (1979) Brief hospitalization two-year follow-up. Arch Gen Psychiatry 36:701–705

Hogarty GE, Schooler NR, Ulrich R, Mussare F, Ferro P, Herron E (1979) Fluphenazine and social therapy in the aftercare of schizophrenic patients. Arch Gen Psychiatry 36:1283–1294

Karon BP, Vandenbos GR (1972) The consequences of psychotherapy for schizophrenic patients. Psychotherapy: theory, research, and practice 9:111–119

Karon BP, Vandenbos GR (1975) Treatment costs of psychotherapy versus medication for schizophrenics. Professional psychol August:293–298

Kayton L (1975) Clinical features of improved schizophrenics. In: Gunderson JG, Mosher LR (eds) Psychotherapy of schizophrenia. Aronson, New York, pp 361–395

Kellam SG (1983) Ward atmosphere, continuity of therapy, and the mental health system. In: Gunderson JG, Will OA, Mosher LR (eds) Principles and practice of milieu therapy. Aronson, New York

Kellam SG, Goldberg SC, Schooler N, Berman A, Shmelzer JL (1967) Ward atmosphere and outcome of treatment of acute schizophrenia. J Psychiatr Res 5:145–163

Klein DF (1980) Psychosocial treatment of schizophrenia, or psychosocial help for people with schizophrenia? Schizophr Bull 6:122–130

Langsley D, Pittman F, Swank G (1969) Family crisis in schizophrenics and other mental patients. J Nerv Ment Dis 149:270–276

Leff JP (1979) Developments in family treatment of schizophrenia. Psychiatr Q 51:216–232

Leff J, Kuipers L, Berkowitz R (1981) Intervention in families and its effect on relapse rate. Unpublished manuscript

Liberman RP (1983) Research on the psychiatric milieu. In: Gunderson JG, Will OA Jr., Mosher LR (eds) Principles and practice of milieu therapy. Aronson, New York

Liberman RP, Falloon IRH, Aitchson RA (1981) Multiple family therapy for schizophrenia, a behavioral, problem-solving approach. Unpublished manuscript

Liberman RP, Wallace CJ, Vaughn CE, Snyder KS, Rust C (1980) Social and family factors in the course of schizophrenia: toward an interpersonal problem-solving therapy for schizophrenics and their families. In: Strauss JS, Bowers M, Downey TW, Fleck S, Jackson S, Levine I (eds) The psychotherapy of schizophrenia. Plenum Medical, New York, pp 21–54

Lindberg D (1981) Management of schizophrenia: long-term studies with special reference to the combination of psychotherapy with depot neuroleptics. Acta Psychiatr Scand 63:Suppl 289

Linn L (1970) State hospital environment and rates of patient discharge. Arch Gen Psychiatry 23:346–351

Linn NW, Caffey EM, Klett CJ, Hogarty GE, Lamb HR (1979) Day treatment and psychotropic drugs in the aftercare of schizophrenic patients. Arch Gen Psychiatry 36:1055–1072

Litwack TR, Wiedemann CF, Yager J (1979) The fear of object loss, responsiveness to subliminal stimuli, and schizophrenic psychopathology. J Nerv Ment Dis 167(2):79–89

Malan DH (1979) Individual Psychotherapy and the science of psychodynamics. Butterworths, London

Mattes JA, Rosen B, Klein DF (1977) Comparison of the clinical effectiveness of "short" versus "long" stay psychiatric hospitalization: II. Results of a 3-year posthospital follow-up. J Nerv Ment Dis 165:387–394

Mattes JA, Rosen B, Klein DF, Millan D (1977) Comparison of the clinical effectiveness of "short" versus "long" stay psychiatric hospitalization: III. Further results of a 3-year posthospital follow-up. J Nerv Ment Dis 165:395–402

Mattes JA, Klein DF, Millan D, Rosen B (1979) Comparison of the clinical effectiveness of "short" versus "long" stay psychiatric hospitalization: IV. Predictors of differential benefit. J Nerv Ment Dis 167:175–181

May PRA (1974) Treatment of schizophrenia: I. A critique of reviews of the literature. Compr Psychiatry 15:179–185

May PRA, Simpson GM (1980) Schizophrenia: evaluation of treatment methods. In: Kaplan JI, Freedman AM, Sadock BJ (eds) Comprehensive textbook of psychiatry III, vol 1. pp 1240–1275

May PRA, Tuma AH (1976) Schizophrenia – a follow-up study of the results of treatment. Arch Gen Psychiatry 33:474–478, 481–486

May PRA, Van Putten T (1974) Treatment of Schizophrenia: II. A proposed rating scale of design and outcome for use in literature surveys. Compr Psychiatry 15:267–275

May PRA, Tuma AH, Dixon WJ (1981) Schizophrenia: a follow-up study of the results of five forms of treatment. Arch Gen Psychiatry 38:776–784

Michaux MH, Chelst MR, Foster SA et al. (1973) Postrelease adjustment of day and full-time psychiatric patients. Arch Gen Psychiatry 29:647–651

Moos RH (1974) Evaluating treatment environments: a social ecological approach. Wiley, New York

Moos RH, Shelton R, Petty C (1973) Perceived ward climate and treatment outcome. J Abnorm Psychol 82:291–298

Mosher LR (1972) A research design for evaluating a psychological treatment of schizophrenia. Hosp Community Psychiatry 23:17–22

Mosher LR (1976) Family therapy for schizophrenia: recent trends. In: West LJ, Flinn DE (eds) Treatment of schizophrenia progress and prospects. Grune and Stratton, New York

Mosher LR, Gunderson JG (1979) Group, family, milieu and community support systems treatment for schizophrenia. In: Bellak L (ed) The disorders of the schizophrenic syndrome. Basic, New York

Mosher LR, Keith SJ (1979) Research on the psychosocial treatment of schizophrenia: a summary report. Am J Psychiatry 136:623–631

Mosher LR, Keith SJ (1980) Psychosocial treatment: individual, group, family, and community support approaches. Schizophr Bull 6:10–41

Mosher LR, Menn AZ (1976) Dinosaur or astronaut? One year follow-up data from the Soteria project. Am J Psychiatry 133:919–920

Mosher LR, Menn AZ (1978) Community residential treatment for schizophrenia: two-year follow-up. Hosp Community Psychiatry 29:715–723

North C, Cadoret R (1981) Diagnostic discrepancy in personal accounts of patients with "schizophrenia". Arch Gen Psychiatry 38:133–137

O'Brien CP, Hamm KB, Ray BA, Pierce JF, Luborsky L, Mintz J (1972) Group vs. individual psychotherapy with schizophrenics: a controlled outcome study. Arch Gen Psychiatry 27: 474–478

Paul GL, Lentz RJ (1977) Psychosocial treatment of chronic mental patients: milieu vs. social-learning programs. Harvard University Press, Cambridge

Rappaport M, Hopkins HK, Hall K, Belleza T, Silverman J (1978) Are there schizophrenics for whom drugs may be unnecessary or contraindicated? Int Pharmacopsychiatry 13:100–110

Rogers CR, Gendlin EG, Kiesler DJ, Truaz CB (1967) The therapeutic relationship and its impact: a study of psychotherapy with schizophrenics. University of Wisconsin Press, Madison

Rubenstein R (1972) Mechanisms for survival after psychosis and hospitalization. Annual Meeting of the American Psychoanalytic Association, Dallas, Texas, 27–30 April 1972. Available through author, Mt. Zion Hospital, San Francisco, CA 14115

Schooler NR (1978) Antipsychotic drugs and psychological treatment in schizophrenia. In: Lipton MA, DiMascio A, Killam KR (eds) Psychopharmacology: a generation of progress. Raven, New York, pp 115–1168

Schooler NR (1980) Neuroleptics and psychosocial treatments: a discussion. Schizophr Bull 7: 131–134

Scott RD (1974) Cultural frontiers in the mental health service. Schizophr Bull 10:58–73

Silverman LH, Levinson P, Mendelsohn E, Ungaro R, Bronstein AA (1975) A clinical application of subliminal psychodynamic activation on the stimulation of symbiotic fantasies as an adjunct in the treatment of hospitalized schizophrenics. J Nerv Ment Dis 161:379–392

Snyder KS, Liberman RP (1981) Family assessment and intervention with schizophrenics at risk for relapse. New Directions in Mental Health Services (in press)

Stanton AH, Boutelle W, Gomes-Schwartz B, Gunderson JG, Katz H, Knapp P, Mintz M, Schnitzer R, Vannicelli M (1979) An evaluation of individual psychotherapy with schizophrenic patients: determinants of engagement in therapy. 132nd Annual Meeting of the American Psychiatric Association, 12–18 May 1979, Chicago

Stierlin H (1982) Delegation und Familie. Suhrkamp, Frankfurt

Vaughn CE, Leff JP (1976) The influence of family and social factors in the course of psychiatric illness: A comparison of schizophrenic and depressed neurotic patients. Br J Psychiatry 129: 125–137

Washburn S, Vannicelli M, Longabaugh R et al. (1976) A controlled comparison of psychiatric day treatment and inpatient hospitalization. J Consult Clin Psychol 44:665–675

West LJ, Flinn DE (eds) (1976) Treatment of schizophrenia progress and prospects. Grune and Stratton, New York

Wilder JF, Levin G, Zwerling I (1966) A two-year follow-up evaluation of acute psychotic patients treated in a day hospital. Am J Psychiatry 122:1095–1101

Wynne LC (1979) Suggestions from recent family research for treatment of schizophrenics. Proceedings of the 6th International Symposium on the Psychotherapy of Schizophrenia, Lausanne, Switzerland, 28–30 September 1978. Excerpta Medica, Amsterdam

Some Preliminary Thoughts on the Psychotherapy of the Schizophrenias

Robert Cancro

The title of this paper encompasses two major areas – psychotherapy and the schizophrenias – where limitations in knowledge contribute to the affective intensity of the associated debates. Schizophrenia has suffered a peculiar fate not unlike that of clothing fashions in which change is the only certainty. Whether it is the conceptualization, diagnostic criteria, prognostic factors, outcome, or treatment; opinions differ regularly and diametrically. This year's cure is next year's fraud. The theoretical etiology of this disorder has been placed on every imaginable factor from teeth, to mothers, to genes, to neuronal malfunctioning, and to family interaction. This list is only partial and inherently limited solely by the imaginativeness or lack thereof of the theoretician.

From the end of World War II until the late 1950s there was an increasing emphasis on sustained individual contact between patient and doctor as the therapeutic modality of choice. There were disagreements as to the appropriate quality of that interaction with proponents arguing the merits of techniques ranging from supportive to direct analytic therapy. There were also arguments about reconstruction upwards versus depth analysis. However, despite these differences over tactics a general agreement existed concerning the value of the strategy of individual contact. Since the early 1960s this approach has fallen into disfavor, partly because of the cyclical nature of professional thinking concerning schizophrenia. There are, however, other and more fundamental reasons. The personal frustrations for the therapist inherent in the long-term individual psychotherapy of schizophrenia contribute in real ways to the disenchantment (Will 1970). Even more importantly, the combination of the increasing demand for patient care and the increasing cost per unit of such care has led to the necessity of devising less expensive ways of treating more people. Finally, the failure of research studies to demonstrate a significant value in the psychotherapeutic approach contributed to a general loss of interest in the method. These various sources of difficulty concerning individual psychotherapy in schizophrenia have resulted in an overreaction in which many professionals now reject this treatment modality as out of date.

The very terms "psychotherapy" and "schizophrenia" refer to broad heterogeneous categories and not to precise and well-defined entities. Truax and Carkhuff (1970) have pointed out very clearly that psychotherapy is not a unitary process, even when adjectives such as psychoanalytically oriented or client centered are used. Just as there is much contention concerning the definition and merit of psychotherapy, there is at least equal disagreement concerning the concept of schizophrenia. The schizophrenias represent a markedly heterogeneous group of disorders that have some features in common (Cancro 1970). It is not even certain that the shared features are the significant ones. Even if these problems were to be solved there would still be the issue of individual differences among therapists as to ability, personality, and training. Strupp and Bergin (1969) have phrased the therapeutic question best. They asked: "What specific therapeutic interventions produce specific changes in specific patients under specific conditions?" This formulation emphasizes the degree of complexity of the problem and it is only in this way that we can recognize how much of the debate concerning treatment in schizophrenia is totally without point.

It may be helpful to review briefly and selectively a very small segment of the literature concerning research in psychotherapy in schizophrenia. Whitehorn and Betz (1954, 1960) did pioneering work to show that certain individuals – the so-called A therapists – were more successful with schizophrenic patients than others. This line of investigation demonstrated that, unlike carburetors, psychotherapists could not be grouped together as interchangeable units, even though they may have trained and worked at the same institution. More recently the research of May and his associates on the hospital treatment of schizophrenia has received considerable attention. Unfortunately, there has been almost an equal amount of disagreement and misunderstanding. May and Tuma (1965) and May (1968) published results which indicated that psychotherapy done by residents – not otherwise differentiated – added very little to drugs alone in the hospital treatment of schizophrenia. The source of misunderstanding has been that some workers have extrapolated from these hospital findings to the conclusion that psychotherapy is of no help in the treatment of schizophrenia. May (1969) never held that position and in fact argued that psychotherapy is likely to be helpful during the outpatient but not the hospital phase of treatment. Karon and VandenBos (1970) reported that experienced psychotherapists are able to influence the course of the schizophrenic illness to the degree that patients receiving such treatment have shorter periods of hospitalization, less thought disorder, and higher overall measures of functioning. They concluded that psychotherapy done by experienced therapists helps the thought disorder. The reply of May and Tuma (1970) took the form of a severe methodological critique of the Karon-VandenBos study which left some doubt about the validity of the conclusions.

In fairness, there are profound problems in all of the existing studies done on psychotherapy. Sargent (1960, 1961) reviewed many of the methodological issues with great skill and clarity. The basic problems that she raised 2 decades ago remain unsolved today. They range from the nature of the psychotherapeutic process itself (Colby 1962) to the extreme complexity and difficulty in identifying that which is done by whom to whom in what context and for what purpose. New research strategies and techniques are being developed and are promising. For example, Chassen (1967) discusses the use of the intensive single case method which offers a potentially powerful research tool. While rigorous studies of different types are necessary and will ultimately answer many of our questions, they cannot be looked to at the present time for such quidance. As so often happens, it is necessary to turn to clinical experience rather than rigorous experimental design. The heterogeneity of the sample labeled schizophrenic is such that it is statistically probable that virtually any specifiable intervention will be useful in some subset of the population. Whatever psychotherapy may or may not be, it is certainly a form of human contact and thereby of potential influence. In a very real sense effective therapy both influences and indoctrinates (Frank 1961). Lennard and Bernstein (1960) go so far as to view psychotherapy as a form of training in socialization. What is common between these and other positions is that therapy is a process in which a human being's attitudes, feelings, beliefs, values, and behaviors are influenced in various ways to varying degrees.

It is not simply anecdotal to report that certain patients, including schizophrenics, respond dramatically to this form of human influence; rather it is a form of clinical evidence. The question then becomes what aspects of the person can be influenced by the therapeutic intervention. If the goal is reduction of symptoms – particularly socially unacceptable behaviors – there are a variety of faster and cheaper techniques than psychotherapy. Pharmacotherapy presently is undoubtedly the most efficient and least expensive way of controlling most schizophrenic symptomatology including the socially unacceptable bahaviors. It is pointless to talk about therapeutic indications in the schizophrenias without specifying the goal of a particular intervention. Individual psychotherapy can only be evaluated as a treatment modality within the context of specified goals. Most workers recognize that schizophrenia as usually defined is chronic and devastating. Yet, the recognition of these realities does not mean that the personality characteristics of the patient cannot be influenced. The goals of individual psychotherapy involve intrapsychic and interpersonal as well as behavioral change. The means for achieving these goals of personality change in individual psychotherapy include the establishment of a relationship with a therapist that is intense, stable, predictable, and nonpunitive. This often is the first such human relationship that a schizophrenic person has experienced and it can foster psychosocial development.

The intrusion of the thought disorder into the patient's associations and the presence of delusions are neither fortuitous nor random. It is a commonplace clinical experience to find the thought disorder most evident – both as to frequency and formal severity – when the patient is discussing affectively charged material. In reducing the patient's conflicts and successfully treating the characterologic and neurotic components of the personality, it may be possible to reduce both the formal severity and frequency of the thought disorder. This is not to deny the efficacy of certain drugs in reducing the thought disorder, but rather to highlight the possible complementary role of psychotherapy in achieving this goal. By increasing the patient's awareness of psychological vulnerabilities, independent of their etiology, it becomes increasingly possible for that person to develop new or to modify selectively old coping devices. Those improvements in psychological adaptation can help to suppress the signs and symptoms of the disorder. In addition, the therapist serves during certain phases of treatment as a reality testing adjunct to the patient's impaired cognitive functioning. In this way the patient may "learn" to recognize characteristic cognitive aberrations, correct them and, thereby, think in a more logical fashion.

This writer's clinical experience has been that the major initial changes in ego functioning in a schizophrenic patient resulting from psychotherapy alone are in the areas of object relations and affect. The quality of the improvement seen initially in a schizophrenic patient receiving psychotherapy alone differs from that seen in a patient receiving only drugs. In many ways the former patient may appear deceptively improved because of better relatedness and richer affect. Even though the thought disorder and delusions may still be present, the patient appears to be in better contact and more "human." It follows then that measures of clinical improvement must take into account different ego functions because improvement can be selective and not global (Bellak 1970).

There have been a number of enormously gifted individuals who have devoted their professional lives to the psychotherapeutic treatment of schizophrenic people. Examples from this group include Federn, Sechehaye, Schwing, Fromm-Reichmann, Sullivan, and Hill to name only a few. These people and others not cited have left a legacy in both the form of their activity and their written record of that activity. It is not surprising that sensitive and articulate clinicians are also convincing authors. The surprise is how much they disagree in basic theory and technique, despite their common denominator of clinical success with the patients. Their efforts to capture the science tend to ignore the art and may even misidentify the proper areas of investigation. Much is said about technique and little about the therapist. Yet, what comes across most clearly in the writings of the unique therapist is the very uniqueness of the therapist. Careful scrutiny of their publications allows certain personal and process variables to emerge as the beginnings of a philosophy of the psychotherapy of the schizophrenic patient.

Perhaps the single most important personal trait is that of honesty. There is a direct and simple honesty – an absence of artifice – that can be observed in the writing of people such as Frieda Fromm-Reichmann. It tells the reader more about the fundamental nature of the therapeutic interaction than do her chapters on technique. The trust that some schizophrenic patients are able to develop in these therapists very likely stems, at least in part, from their ability to sense the therapist's basic honesty.

Another characteristic which emerges with great vividness is that of flexibility. This is both a personal and a process variable. The therapists who are able to transcend the limitations of the standard technique do better with these patients. The great therapists are not wed to theory as a dogmatic doctrine but rather use it as a cognitive crutch. Unfortunately, their writings often emphasize the cognitive crutch rather than the personal qualities which are critical to the development of an effective psychotherapeutic relationship with the schizophrenic patient.

One of the process variables, which of course also reflects the personality characteristics of the therapist, involves persistence. The psychotherapy of a schizophrenic patient is usually neither short nor straightforward. There must be a commitment on the part of the therapist which continues over time and often in the face of extreme resistance. The therapist must be able to defer, perhaps indefinitely, the gratification of experiencing positive growth in the patient. This form of psychotherapeutic intervention cannot be time limited. The consequences of this temporal uncertainty can be disruptive for certain therapists who need to anticipate and plan their professional time well into the future.

It is important that the emotional commitment of the therapist not take a form of overinvolvement with the outcome of treatment which reenacts the parental aspirations for the patient. Jan Frank (1957, personal communication) emphasized the importance of what he called "desirelessness" on the part of the therapist. By this term he recognized the danger of overinvolvement which could lead to excessive and destructive zeal. Conversely, the therapist cannot be totally neutral or a passive blank screen. It is a difficult channel to steer between the Scylla of indifference and the Charybdis of overinvolvement.

The therapist must have an excellent tolerance of uncertainty if not an actual ability to enjoy it. The psychotherapy of these patients is a journey into profound uncertainty. Even the most sensitive person simply does not understand a major portion of what the actively schizophrenic patient is saying, let alone why. It is very difficult for some therapists to do psychotherapeutic work when they do not know what the patient is talking about. The therapist who is talented in this sort of work is able, nevertheless, to continue to build a relationship that transcends and ultimately may even bridge the communicative gap produced by the schizophrenic patient's use of language. It is undoubtedly important to be able at times to understand the schizophrenic's speech but it is perhaps even more important to be comfortable with the patient *without* understanding the content of the communication. This is not something which all therapists are able to do. It is perhaps only those who are willing to trust their patients to quide them safely through the morass of a schizophrenic illness who can do good psychotherapeutic work with them.

If tolerance of uncertainty is important, tolerance of error is essential. The therapist's effort to clarify and translate into, the language and frame of reference of the nonschizophrenic is doomed to fail. There will be repeated distortions and misunderstandings on the part of the therapist. Yet, the response of the therapist to error and how the therapist deals with the frustration and narcissistic injury of repeated error reveals to the patient essential information about the therapist. There can be more revealed truth in an illtimed and/or incorrect interpretation than in a correct one. The schizophrenic may find that he is in more need of information concerning his therapist than concerning his unconscious.

Summary

The advent of the age of pharmacotherapy contributed to a diminution of interest in the psychotherapy of the schizophrenias. Recent increasing concern over tardive dyskinesia and other dangerous consequences of drug management suggests the utility of a reassessment of psychotherapy. Psychotherapeutic approaches to schizophrenic patients differ greatly and this variability contributes significantly to the methodologic problems inherent in their evaluation. The search for the common factors in the different but successful psychotherapies is essential for adequate evaluation research. This paper suggests that this commonality may be in the therapists' attitudes and character structure rather than in the theories and/or techniques of the various schools of psychotherapy. The full identification and articulation of these personal factors would create a philosophy of the psychotherapy of the schizophrenias as opposed to the development of one more theory about its conduct.

References

Bellak L (1970) The validity and usefulness of the concept of the schizophrenic syndrome. In: Cancro R (ed) The schizophrenic reactions: A critique of the concept, hospital treatment, and current research. Brunner/Mazel, New York, pp 41–58

Cancro R (1970) A review of current research directions: Their product and their promise. In: Cancro R (ed) The schizophrenic reactions: A critique of the concept, hospital treatment, and current research. Brunner/Mazel, New York, pp 189–196

Chassen JB (1967) Research design in clinical psychology and psychiatry. Appleton-Century-Crofts, New York

Colby KM (1962) Discussion of papers on therapist's contribution. In: Strupp H, Luborsky L (eds) Research in psychotherapy. American Psychological Association, Washington, D.C., pp 95–101

Frank JD (1961) Persuasion and healing. Johns Hopkins Press, Baltimore

Karon BP, VandenBos GR (1970) Experience, medication, and the effectiveness of psychotherapy with schizophrenics. Br J Psychiatry 116:427–428

Lennard HL, Bernstein A (1960) The anatomy of psychotherapy. Columbia University Press, New York

May PRA (1968) Treatment of schizophrenia: A comparative study of five treatment methods. Science House, New York

May PRA (1969) The hospital treatment of the schizophrenic patient. Int J Psychiatry 8:699–722

May PRA, Tuma AH (1965) Treatment of schizophrenics: An experimental study of five treatment methods. Br J Psychiatry 111:503–510

May PRA, Tuma AH (1970) Methodological problems in psychotherapy research: Observations on the Karon-VandenBos study of psychotherapy and drugs in schizophrenia. Br J Psychiatry 117: 569–570

Sargent HD (1960) Methodological problems of follow-up studies in psychotherapy research. Am J Orthopsychiatry 30:495–506

Sargent HD (1961) Intrapsychic change: Methodological problems in psychotherapy research. Psychiatry 24:93–108

Strupp HH, Bergin AE (1969) Some empirical and conceptual bases for coordinated research in psychotherapy: A critical review if issues, trends, and evidence. Int J Psychiatry 7:18–90

Truax CB, Carkhuff RR (1970) Toward effective counseling and psychotherapy: Training and practice. Aldine Press, Chicago

Whitehorn JC, Betz BJ (1954) A study of psychotherapeutic relationships between physicians and schizophrenic patients. Am J Psychiatry 111:321–331

Whitehorn JC, Betz BJ (1960) Further studies of the doctor as a crucial variable in the outcome and treatment of schizophrenic patients. Am J Psychiatry 117:215–223

Will OA (1970) The psychotherapeutic center and schizophrenia. In: Cancro R (ed) The schizophrenic reactions: A critique of the concept, hospital treatment, and current research. Brunner/ Mazel, New York, pp 153–167

Possibilities and Limits of Individual Psychotherapy of Schizophrenic Patients

G. Benedetti

I should like to present my thoughts concerning the possibilities and limits of individual psychotherapy by relating one case history, where paintings made by the patient illustrate from the inner being of the patient that which I objectively experienced as an individual psychotherapist. I should like to begin by presenting a poem, written by the patient, in order to help you to understand the intensity of her transference through all the psychosis.

They understood nothing, nothing,
And so, therefore, I became filled with hatred.
I wanted to spit out my hatred
But they forced me,
Spoonful by spoonful,
To swallow what I had vomited.
Then my body enlarged
In all directions.
The hatred in me swelled my body.
I became misformed.
Why are you so fat?
You aren't like the other children.
They put a corset on me,
Bound my body,
And the hatred pressed itself together,
Atom into atom,
Till it fit into the corset.
But the mass of hatred
Had not changed
Neither its weight.
In your house there is no air,
Oxygen is missing;
Lack of breath oppresses me.
Fists are hanging in the air,
The dead eyes,
The screaming eyes,
Into whose whirlwind one is sucked,
Don't they see
That their owner is suffocating,
Even if the mouths

No longer speak
And have not, for ages?
This house
Is like blows upon the head.
Despair thrusts itself
Mockingly laughing
Out of the nooks and crannies.
You do not see the ghosts
Who, with drawn knives
Crawl up my legs.

There,
A millimeter away,
Hell is laughing.
Who will murder me?
Am I a murderer?
The light in the house is cold.
Upon my return
Glittering gloom races towards me.
Where is my head
Where are my feet
The hands
Which are still carrying the milk pail?
Darkness inside and out
Surrounds my senses.
Inside the house
The mother of horror is waiting.
Stinking,
The unconscious hatred
Of a family
Ripping itself to shreds
For hundreds of years
Spreads
With the ringing of the bell.
I, however, was struck with fear
And knew
That the ghosts
Were hanging behind me.
The light
Became a bad omen
I became a murderer
The corpse,
Which I could only see,
Lay there.
I screamed,
And no one understood
What I had seen.
Horror shook me

And I cursed the day
On which I had come upon the world.
They called it sickness
And gave it an ugly name
Madness!
The grating of the door
Is eternal damnation.
A color
Which is no color
A sound and a smell
A swallow of everything
But not describable
And in everything
An endless feeling
Where I, who determine
No longer exist.
Below
Fear is hanging
Like a giant drop
Encompassing the world
And the monstrous depths
Of nothingness
Into which I am falling
On the way down
Accompanied by multicolored rage
And the loss of solidity
And the decay into undefined gravel.
Always and again this hated presence
While the rage
Like a transparent bomb
Ticks on.

A picture of violence painted by the patient (Fig. 1) gives a glimpse of what she and her psychotherapist went through during the first 3 years of treatment. Her fits of rage during some psychotherapeutic sessions were only the outer expression of what she often experienced within herself, even when quietly alone. What this picture cannot, however, convey is the patient's feeling that she had to identify with something destructive; this filled her with deepest dismay. This "principle of hatred," as we have often called this inner demon, represented an absolute negation of her fellow humans, and of her own feelings. The patient's sickness seemed to be an ever necessary confrontation with a demon of hatred, which she herself had to personify against her own wishes. This demon constantly depersonalized both her and her fellow men, whom she then characterized as "not real."

After one particular crisis of violence had died down somewhat, and the patient was able to regard it at a distance, she visualized her destructive drive in the form of most horrible faces. She also saw it in the form of a malignant tumor which filled her belly and devoured it; and also in the form of a mysterious destructive woman who

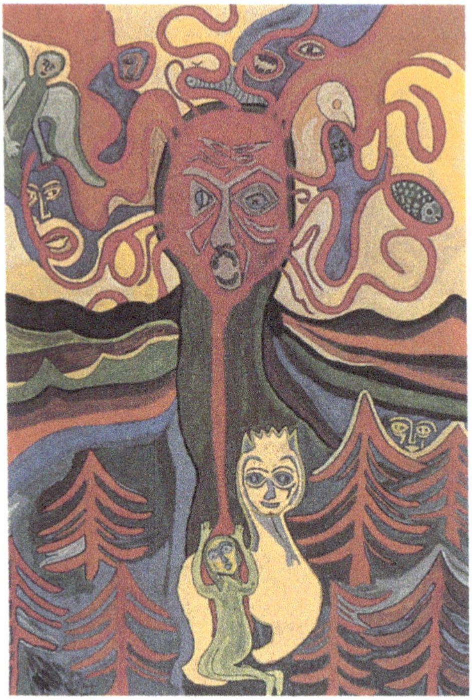

Fig. 1.

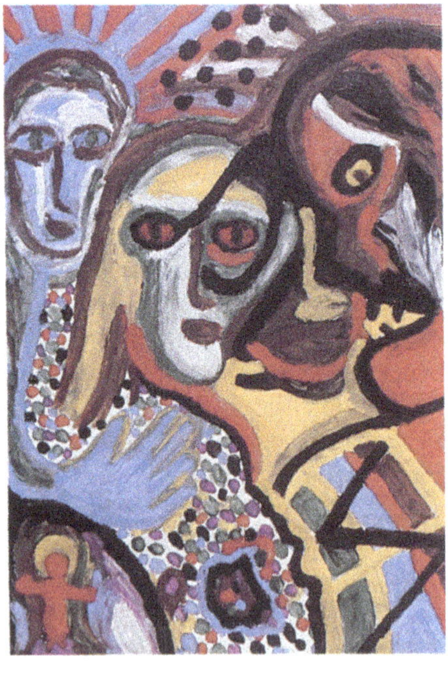

Fig. 2.

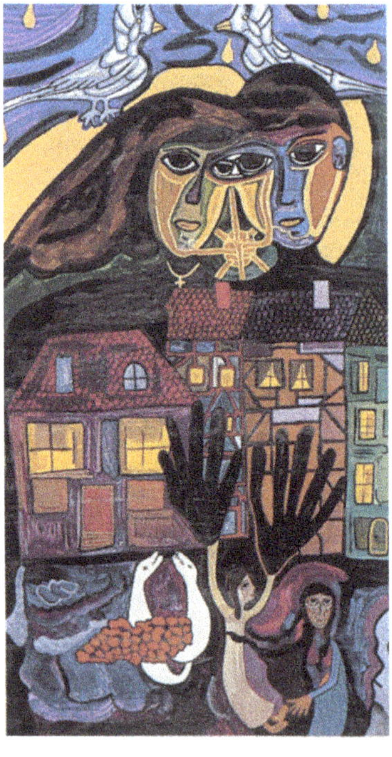

Fig. 3.

dwelled at the source of her being. She was not even able to see her face to face. The awful sight of her legs alone, seen at a distance, was unbearable for the patient. It was for her an inexpressibly terrible thing to be both symbiotically and bodily fused together with this "witch," whose absolute evil caused the patient to experience a metaphysical distance from humanity.

She attempted to express this symbiosis metaphorically in a picture (Fig. 2), showing herself connected bodily, like Siamese twins, with this overwhelming demon. Only after 3 years of psychotherapy was the malignant symbiosis with the "witch" substituted by that with her psychotherapist (Fig. 3).

In order to become herself, she had first to die. Dying signified not only denial of herself, but of every word, of every movement, of her "pseudonormal" previous existence, of the structure of space, of time, the meaning of every sentence. Dying was for her an endless sinking into something which life or truth could have been, but which could only come to her, during that time, as decay, dissolving, "acidity," fragmentation or pulverization, so that, finally, the demon would cease to exist.

The most impressive aspect of our relationship was not her loud and passionate accusations during her hours of rage, when she branded me a murderer, when she beat me. The most shattering experience for me was when my patient, between her fits of violence, feared nothing more than she did her own violent anger. She would then beg me to be careful; she feared for my life; she hung signs on the walls of her room, warning herself not to attack me, as I was fragile. And then again, in her rage, it was exactly with her very worst enemy that she had to identify, and so become an enemy of both herself and myself.

I like to characterize my work by the word "dualization," which expresses a process that makes psychotherapy possible, but also transcends it dialectically. The word dualization signifies a "jumping into" the situation of the patient, which, in effect, makes me a kind of fellow patient. The first thing I noticed about my patient was her total helplessness in her attempts to give herself any direction in her thinking, her caring for herself, her motions. It seemed to me that a demonic past source of her visible existence would have to return as a destructive drive so that it could be overcome by a loving working through together. Dualization here meant that I participated in the helplessness of the patient by the working through of her endless misery. I identified with the conviction of the patient that her rage must return in its moments of unavoidability, and the only difference between insane repetition and healing return lay not only in catharsis or in interpretations, but primarily in the freedom coming from human acceptance. The psychotherapist was supposed to, in the words of the patient, create something on the peak of her rage which would then transcend it. In this sense I attempted to take this embittered and malignant violence into me with benevolent calm, which sprang from my connection with the inexpressible human substance of this psychotic person.

I have often realized, in my countertransferences, that there is a discrepancy between that which a psychotherapist tells himself during reflection and that which actually happens to him. How often was I overcome by aggressive feelings towards my patient; at such times I had to experience myself almost literally as two persons in one, alternating between insight and anger, a copy of the helpless torn apart condition of the patient repeating itself in my own still healthy model, until I realized that my failure to solve this splitting contradiction was not a basic barrier blocking the way towards

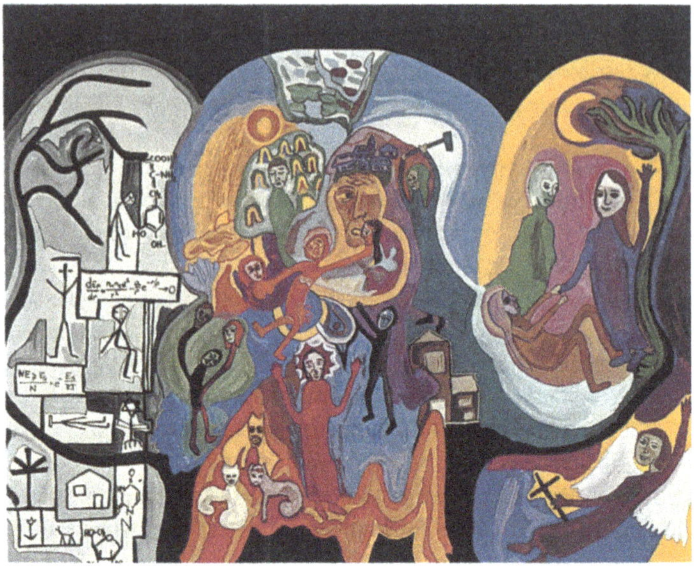

Fig. 4.

healing, but was, rather, a proof of my unconscious willingness to step into the world of the patient and to bear the many sides of her being as an inner contradiction. I sensed an identification with the patient in the possibility of suffering with her and so taking upon myself some of the weight of suffering which was pressing down upon her.

After this, the patient's "chaotic" encounter with me became real in the midst of the depersonalization. She pictured her life in three stages (Fig. 4); in a prepsychotic one of "pseudonormality" in which she was a brilliant biologist working with mathematical formulas, while hiding the death of her being from herself, expressed in the gray colors of the drawing; the second stage was one of the chaos of madness in the encounter with me, which in the creation of the patient appeared to have a double significance – the end of everything and at the same time the exclamation: "What luck that I have become mad." The third stage is shown as a freedom sensed in the future, only made possible by the compassionate response of the psychotherapist.

What particularly impressed me in the second section of the picture was the ability of the patient to dare the impossible in the shadow of the psychotherapist, to willingly allow her madness and its violence to arise. The patient expressed this in the constantly repeated words: "to let oneself fall into that which destroys," and thus to overcome it, for in this decision was something which for the patient represented a beginning of herself, whereas in attempting to adjust to our normal world she had only become unreal, without ego, "pseudonormal." The "controlled explosion" seen in the picture, which the patient could only paint, as she had so many of her paintings, with tears in her eyes and while afraid, led, in the third part of the picture, to a transcendence of her violence. The peacefulness, which the patient was not yet able to experience, appears to us as a metaphor of her future healing. "One must go through all of hell to reach the other side." The violence of the patient becomes, in the psychotherapeutic dualization, the violence of a hell which is to be overcome together.

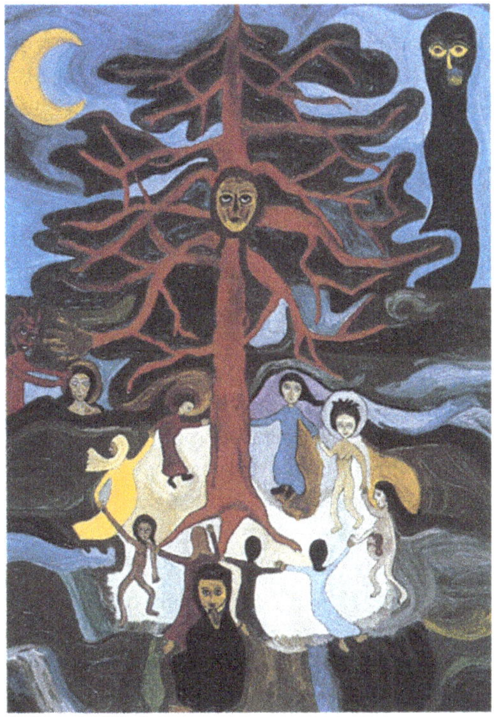

Fig. 5.

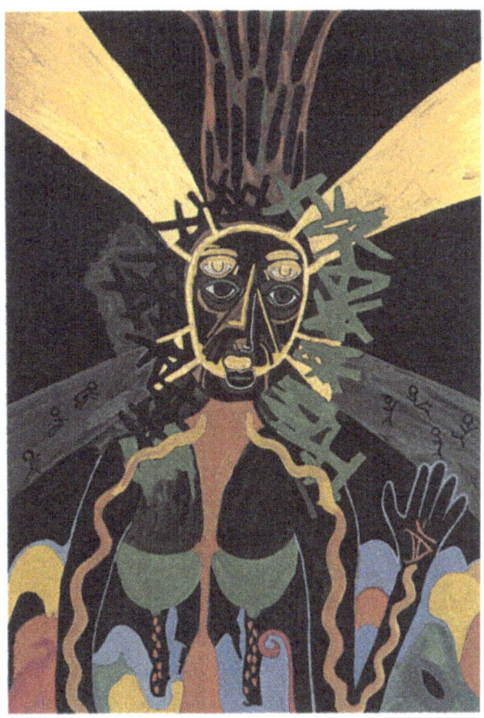

Fig. 6.

Here there arose for the patient the narrow crevasse in her desert out of which the tree of life could grow (Fig. 5), and where she felt herself pregnant by her own future self. The dance in the painting was the result of the patient's once hearing, during psychotherapy, how the therapist experienced different persons in her being as future partial aspects of her unified being mutually offering each other their hands under the yellow eyes of the threatening snake.

A later picture (Fig. 6), entitled by the patient "The Mother of Pain," was a self-portrait. In the two lower stripes, which surround the head of the woman in pain like ghostly rays, little black humans are indicated; to the patient they signified her pre-psychotic life. How incredibly large and alive the mother of pain appears in comparison with such marionettes! She became such a figure not only because of her suffering, because of the crown of thorns, but because of her therapeutic symbiosis, or, as she expressed it, because of her being someone with four eyes. She saw herself as I saw her, with the eyes of the therapist; his eyes had become her eyes, in this way becoming "three dimensional," that is, they discovered the positive sides of her being, as I tirelessly told her. The facial features of the woman have been drawn over with the light features of the psychotherapist; over her sad eyes are the open ones of her therapist.

Her new identity formed itself so that her therapist not only gave her life, but also death (Fig. 7); but not as persecutor! He appeared to the patient as executor of our own negative potential, so that it would receive positive aspects in the mirror of the therapist. A "positive" relation in negation is what I call an occurrence in individual psychotherapy which, although it remains negative in its dual repetition of destruction, nevertheless, by exchanging the persecutor with the positively experienced, and even loved therapist, unfolds a positive dynamic although the terrible content remains the same.

The patient stated that the knights were the words of her psychotherapist, which were paradoxically killing her. This did not happen because these words offended her

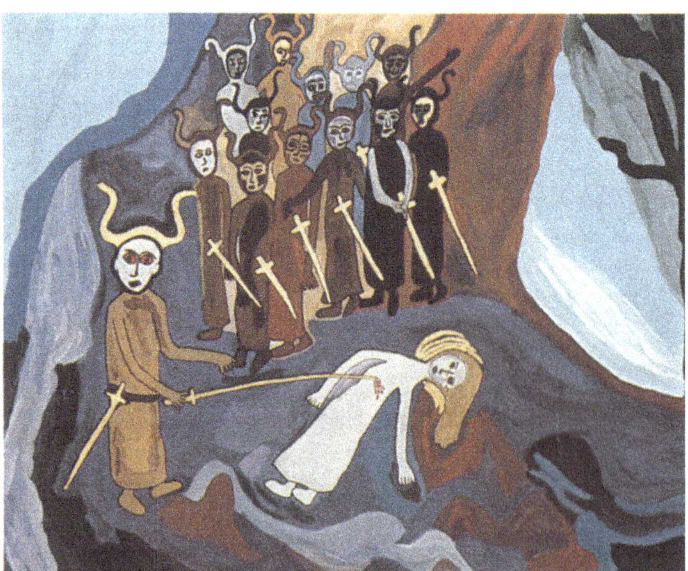

Fig. 7.

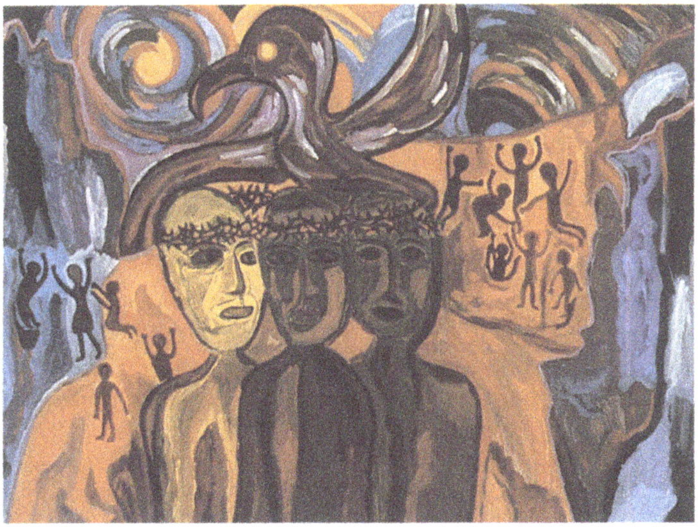

Fig. 8.

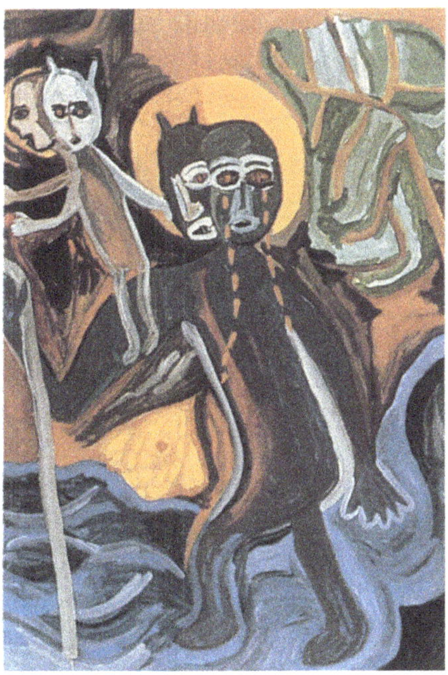

Fig. 9.

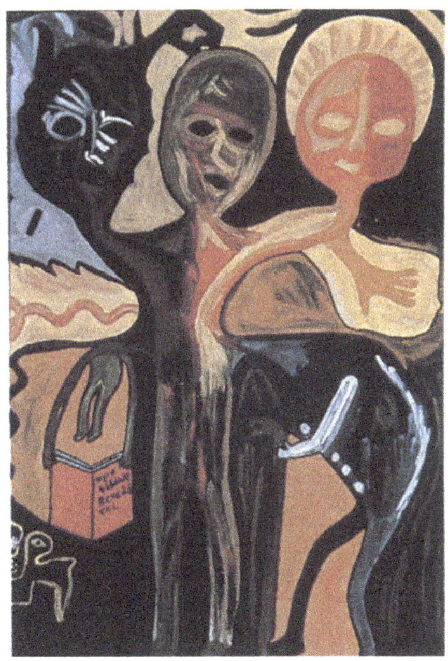

Fig. 10.

in a narcissistic way. On the contrary, exactly those words which gave her most strongly the feeling of being alive brought her the "second death," which overcame the first death. The deeper meaning of the symbol expressed in words and pictures was that the psychotherapist had been made able, by the patient, to fill that place which had been taken by the persecutor. Instead of his trying to protect – perhaps helplessly – his patient from the all-powerful persecutor, he himself took over and filled the persecutor's place. In the patient's words, she had to, at first, accept existence as death, without defenses, because something had destroyed existence in her. The woman killed by the knight is also, however, in reverse, the therapist who was sometimes threatened by the rage of the patient. The danger consisted of death impulses.

The identity of the patient and therapist which arose in this way was expressed in a painting with a shared crown of thorns (Fig. 8), and also in a remarkable Christophorus picture (Fig. 9) where the therapist, splitting himself, takes over the demonic features of the patient, also wearing the devil's horns next to the aura around his head, so that the patient can experience her splitting positively, progressively, and so, on her part, also take over the features of the therapist, his aura. The identity is shown in the splitting of the therapist (Fig. 10) which stands parallel to that of the patient (Fig. 11), thereby dualizing the psychopathological symptom.

In that both splittings are symmetrically correlated, the psychopathological picture becomes filled with progressive meaning. The splitting of the therapist is more than a fantasy of the patient, for it was through her words that I stepped into the contradictions of opposites; for example, the contradiction between objective countertransference and subjective identification with her suffering; between my partial inability to understand all of her language and my empathic ability to understand her entire being; between my despair in a situation of heplessness and my feeling of therapeutic power which was given to me by the patient herself through some picture (Fig. 12 a symbol of individual psychotherapy).

Only a countertransference which includes the suffering of the patient can make possible the human exchange, the therapeutic symbiosis, the identification and counter-identification, the reversal of identity, the dualization which, more than any interpretation, can overcome the psychotic imprisonment. After this example of my individual

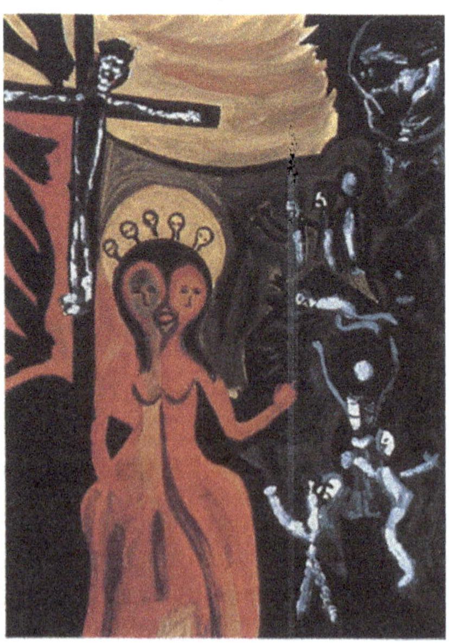

Fig. 11.

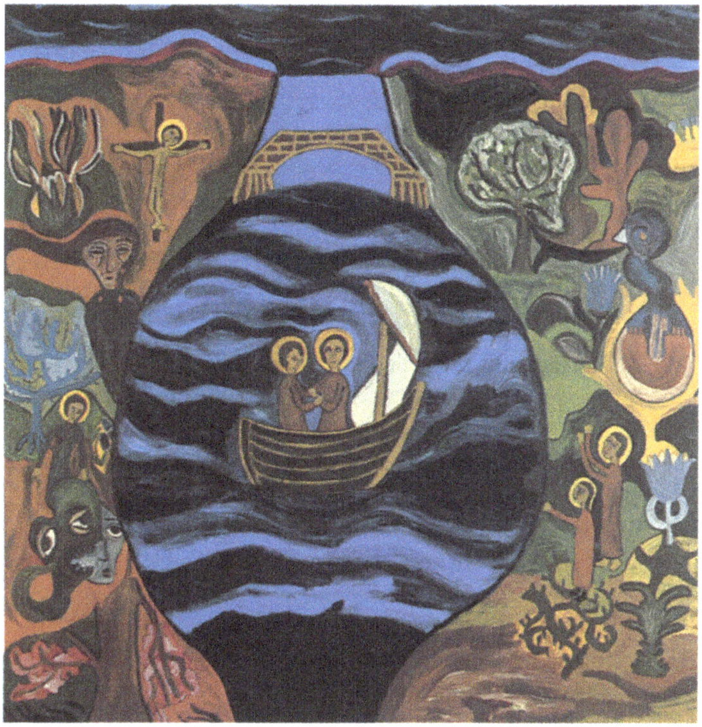

Fig. 12.

work with schizophrenic patients I should like to say which sort of indications permit and which limit, by their absence, this kind of encounter according to my experience:

1. Autistic delusions which are in no immediate contact with the social world of the patient; they seem to be out of touch with reality, they seem rather to symbolize universal entities, like the "symbiosis with the sun," or the "split between evil and goodness," the identification of the patient with the savior of humanity, and even more abstract and existential things, as in the words of my patient:

My illness somehow seems to arise from two opposite facts crashing into each other and cumulating – the fact that doing all things is terribly wrong, "pseudo," irreal – and at the other hand the fact that there might be an existential "weight" in it that cannot get hold of and neither know what it is, which I am afraid of, because it seems to bear unbearable risks.

Even if social experiences *may* lay at the roots of such delusions, they cannot be easily recaptured into the dynamics of present psychotic thinking. What the patient in such cases needs is not, in my experience, the causal reduction of his "delusions" to group transactions, but first of all the "entrance" of his therapist into his symbolic world along a dimension of mutual identifications and counteridentifications, where "delusions" appear to the psychotherapist *progressive* symbols of the patient's truths. "Normals," says my patient, "are calming themselves down by calling my states 'delusions,' which increases my panic and drives me to utmost despair." In the mirror of my listening and participating, psychopathology becomes creativity. The greater the creativity, the more positive the therapeutic indication.

2. A *motivation* of the patient to individual psychotherapy, to the encounter with the uniqueness of partnership, to what my patient calls "a shared travel through hell" is of fundamental importance. Motivation for treatment is not frequent in schizophrenia, but, if present, as in my case, is always a main source of progress.

3. A corresponding motivation of the therapist is necessary, whose narcissistic gains depend then more upon the *experience of duality* than upon group interaction.

4. Individual therapy presupposes collaboration with at least one significant member of the patient's family, who can be counted on for support and continuity of treatment.

After these four *direct* indications, may I mention four *indirect* ones:

1. The patient's radical refusal of every kind of familiar talks.

2. The great fragility and narcissistic vulnerability of some family members, who would prefer to give up the psychotic object of their projections, that is, to let the patient go his therapeutic way, rather than to permit the therapist to enter the family member's own disturbed world.

3. Poor affective resources of the family, which are also not sufficient to permit new existential experiences of the patient, and which only permit some kind of clarification of transactional "bookkeeping."

4. A patient's psychopathology which is not reproduced by actual perverse family transactions, filled up again and again by the family with actual conflicts, reproaches, and transmissions of culpability.

These short remarks can only give, of course, a brief glimpse of the importance of this old problem.

The Establishment of Transference in the Psychoanalysis of Schizophrenics

Paul Matussek

The following statements deal with the establishment of transference in schizophrenics as we observe it in the Research Institute for Psychopathology and Psychotherapy of the Max Planck Society. The data are provided to illustrate the ideas put forward.

I myself have been working since 1950 psychotherapeutically with schizophrenics. However, only since the end of the 1950s have I had the assistance of two co-workers and only since 1965, when an Institute for Psychodynamic Psychiatry was established by the Max Planck Society, has the number of therapists dealing with individual therapy of schizophrenics multiplied. The majority of my colleagues stayed more than 5 years before going into private practice or accepting a teaching position.

During this time, the concepts of technique – including the handling of transference in the psychoanalytical treatment of schizophrenics – have undergone considerable change. Even today, a consensus on the international level is still far off. This has to do not only with the therapist's level of experience and training but, to a large degree, also with his personality, and above all his sensitivity, tolerance of frustration, and narcissistic stability. For the past 15 years, we have always had a relatively large group of analytically trained individual therapists, which enabled us to compare their personalities, experience, and techniques.

The success or failure of psychotherapy, however, does not solely depend upon the psychotherapist's experience and personality. Aside from the duration and course of the illness, schizophrenia is not simply schizophrenia. Today clinicians speak of the group of schizophrenias more frequently than they did 30 years ago, and when they do so they are making a diagnostic differentiation which increasingly affects psychotherapeutic work. Such diagnostic differentiations are not to be confused with the shifting of labels practiced for a long time. They ought to be regarded, rather, as efforts to understand the symptoms hiding behind the term "schizophrenia" so that their psychodynamic interpretation can be verified. This interpretation should be more than a habit depending upon a particular school of thought.

In conformity with these considerations, the psychotherapist is faced with the necessity of reconstructing his patient's life story during years of therapy and understanding him better and better. A one-sided or premature reconstruction will lead to misinterpretations as we have known them to arise from the terms "schizophrenic family," "schizophrenogenic mother," the "double bind," the "absent father," or similar clichés. In a study done jointly with Triebel (Matussek and Triebel 1974), we were able to prove that the family constellation of schizophrenics is by no means uniform but that constellations of considerable diversity lend themselves to the development of a future psychosis. For the past 3 years, our investigation has been conducted with detailed clinical and statistical methods, and one of the questions we have been examining is that of the dependence of successful therapy upon the family constellation and course of the illness, as well as upon the therapist's technique and personality.

During this time period, a total of 18 co-workers have been treating nearly 100 schizophrenics with individual therapy. It will take years to verify statistically the numerous issues involved. Now I would merely like to point out a fact which prompted me to make the establishment of transference in psychoses the subject of my statements. In view of the present state of our analysis, I can already say this much: The success of the psychotherapy of psychoses – independently of their duration and symptoms – depends above all upon the successful establishment of transference. In addition I would like to make the distinction between a labile transference and a stable one in order to indicate that the initial transference, as impressive as it may seem, is still no guarantee of successful therapy.

The emphasis upon transference is nothing new to the analyst. Freud had believed the psychoanalysis of psychotics to be impossible because he considered them incapable of transference. He expressed some hope, however, that refinements and adaptations of psychoanalytic technique might prove fruitful (Freud 1933). This leads us to the following question: Which change made in regard to the process of transference within the past 3 decades is of special significance? In this connection, let me stress only two points: psychotropics, on the one hand, and the development of psychoanalytical theories, on the other.

As for psychotropics, the combination of psychotherapy and drug treatment has been and still is controversial. There have been and still are psychoanalysts who reject drug therapy not only on the basis of its alleged inefficacy. They consider drug treatment useless, even harmful. When tested, neither view can hold its ground. Psychotropics have meanwhile gained an undisputed position in the treatment of schizophrenics, even among psychotherapists working with psychoanalysis. But that is a subject of its own that I can only briefly touch upon to shed light on our point of view.

As concerns the change in psychoanalytical theory, it, for the sake of brevity, can be illustrated only through its practical effect. Our modern standpoint lies between the poles of the orthodox analysis of schizophrenia as represented by such names as Federn, Fromm-Reichmann, Rosen, Sechehaye, and Rosenfeld, and the social psychiatric position that feels responsible not only for obtaining work and housing but also for taking care of the patient's personal problems.

To illustrate this standpoint, I will try to outline our initial impressions which show a rough distinction among the following processes of transference and improvement:

1. Patients with a relatively swift and easily established positive transference and a clear improvement.

2. Patients with whom, in spite of the greatest effort and variation in technique, a positive and stable transference could not be established. The therapy accordingly met with little success. An essential reason for the failures in our cases was either the presence of a narcissistic self-object (as of father or mother) against which the therapist was powerless, or the ideological consolidation of a narcissistic protective strategy such as an absolute refusal to pursue an occupation.

3. Patients whose initially labile transference changed into a clearly negative one, which did not necessarily mean that the therapy had to be broken off. The patients

occasionally enjoyed coming to a session. They were punctual and showed great interest in their therapy, which for a long time was considered the expression of a positive transference not only by some of our therapists but also in the literature. But that was a mistake. Behind the apparent willingness to participate in therapy, there was an attitude of rejection. We nevertheless succeeded, in a considerable number of cases, in turning the negative transference into a positive one, which was often quite difficult to do.

This means that with a schizophrenic – in contrast to a neurotic – transference does not develop spontaneously. Ever since M. A. Sechehaye (1955), we have known that transference has to be induced. In agreement with her, we have ascertained – often after many detours – that a negative transference, even after a relatively long time, can be changed into a positive one through a variation in technique. Obviously I cannot discuss in detail the changes in methods involved. I would like to select only three of them as they are fairly easy to describe: the setting, the significance of dreams, and the symptoms.

Even if today the outer setting of psychotherapy is no longer considered as important as it was at the beginning of the psychoanalytic era, its demarcation from that used in the psychotherapy of neuroses is not insignificant. Whereas for the latter the classical position – lying on the couch, turned away from the therapist – is still regarded as optimal, it is used only in exceptional cases in the psychoanalysis of schizophrenics.

The frequence of sessions has also changed. The principle of a close session frequency, justifiable in neuroses, has proven to be decidedly wrong in schizophrenias. There is no general rule other than adjusting the frequency to each individual case as I described (Matussek 1959). In some cases, one session per week is sufficient, as a greater session frequency can complicate the establishment of transference due to the fear of confinement and proximity involved. A stable positive transference, the agent most conducive to successful therapy, can thus not be established.

Our attitude toward dreams and ideas, too, has changed considerably. Today we are convinced that the closer the beginning of treatment is to the acute phase, the less one should insist upon report and analysis of dreams. It is best to let the patient tell his dreams only at his expressed wish. Furthermore, no interpretation, which is possible only with detailed associations, is performed. If the necessary associations are sought from the schizophrenic too early, they will lead to confusion which makes an integrating insight into the dream experience impossible. If there is dream interpretation at all, it should be more of a description of images rather than a detective search for a hidden dream meaning and its more or less arbitrary interpretation.

Concerning the content of dreams, schizophrenics who report having dreams do not have regular dreams of transference until during a relatively late phase of their treatment. But if these should occur sooner or even if there are verbal manifestations of transference independent of dreams, one should be careful with interpretations. Accepting is better than interpreting, at least during a stage in which transference has not stabilized.

The same principle applies to the third aspect, the interpretation of symptoms. Whereas in the 1950s almost all analysts – myself included – wanted to interpret the significance of individual symptoms, we have had to convince ourselves with time that such an atomistic interpretation is meaningless. Worse than that, it is harmful to the establishment of transference. Not only does the old technique smack of artificialty and ideology, it also places too great a burden on the patient's capability of reflection. A weak ego, such as the one found as a rule in schizophrenics, is not capable of the degree of insight which would be therapeutically necessary. Furthermore, the old techniques had another flaw. The advocates of these techniques believed that – in a similar manner as in neuroses – the decisive step toward recovery, that is the resolution of symptoms, could be reached only through interpretation, whether it be that of a hallucination, of a delusion, or of a catatonic attitude.

The representatives of the English school – from which H. Rosenfeld has been working on schizophrenics for decades with basically unaltered technique – have gone the farthest in this respect. He and his colleagues from the Melanie Klein school remain skeptical to this day of supportive and educational measures which are supposed to form a basis for a positive life-style. A. Rosenfeld (1952) sees the basic healing effect in the psychotherapy of schizophrenics in the detailed interpretation of the positive and negative transference and the unconscious materials of the fantasies, which are mainly expressed in the behavior, gestures, and dealings of the patient. According to Rosenfeld (1952a) the development of a so-called transfer psychosis is made possible by following a central interpretative direction which concentrates on the manifest and latent anxieties of the patient, and therapy trying to control the symptoms. The relief and effectiveness of this kind of interpretation can be observed in that the distortion in the acceptance of the destructive and aggressive struggles of the patient can be relieved on a step-by-step basis.

We hold the view today that symptoms – whether they be experiences or modes of behavior – must not be examined for their inner structure in their acute stage. Such intepretations are always done only retrospectively, just as a dream is not interpreted during the dreaming itself but the following day from a totally different level of consciousness. The fuller and more uniform our consciousness, the more effective the interpretation of the dream. The fact that the contents of a dream elude interpretation can be observed through the phenomenon of awakening. If one wishes to remember a dream before waking up, it will evade our grasp. The dream image must first be present without being interpreted in order to be remembered completely and then be subjected to interpretation. This is also true of a psychosis. Acute as well as chronic modes of behavior resist a healing insight if they are interpreted prematurely. Not until the ego is stable enough for the appropriate interpretations, are these admissible and therapeutically effective. They promote transference to a higher degree than the early direct interpretations proclaimed by Rosen (1968) or Rosenfeld (1954) among others.

These remarks concerning setting, dreams, and interpretations have the purpose of pointing out the changes in technique in a number of cases that have already resulted in a clear improvement of transference. They illustrate the difference between modern therapeutic efforts and those of the 1950s, as they have been made by us as well as by published reports by other therapists. The early efforts were characterized by grotesque experiments that now seem ridiculous to many younger therapists, such as granting oral wishes that had remained unfulfilled by means of apples and balloons. In retrospect one is struck not only by the grotesque element which includes my early wrestling matches or my feeding a patient his favorite dish, but also by the rigidity and narrowness of the theory. My wrestling was meant as a controlled release of aggression acted out on the therapist. The apples of Sechehaye (1955) represented the late satisfaction of oral wishes. And Rosen's grabbing at his patient's penis was motivated by his hope to thus reduce the patient's fear of castration (cit. Matussek 1959).

This demonstrates that all of us were searching for the technique that would be the best possible for schizophrenics just as the traditional techniques seemed to be for neurotics. In doing so, those of us whose papers were published, however, adhered to Freud's theory of libido in principle. Concepts such as the id, the superego, repression and splitting-off, displacement and condensation, and projection and introjection were the fundamental principles that made us feel safe under the protective roof of psychoanalysis in spite of the subjective variations in technique.

Today the psychoanalytical work with schizophrenics has by no means decreased in volume but it has become less noisy and is no longer bombastically stylized. On the contrary: It is growing within the framework of the old classical theory. If one interprets the earlier efforts within the framework of the modern theories of narcissism, the "successes" attributed to the pioneers can be better understood.

Let us say this for our own cases from the 1950s: My successful treatment of patients was largely due to my misinterpretations, for I owe the actual reason for positive transference and the successes involved to the fact that I did not understand and therefore could not interpret the actual reason for positive transference. I adhered to common psychoanalytical clichés. Consequently I could neither recognize nor interpret the actual reason for the establishment of transference, namely a contribution to the stabilization of the patient's damaged narcissism. In the 1950s I and many of my colleagues were at a loss for the correct concept, which proved to be an unexpected stroke of luck in the cases I successfully treated. My interpretation could not concentrate on the one point which, according to recent experience, must remain silent. What we call narcissistic need today was then termed the need for dependence. We believed then that it, too, had to be interpreted. The recovery depended, as Searles (1956) crassly put it, upon the insight into this need for dependence.

Today we tend to formulate the other way around: In the interest of the establishment and preservation of a positive transference, the need for dependence must not be interpreted during the psychotic processes. It must remain silent. Only in this manner can the ever-present impulse toward a positive transference be activated for recovery.

The basic concept behind this idea can be summed up as follows: The traditional structural doctrine of schizophrenia lends itself less to the formulation of therapeutic principles than does the modern theory of narcissism. The damaged self-structure of the schizophrenic causes the patient to experience the therapeutic situation initially as a trial situation. He feels pushed into it and reacts with fear, distrustful tension, rejection, and delusory interpretation of the situation, in short, with schizophrenic dysphoria. This is the stage that I used to call the stage of labile transference. Here the therapist must correctly understand the situation, and his conduct must contribute towards the development of the labile transference into a positive one. If the therapist's conduct is ill-advised or if he acts in the sense of a therapy of neuroses, he contributes to the patient's insecurity and, at the same time, deepens the negative transference. It is therefore necessary to form a clear picture of the tendency to transference and to counteract it purposefully, e.g., by adjusting to the patient's sociableness which varies with the individual and is still preserved. The therapist must casually mobilize the remainders of emotionality, which occasionally means taking over the conversation, avoiding moments of silence, and not insisting on unpleasant themes. In other words, he must avoid everything that might provoke a negative transference.

A negative transference is changed into a positive one when the patient realizes the narcissistically stabilizing function of this relationship with the therapist. Subsequently the patient courts the therapist, so to speak. He strives to present himself in his positive aspects and values and to identify with the therapist whom he has positively experienced and idealized. He makes the therapist his self-object, thus initiating a maneuver toward the stabilization of the narcissistic balance. The empathic and encouraging attitude toward this process of transference is the principal therapeutic factor in the psychotherapy of psychoses. It practical, needs no verbalization, and does not hinder "analysis." It rather creates or improves the basis for it. It is a matter of making up for the process of consolidation of the self, denied the patient in his childhood, which exerts a liberating influence upon his social contacts and activities outside of therapy. There he initiates a similar process. The analysis of negative reactions to transference can only be conducted on the basis of a firmly established positive relationship of transference as, otherwise, offers of interpretation fall victim to negative transference which is experienced as lack of understanding, aggression, hurt feelings, and so forth. This structural factor in the patient can generally be best treated with the aid of findings from outside the therapeutic situation.

Mistaking an erotically tinted positive narcissistic transference for a sexual – especially oedipal one – is a marked danger frequently facing beginners. Doing so as well as an interpretation in this sense or an acceptance of the erotic offer will inevitably lead to narcissistic crises. One refuses narcissistic mirroring and creates the trial situation which the patient is afraid of, as mentioned earlier. From this point of view, the lack of transference becomes understandable. It is a form of negative transference consisting of an unconscious lack of motivation to establish contact with the therapist. This lack becomes most noticeable in the patient's indifference even when he regularly participates in the therapeutic sessions. The one essential difference between previous attempts at analytical therapy with schizophrenics and our present experience can be summarized as follows: The gist of psychosis psychotherapy is neither instinct gratification (Sechehaye 1955), nor encounter discussion, nor for that matter symptom or dream interpretation. Also the transference is not a technique-imposed transference neurosis, or transference psychosis (Rosenfeld 1952), for which regression is a necessary prerequisite. On the contrary: The schizophrenic, who finds himself in a rather more or less marked regressive state, has to be led out of the regressive position via transference so that he can open himself up to the outside world. In other words, the schizophrenic needs less insight at the beginning; rather he needs a structure to be created via the transference, whose secondary effect is to facilitate such insight.

To conclude: This brief sketch cannot contain more than glimpses at the differences in technique between the psychoanalysis of neuroses and that of schizophrenics as practiced during the past 3 decades. Given an abundance of hypotheses, I was forced to dispense with the necessary empirical evidence that would support our point of view. We hope to submit it in a few years. We will attempt to demonstrate the connection between manifested defects in the self experienced in childhood and the family constellation, and to present the course of the illness as dependent upon them. Finally, succesful or unsuccessful therapeutic efforts are to be shown in their dependence on the factors mentioned. We hope to arrive thus at the necessary verification or disproof of our tentative hypotheses.

References

Bateson G, Jackson DD, Haley J, Weakland J (1956) Toward a theory of schizophrenia. Behav Sci 1:251–264

Benedetti G (1955) Möglichkeiten und Grenzen der Psychotherapie Schizophrener. Bull Schweiz Akad Med Wiss 11, Fasc 1/2:142–159

Bowen M (1960) A family concept of schizophrenia. In: Jackson DD (ed) The etiology of schizophrenia. Basic Books, New York

Boyer LB (1961) Provisional evaluation of psycho-analysis with few parameters employed in the treatment of schizophrenia. Int J Psychoanal 42:386–403

Freud S (1933) Neue Folge der Vorlesungen zur Einführung in die Psychoanalyse. G.W., Bd. XV.

Fromm-Reichmann F (1939) Transference problems in schizophrenia. Psychoanal Q 8:412–426

Fromm-Reichmann F (1942) A preliminary note on the emotional significance of stereotypies in schizophrenics. Bull Forest Sanatarium 1:17–21

Fromm-Reichmann F (1948) Notes on the development of treatment of schizophrenics by psychoanalytic psychotherapy. Psychiatry 11:263

Fromm-Reichmann F (1952) Some aspects of psychoanalytic psychotherapy with schizophrenics. In: Brody EB, Redlich FC (eds) Psychotherapy with schizophrenics. International University Press, New York

Fromm-Reichmann F (1953) Principles of intensive psychotherapy. George Allen and Unwin, London

Heimann P (1957) A combination of defence mechanisms in paranoid states. In: Klein M, Heimann P, Money-Kyrle RE (eds) New directions in psycho-analysis. Basic Books, New York

Lidz RW, Lidz T (1952) Therapeutic considerations arising from the intense symbiotic needs of schizophrenic patients. In: Brody EB, Redlich FC (eds) Psychotherapy with schizophrenics. International University Press, New York

Lidz T (1959) Schizophrenie und Familie. Psyche 13:257–268

Lidz T, Fleck S (1960) Schizophrenia, human integration, and the role of the family. In: Jackson DD (ed) The etiology of schizophrenia. Basic Books, New York

Matussek P (1959) Psychotherapie bei Schizophrenen. In: Frankl VE, v. Gebsattel VE, Schultz JH (eds), Handbuch der Neurosenlehre und Psychotherapie, vol IV, pp 385–417. Urban und Schwarzenberg, München Berlin

Matussek P, Triebel A (1974) Die Wirksamkeit der Psychotherapie bei 44 Schizophrenen. Nervenarzt 45:569–575

Matussek P (1976) Psychotherapie schizophrener Psychosen. Reader. Hoffmann und Campe, Hamburg

Matussek P, Triebel A (1980) Die Ausgangssituation des Schizophrenen als Ansatz zur Psychotherapie. Hexagon Roche 8:18–24

Rosen JN (1964) Psychotherapie der Psychosen. Hippokrates, Stuttgart

Rosen JN (1968) Direct Psychoanalysis. Grune and Stratton, New York

Rosenfeld H (1950) Note on the psychopathology of confusional state in chronic schizophrenia. Int J Psychoanal 31:132–137

Rosenfeld H (1952) Notes on the psychoanalysis of the superego conflict on an acute schizophrenic patient. Int J Psychoanal 33:111–131

Rosenfeld H (1952a) Transference-phenomena and transference-analysis in an acute catatonic schizophrenic patient. Int J Psychoanal 33:457–464

Rosenfeld H (1954) Considerations regarding the psycho-analytic approach to acute and chronic schizophrenia. Int J Psychoanal 35:135–140

Searles HF (1956) Die Verlaufsformen der Abhängigkeit in der Psychotherapie von Schizophrenen. Psyche 10:448–481

Searles HF (1960) The nonhuman environment in normal development and in schizophrenia. International University Press, New York

Searles HF (1961) Phases of patient-therapist interaction in the psychotherapy of chronic schizophrenia. Brit J Med Psychol 34:169–193

Sechehaye MA (1955) Die symbolische Wunscherfüllung. Huber, Stuttgart

Sechehaye MA (1961) Introduction. In: Burton A (ed) Psychotherapy of the Psychoses. Basic Books, New York

Sullivan HS (1924) Schizophrenia conservative and malignant features. Am J Psychiatry 81:77–91

Sullivan HS (1927) Affective experience in early schizophrenia. Am J Psychiatry 6:467–483

Sullivan HS (1947) Therapeutic investigations in schizophrenia. Psychiatry 10:121–125

Therapists Who Treat Schizophrenic Patients: Characterization

James P. Frosch, John G. Gunderson, Roger Weiss, and Arlene Frank

Introduction

This is the first in a series of reports on a project designed to characterize the theoretical orientation and relevant personality variables of two groups of psychotherapists who are participating in a study of the effects of psychotherapy on schizophrenia. We believe that such characterization is critical in interpreting the results of outcome studies, and that prior studies have been hampered by inadequate analysis of who the therapists were and what they believed. This has been true both in the studies of the efficacy of psychotherapy with schizophrenic patients, and in more general studies of psychotherapy. Only by developing valid, reliable instruments to describe the therapists' theoretical model of treatment and to isolate important personality variables can the researcher speak with confidence about the nature of the treatment administered and the factors that influenced outcome.

Of the previous attempts to characterize therapists who worked well with schizophrenic people, (Whitehorn and Betz 1954; Shader 1971; Rogers 1967; Mosher 1973), only two studies seemed promising enough to incorporate into our study. The first is that of Karon and VandenBos. Starting with the hypothesis that therapists who consciously or unconsciously utilize dependent individuals to satisfy their own personal needs would have poor results in their work with schizophrenic patients, Karon developed a measure of this quality, which he termed "maternal pathogenesis" (VandenBos and Karon 1971). He scored the TATs of ten inexperienced therapists and found that the presence of this characteristic did correlate with negative outcome. This is a promising finding, but, pending further confirmation, the small number of therapists in the study makes it difficult to evaluate its significance.

The second study we relied on was that of Gunderson and Feinsilver. They developed a rating scale consisting of ten dimensions assessing certain characteristics of therapists working with schizophrenic patients (Gunderson 1978). In Gunderson's initial study the qualities most predictive of positive outcome boiled down to the therapist's comfort with strong affect, his composure in the face of strong feelings, both his own and the patient's. In practice this was an attempt to rate systematically how well therapists had resolved for themselves the issues with which schizophrenic patients inevitably struggle. Figure 1 contains a list of these traits. However, this procedure was not part of a controlled, prospective study and has been included more systematically in the current research reported here.

In addition to personality traits, we have been interested in studying the impact of the theoretical model the therapist uses in psychotherapy. Some have questioned whether it matters what therapists think they are doing. Gomes-Schwartz, in her extensive 1978 review of the psychotherapy outcome literature, concluded about this issue: "It remains to be demonstrated that what the therapist does has an impact over and above the effects of a supportive relationship (which therapists of varying orientations may be capable of providing)" (Gomes-Schwartz 1978). On the other hand, many experienced therapists believe, although it has not been proven, that whatever the contribution of nonspecific factors common to any therapeutic relationship, these alone are insufficient to effect deep and lasting change. They contend that while warmth and acceptance may be the necessary underpinning for establishing therapeutic atmosphere, specific approaches based on theories of etiology and treatment have a greater effect.

In designing our study the hypothesis was that both specific and nonspecific factors are important and must be considered in interpreting the results when a given therapist is at work. Both the theoretical approach and the personality of the therapist may well influence the outcome of treatment, and, furthermore, there may be an interplay between these two variables. However, an additional possibility is that having a theory is more important than which theory it happens to be. A theory of treatment provides a framework with which to organize the intellectually confusing and emotionally overwhelming data of therapy sessions. Ultimately the patient too is helped because he is given a framework with which he can better understand himself and his behavior. This reduces the chaos of the schizophrenic person's experience of the internal and external worlds. If this hypothesis is true, positive results would correlate with the degree to which a therapist was theoretically minded, regardless of the specific content of the theory.

The aim of this project, then, was to characterize two groups of therapists participating in a larger outcome study in the following respects: first, their ideas about schizophrenia and its treatment; second, relevant personality factors, such as those previously studied by Gunderson and Karon; and third, the degree to which they were theoretically minded. In later reports we will focus on the relationship between these factors and therapist behavior as recorded in transcripts of taped sessions, and the relationship to overall outcome.

Methods

The subjects of this study are two groups of psychotherapists who are participating in the Psychotherapy Outcome Study at McLean Hospital. In this study two distinct types of psychotherapy are being compared while other factors, such as medication and milieu, are controlled. One type is called EIO, exploratory intensive psychotherapy (EIO), in which the patient and therapist meet at least three times weekly with the aim of increasing the patient's knowledge of himself and why he became psychotic. The other type, RAS, is restorative supportive psychotherapy, with a maximum frequency of 1 h/week and a goal of restoring the patient quickly to his premorbid level of functioning, and helping him maintain it. Both groups of psychotherapists are experienced in treating schizophrenic patients and believe that their modality is the treatment of choice. The EIO therapists have had a minimum of 3 years experience working intensively with

Table 1. Demographic data

	EIO	RAS
Number	22	15
Age	46	41
Years experience	15	11
Sex	15 M/5 F	15 M/0 F
Personal analysis	20	2
Analyst	10	0

Table 2. Areas covered by questionnaire

Theory of the problem of schizophrenia	Q1	Defense vs defect
	Q2	Reversibility vs irreversibility
	Q3	Etiology: developmental vs hereditary
	Q4	Reconstruction – is it a necessary part of treatment
Technique in therapy	Q5	Transference
	Q6	Structure of session
	Q7	Self-revelation of therapist
	Q8	Gratification of patients' wishes
	Q9	Patient/therapist match
Mechanism of change	Q10	Medication
	Q11	Regression – is it necessary?
	Q12	Mechanism of change

schizophrenic patients, and they must have treated a schizophrenic patient who greatly improved over the course of the psychotherapy. Table 1 compares the mean age, number of years experience, sex, number of therapists who have had personal analyses, and the number who are psychoanalysts themselves in each group. In the study a variety of outcome measures are used to assess both functioning and growth of self-awareness, and the follow-up raters are blind to the type of therapy employed. The patients are schizophrenics with minimal prior psychotherapy who are randomly assigned to one of the modalities after acceptance into the study. A number of diagnostic criteria were used, including the World Health Organization criteria, and the clinical impression of the admitting psychiatrists initially based on DSM-II and subsequently on DSM-III. This was not a chronic population, since one requirement for inclusion in the study was that the person had functioned well (i.e., job, school, etc.) for at least 4 months in the prior 2 years.

The initial step in characterizing these therapists was to write a questionnaire aimed at eliciting their opinion in 13 areas of theoretical importance and controversy in the psychotherapy of schizophrenia. These variables were selected from the literature and from previous surveys of differing approaches among those therapists who specialized in the treatment of schizophrenic patients (Gunderson 1973). The first set of questions (Q1–Q3) (see Table 2) concern the therapist's formulation about the nature of the psychopathology in schizophrenia, its etiology, and reversibility. The second set of questions (Q4–Q9) concern specifics of technique with schizophrenic patients, while the final set (Q10–Q12) concerns the therapist's beliefs about the mechanism of therapeutic change and the relative importance of ancillary modalities, such as medication and milieu. Each therapist was asked to rate himself on a seven-point scale with the one, four, and seven positions anchored. The one and seven positions represented extreme points of view. In general, low ratings indicate adherence to a strict psychoanalytic approach, while high ratings indicate a supportive, maintenance approach. Twenty-two (22) EIO and fifteen (15) RAS therapists filled out the questionnaire.

We developed this method of characterizing the therapist's theoretical beliefs by conducting semistructured interviews with therapists who were not participating in the study. Initially two research psychiatrists (John Gunderson and James Frosch) were present and both rated the therapist's responses. This allowed us to develop reliability and to refine some of the variables, but it also became clear that some therapists would be anxious in the interview situation or needed more time to consider the issues fully. Because of these considerations it seemed preferable to give the questionnaire directly to the therapist before an interview with one researcher (James Frosch), during which he was encouraged to elaborate on his responses. This interview was taped, and another researcher (Roger Weiss) listened to the interview and independently rated it. A *t*-test revealed no significant differences between the therapist's self-rating and the ratings of the two researchers. Furthermore, the independent ratings of the two researchers were within one (1) point of each other 88% of the time. This indicated that the therapists rated themselves in the same way another knowledgeable person listening to them would, and that the therapist self-ratings had at least the validity of external ratings.

In addition, each of the two researchers rated the therapist for "theoretical mindedness." This quality was defined as the extent to which the therapist's work with patients was informed by a clear and coherent theory of etiology and treatment. For these ratings a consensus was used between the two researchers (James Frosch and Roger Weiss). The therapists were also rated on the Gunderson-Feinsilver scale by two researchers familiar with their work (John Gunderson and James Frosch). If in these ratings there were differences of more than one point on a five-point scale, a consensus was used; otherwise the simple mean score was used. It was necessary to use a consensus score in only 16% of the ratings. Finally, in order to test Karon's hypothesis about maternal pathogenesis, each therapist was given a self-administered, anonymous TAT test.

As part of the Psychotherapy Outcome Study a group of seven clinicians meets to review and rate transcripts of therapy sessions. Each researcher independently rates the sessions on a variety of scales, some descriptive and some evaluative. The group rates three successive sessions occurring at 6-month intervals in the psychotherapy. Where there are disagreements between any two raters of two or more points on a ten-point scale, the rating is discussed by the group and a consensus arrived at. In this report we have correlated a few of the areas surveyed in the questionnaire with ratings of similar qualities by the process group.

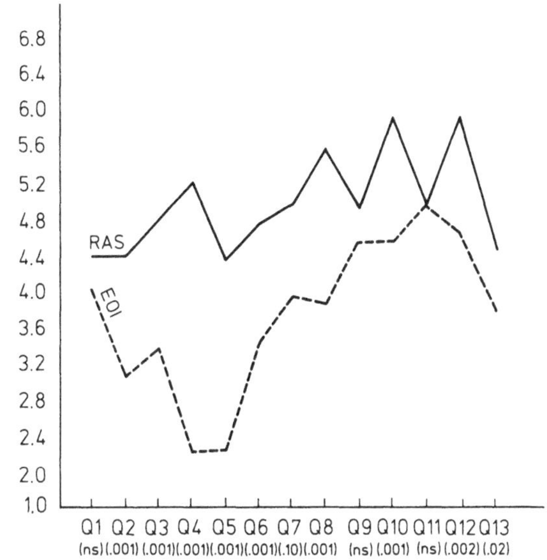

Fig. 1. Theoretical orientation: mean scores of EIO and RAS therapists

Results

Figure 1 compares the mean responses of the EIO and RAS groups as a whole. In all except three areas the differences are significant and in the expected direction. That is, the RAS therapists viewed schizophrenia as an illness with a hereditary component resulting in ego deficits. They advocated a therapeutic approach incorporating major modifications of psychoanalytic principles in keeping with this view. Generally it was an approach stressing the real relationship as opposed to transference, the present as opposed to the past, and a structured session as opposed to free association. They also found self-revelation of the therapist and, at times, direct advice, useful, and they relied heavily on ancillary treatments such as medication and milieu. These responses are not surprising; in the United States they have come to represent the conventional wisdom about schizophrenia and its treatment. The EIO therapists agree that ego deficits are present, but place more stress on developmental than hereditary factors, and are more optimistic about the efficacy of a psychoanalytic approach. They believe that transference occurs and is workable in the therapy of schizophrenic people, and that the patient's understanding and appreciation of his own past is crucial. They described themselves as less active within the session, tending to follow the patient's lead, and were somewhat more reluctant to reveal their own feelings and personal data about their lives, although most felt that there was a place for this in the treatment of schizophrenic people. They agreed that medication and milieu were useful, though they were less convinced than the RAS group about the benefits of medication. It is interesting that both groups believed in the presence of nearly equal components of defense and defects, thought the personality match between therapist and patient is important, and neither group believed therapeutic regression was necessary or useful. The greatest differences between the two groups were on the issues of trans-

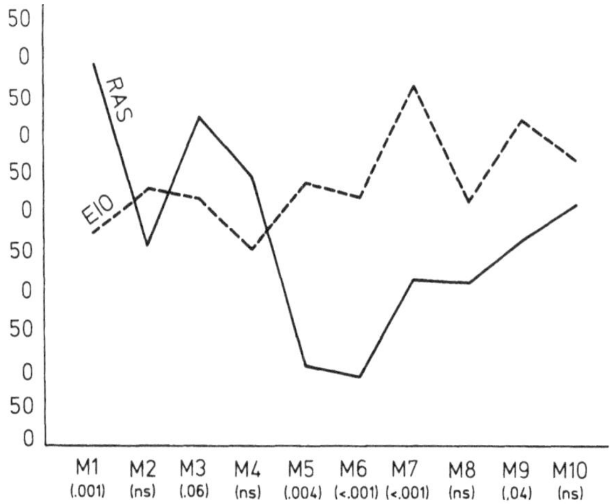

Fig. 2. Personality variables: mean scores of EIO and RAS therapists

ference and the importance of an in-depth understanding of the past. These two issues polarized the groups, with the EIO group strongly advocating the importance and possibility of transference work with schizophrenics and an understanding of the past. It is important to notice the absolute scores as well as the relative differences between the two groups. The overall EIO profile reveals a moderate group of therapists, with few scores in the low range.

Figure 2 compares the ratings on the Gunderson-Feinsilver dimensions for the two groups. The RAS therapists were more active; they were "doers." On the other hand, the EIO group scored higher on comfort with patient seductiveness, comfort with depression, and composure. They were also gentler. The two groups were not significantly different on comfort with aggression, optimism, comfort with dependency, and externalization. In Gunderson's previous study the four dimensions having to do with comfort in the presence of affects (M2, M7, M6, M10) were the best predictors of positive outcome. In this study the EIO group scored higher on comfort with patient's seductiveness and depression, but not on comfort with aggression and dependency.

In order to investigate the interplay between the two sets of variables we looked at the intercorrelation between the responses to the questionnaire and the ratings of personality. In other words, the question was: "Did particular personality traits match with certain theoretical approaches?" There were a number of statistically significant correlations, some of which were predictable and others quite difficult to explain. For RAS therapists the characteristic of activity correlated with a theory stressing the presence of defects, a hereditary cause, an emphasis on the present, self-revelation, gratification, the use of medication and a belief that regression is counterproductive. This makes sense: those RAS therapists who are active people actively embrace non-analytic techniques stressing support rather than exploration. For the EIO group activity as a personality trait correlated with a belief in the existence and workability of transference with schizophrenic patients. This means that EIO therapists who are active people actively embrace an analytic framework. For EIO therapists gentleness, grandfatherliness, and composure correlated with a belief in more supportive techniques such as medication, self-revelation, gratification, and a stress on the real relationship.

For the EIO group the personality characteristic of therapists who were judged to be the most and least theoretically minded were compared. The most significant difference was that therapists who articulated a clear and coherent theory were more composed and more comfortable with patient seductiveness.

Because the Psychotherapy Outcome Study is still in progress, we cannot at this point correlate the above findings with outcome. We have begun to examine the ratings of the process transcripts and would like to present a few impressions based on the ratings of the process group. First of all, although nearly all EIO therapists profess to be interested in the past, most emphasize the present in their actual work with patients. Second, few EIO therapists emphasized exploration of the transference, whatever their theoretical belief about the issue. The third impression, a somewhat disheartening one, is that process ratings of overall skill are not consistently correlated with theoretical mindedness.

Discussion

The emergence of two distinct profiles on the survey of theoretical approach supports the validity of the Outcome Study design as a test of two distinct types of psychotherapy. The EIO therapists, as might be predicted, put more stress on psychological aspects of etiology and treatment. However, combining all the results, this group may be characterized as somewhat passive in style and moderate in beliefs. They tended to be rather supportive, both in personality and in their reliance on ancillary measures, such as medication. This approach differs from those advocated by, for example, Searles (1965) or Semrad (1969). Searles emphasized the importance of reviving a regressive, symbiotic relationship in the transference, while Semrad saw psychotic symptoms as defense against intolerable affect. The McLean EIO group had few therapists strongly identified with these views. This may result from a tradition at the hospital stressing cognitive and social approaches to the schizophrenic patient. This will be important in interpreting the results of the study, since it represents a different brand of intensive psychotherapy than one might find in a sample of therapists from, for example, Chestnut Lodge. While this EIO group strongly believed in analyzing transference and a focus on the past, transcripts of actual sessions indicate that they are not very active in pursuit of these issues.

The fact that the more theoretically minded EIO therapists were more composed and comfortable with affect lends support to the hypothesis that a firm theory may provide some peace of mind on the firing line. Unfortunately, the suggestion that this does not seem to correlate with ratings of overall skill indicates that, while the therapist may feel more composed, he is not necessarily more effective. In fact, the impressions about the lack of exploration of transference and the past raises the possibility, so often suggested previously in the literature, that there is not a clear relationship between theory and practice.

In future communications we will report more extensively on correlations with process and outcome data, as well as with the TAT responses of the therapists. In addition we will discuss more extensively some of the methodological difficulties in research on the therapist variable.

References

Buckley P, Karusu TB, Charles E, Stein SP (1979) Theory and practice in psychotherapy, some contradictions in expressed belief and reported practice. J Nervous and Mental Disease 167(4): 218–223

Glover E (1955) Common technical practices: Questionnaire research in the technique of psychoanalysis. International University Press, New York

Gomes-Schwartz B, Hadley SW, Strupp HH (1978) Individual psychotherapy and behavior therapy. Ann Rev Psychology 29:435–471

Gunderson JG (1973) Controversies about the psychotherapy of schizophrenia. Am J Psychiatry 130:677–681

Gunderson JG (1978) Patient-therapy matching: A research evaluation. Am J Psychiatry 135: 1193–1197

Mosher LR, Reifman A, Menn A (1973) Characteristics of non-professionals serving as primary therapists for acute schizophrenics. Hospital and Community Psychiatry 24(6):391–396

Razin AM (1971) A-B variable in psychotherapy: A critical review. Psychol Bull 75(1):1–21

Rogers CR (1967) The therapeutic relationship and its impact: A study of psychotherapy with schizophrenics. University of Wisconsin

Searles HF (1965) Collected papers on schizophrenia and related subjects. Int University Press

Semrad EV, Van Buskirk D (1969) Teaching psychotherapy of psychotic patients. Grune and Stratton, New York

Shader RI, Grinspoon L, Harmatz JS, Ewalt JR (1971) The therapist variable. Am J Psychiatry 127:1009–1012

Sloan RB (1975) Psychotherapy vs. behavior therapy. Harvard University Press, Cambridge

Strupp HH (1958) The performance of psychiatrists and psychologists in therapeutic interviews. J Clin Psychology 14:219–226

Van den Bos GR, Karon BP (1971) Pathogenesis: A new therapist personality dimension related to therapeutic effectiveness. J Personality Assessment 35:252–260

Whitehorn JC, Betz BJ (1954) A study of psychotherapeutic relationships between physicians and schizophrenic patients. Am J Psychiatry 111:321–331

IV. Family Therapy

Introduction

The beginnings of family therapy in the decade following World War II interwove with new attempts to understand and possibly treat schizophrenia. Pioneering researchers and therapists, such as Gregory Bateson and the Palo Alto group, Ted Lidz, Lyman Wynne, Murray Bowen, and their teams, began to study the family of the schizophrenic patient. As a result, they came to challenge traditional medical as well as psychoanalytic notions concerning schizophrenia. Freud, for example, in assessing the treatment possibilities for such patients, had written in 1917: "... they give no evidence of transference and are therefore beyond the scope of our efforts, incurable from our point of view." Within this new approach such assessment appeared rather a consequence of restricting observations and concepts that filtered out those powerful relational forces that operate within the schizophrenic's family which subdued any individual member's transference, as it were. In fact, probably no other psychiatric research and treatment endeavor has alerted us so much to how differing basic premises and differing observational tools entail differing therapeutic perspectives and strategies.

This may, therefore, be seen as the main lesson the chapters of this section could offer: Each author treats, in his or her own way, the therapeutic implications of a family view or a systems view of schizophrenic dynamics. The positions differ also as to the desirability and feasibility of integrating individual-centered (primarily psychoanalytic) and family-centered (or systems) approaches. Whereas Christian Müller speaks as an advocate of such integration, Mara Selvini and Giuliana Prata make claims for the "curing power" of a pure systems approach – and back such claims with impressive data from their innovative work. Helm Stierlin reflects on the need for therapeutic approaches which may mobilize, in each family member, motivations to individuate while they take account of, and even try to utilize, the formidable systems forces which so far have blocked any such individuation. Paul Watzlawick examines how certain basic premises and preconceptions may not only block attempts to "cure" schizophrenics but also may have fundamentally shaped (and restricted) our notions as to what "cure" is or should be. Norman Paul shows how the chronic schizophrenic disturbance of one family member and a whole family's misery and blocking of communication may be due, in major part, to several generations' collective denial and collective avoidance of grief work in the context of one member's early and tragic death. Carol Anderson reports on psychoeducational approaches to schizophrenics and their families which have been tried and studied during the recent past in various parts of the English-speaking world. Finally, this section reproduces a major part of the discussion held at the panel on Family Therapy during the 7th International Symposium on the Psychotherapy of

Schizophrenia. This discussion, in particular, may convey some of the excitement, the promise, but also the as yet unanswered questions and the controversies which presently revolve around the family therapy of schizophrenia.

Helm Stierlin

The Schizophrenic and His Family

Christian Müller

Each of us has his own opinion of what schizophrenia is or is not. This term, coined by Eugen Bleuler (1912) and which has replaced the even more shocking *dementia praecox*, awakens in each of us, according to his experience, his level of knowledge, and his profession, associations which turn on mental alienation, derangement, and insanity, but also loss of a sense of reality, paralogical thinking, and autism (Bleuler 1911). Schizophrenic existence is a dramatic distortion, misfortune, and loss, and words such as benightedness may justifiably be used to describe such an existence.

What about the schizophrenic's family? Is it possible that this word has the same significance for each one of us or would it not be more pertinent to inquire whether, depending on our background, knowledge, and activity, a wide variety of conceptions revolves around this word? One is tempted here to digress and speak of the history of the notion of family and the changes time has wrought on it. Briefly, for centuries the family has been, on the one hand, fact and reality and, on the other, ideal and wish dream. It is no mere coincidence that the Holy Family is constantly illustrated in forms sometimes approaching sugarcoated kitsch. More than a hundred years ago, a natural history of the people was published in Stuttgart to serve as the basis for a German social policy. In the volume devoted to the family, Riehl, the author, outlined (1862) the family as he believed it would be in the twentieth century. He wrote as follows:

The whole family will stick together; cousins will drop in frequently and find a cordial welcome. The family feast days will once more be red-letter days, being celebrated more cheerfully than a hundred years ago. Grandfather, in his attic, will be at special pains to bring to light once more the old German customs, to adapt them if necessary to 20th century requirements and, in his capacity as head of the house, to ensure their observance.

Today we are amused by such touching ingenuousness whose keyword is intimacy. But does not this intimate family idyll still haunt many of our contemporaries? And we must go on to ask if this discrepancy between dream and reality does not cause suffering precisely in the case of the schizophrenic. There is a great deal of evidence to the effect that the families of schizophrenics adhere to a perverted form of family intimacy.

We have acquired considerable knowledge of psychic sickness, particularly of the psychoses, the paths that led to this knowledge were paved with renunciation. We were forced to renounce the dream of the intimate family. The vast process of demystification brought about by psychoanalysis stopped neither at schizophrenia nor at the basic structure of the family. On the territory, to quote Freud, recovered from popular superstition and mystic a new form of humanism was to be created. No less a person than Thomas Mann (1936) spoke prophetically on Freud's 80th birthday of a humanism that would stand in a bolder, freer, more cheerful, and artistically maturer relation to the powers of the underworld, the subconscious, and the id than had been granted an earlier humanity travailing admist neurotic fears and all the hate these engendered. And at the end of his speech he said:

The discernment psychoanalysis has achieved will revolutionize the world. It has brought a degree of cheerful mistrust, an unmasking suspicion in regard to the secretiveness and general carryings-on of the soul which, once awakened, will never disappear. It infiltrates all of life, undermining primitive ingenuousness, abolishing the pathos of uncertainty, bringing about its "depatheticizing" by encouraging a taste for understatement and cultivation of a more subdued mode of speech which seeks its strength in moderation.

There is no doubt that the family today is having to face revealing mistrust which, once aroused, can never be completely banished. The dream of the intimate family has come to an end. And if interest in many countries has become focused on research into family life it cannot be denied that a certain element of nostalgia plays a role here. The more liberated attitude towards the family that we adopt today allows us to consider more frankly the relation between schizophrenics and their families.

What does it mean, therefore, to have dealings with the schizophrenic and his family, rather than being a mere bystander, to play a central role, to be drawn into the whirlpool of events? And what about our own well-nigh schizophrenic past? I once proved in a brief study that 25% – *one quarter* – of all specialists in psychiatry have one or more schizophrenics in their immediate family, that is among father and mother, uncles, aunts, brothers, and sisters. This is a point that must be borne in mind when we venture into the difficult territory of trying to understand and treat this condition. *Mea res agitur*. The schizophrenic is not the "totally different one." He is one who has gone farther than we have in his encounter with nothingness or, better, with non-existence. Shakespeare said (Macbeth I, 3):

Present fears are less than horrible imaginings:
My thought, whose murder yet is but fantastical,
Shakes so my single state of man, that function
Is smother'd in surmise; and nothing is
But what is not.

And Racamier (1980), a psychiatrist who devoted his life to understanding and treating the schizophrenic, said:

The schizophrenic has paradoxical solutions in regard to the relation between the object and himself: object, subject and relationship exist only in so far as they be non-existent. If they exist it is only in as much as they do not exist. If they are non-existent, then they exist. The schizophrenic cannot escape from this unsolvable paradox and in one's dealings with him, one does not have the impression that there is a way out. He must be non-existent in order to exist.

And, finally, let me quote to you what a patient said (Finzen 1974). This schizophrenic writes as follows within the context of a self-analysis:

We must not forget that everyone is prone to inward-outward personality splits and none of us knows when the hour will come to lose control of mind and consequently also of thinking and action. The mentally sick person exists in an inner hell where he is deprived of freedom of spirit, his mind lies under a fateful enchantment and freedom is totally excluded. Inside this person whole films – complete with sound-

track – are projected. In the course of the years the sufferer experiences the entire history of the world, becomes acquainted with the life of the gods, thus penetrating the possibility and reality of primordial conditions, pre-history and the origins of God, while himself becoming non-existent. Inside himself the sufferer is led into hell by means of fearful spectacles, mystical signs and occult experiences.

So – to be or not to be – the struggle for survival against a background of enraptured playing with grandiose imaginings, a yielding to the narcissistic seduction into a galaxy where the traveller is all-powerful. Not infrequently the therapist will find himself acting out the part of Daedalus holding back his son from flight into the allconsuming fire of the sun, warning him against his all-or-nothing attitude – Daedalus who knows the melting point of wax and who attempts to moderate his son's passion and keep it within limits. For it is in this limitlessness that the schizophrenic differs from other people. The limited object represents for him a danger and a threat; he will try to avoid it in order not to be at its mercy and, for this reason, he will at first also see the therapist as an enemy – he who desires to throw him back, tie him down, and restrict him – not to say, throw him into the melting pot and soak him up.

On first acquaintance the therapist is not, in the eyes of the schizophrenic, an understanding partner. Rather, he is someone lacking credibility who is trying to draw the patient into a world that, for him, does not exist in the first place, and must not be allowed to exist in the second. Once, in total despair, I cried out to a patient I had been treating for years: "Wake up from your dream, look around you – the world is not a bit as you think it is!" And his answer, the answer of a simple, unschooled laborer, given in a tone of deep sadness, was: "If I waken, I shall be dead." It was then that I discovered for the first time the paradox of which Racamier spoke – the nonexisting in order to exist. To repeat the words of Shakespeare, that, in the end, "... nothing is but what is not." Patient and therapist thus confront each other in mutual helplessness and it is often this state of affairs that initiates their true meeting. The therapist understands the schizophrenic; he *wants* to understand him, but is unable to follow him into his galaxy. The patient, for his part, understands the therapist's intent or, at least, obscurely perceives it, but is unable to approach him more closely. On the contrary, as Searles (1965) has described, the patient sometimes even attempts to draw his therapeutic partner into the realm of madness.

These are just a few fragmentary remarks in regard to the encounter between schizophrenic and therapist in the course of individual treatment. But this is not the main gist of my discourse. Let us now consider the question of the pathologenesis of schizophrenia within the context of the family.

I have already said that it took decades and the influence of Lidz, Wynne, Stierlin, Kaufmann, and others to give shape and clarity to that of which a kind of preperception existed in us – namely the knowledge of the complicated process of interaction among the members of the schizophrenic's family. I have also referred to the old myth of Daedalus and Icarus. It would, however, be quite wrong to assume that events in a schizophrenic family would inevitably take place in accordance with this blueprint. It will seldom occur that a parent will clearly see the increasing eccentricity, isolation, and grandiose-fatal extravagances of a child. Scott (1976) was undoubtedly right when, in 1975, at one of our symposia, he drew attention to the fact that the family diagnoses the trouble long before the doctor. There is no question of finding a coarse lack of sensitivity or of instinctive feeling in schizophrenic families. Scott

(1976) has also described how relations gradually deteriorate and how a relationship loses its meaning long before any intervention on the part of a psychiatrist, and how, only after the intervention, this depersonalized relationship is labeled as a disease. "What should be relationship becomes inner states of disturbance in the patient."

This then leads to the situation described by Scott (1975) as "closure." The die has been cast. He who had once been accepted as a member of the family is no longer regarded in the same light; now he is a patient. And it is here that the doctor plays an eminent role. He confirms; he gives shape to the family's nameless suspicions and initiates the ritual. His is the important function of attenuating the family's massive sense of quilt and this he does in the formulation of his diagnosis. The psychiatrist is frequently summoned not by the patient but by the family. It is not a rare circumstance that the family urges the sufferer to consult a psychiatrist. It thus becomes clear that, whether he wants it or not, the psychiatrist is drawn into the family tragedy right from the start and has his role to play. Woe betide him if he attempts to take up the position of being a servant of the truth, of being a neutral party personifying objectivity. This is, of course, his major aim and one which, to a certain extent, he pursues. But it is beyond doubt that the family will immediately attribute to him the role of judge and witness in one and the same person, the role of participant, conspirator, and the administrator of the secret anxieties, desires, and imaginings that run rife in the family.

The mother-child symbiosis has been mentioned – a mutualism which creates pathological preconditions. Racamier and Conran have both shown that this is an inadequate characterization. I agree with Conran when he says that only two mutually independent beings can enter into a symbiotic relationship to the advantage of both. But the schizophrenic and his mother are not in reality separate beings. Their nondifferentiability is the only salvation from destruction. On the one hand it is a question of incest and, on the other, the fear of destruction. Fears such as these are alive in both mother and child. The maternal imaginings of parthenogenesis correspond to the fantasy of the schizophrenic son of having fathered himself. The only answer to this unsolvable dilemma, this deepest of secrets, is ultimately the "blinding" wrought by psychosis and thus the schizophrenic staggers along his fateful path like the blinded Oedipus. He also appears as blinded to his therapist.

It is therefore no wonder that the schizophrenic experiences his own body as something foreign, against the background of this early disturbed emotional relationship. He experiences it frequently as a machine, as separate from any emotional relation to concrete reality. Racamier shows this clearly in his recently published book on schizophrenia.

If we now accept that the disturbance of the schizophrenic's emotional life, his thinking, and physical sensations derive from experiences undergone during childhood and if we also assume that that which took place in the family before the commencement of his existence as a chronic schizophrenic was a continual repetition, we are forced to ask ourselves how such distorted and life-rejecting anomalies in communication can ever have come about. One hypothesis is that the parents' behavior can be traced back to the disrupted relationship they had with their own parents, the patient's grandparents. I shall not go further into this hypothesis here but should like to consider another aspect. I want to examine the existence in these families of massive repression of both the past and the present. There is no doubt that those members of the family concerned are not conscious of most of these motives. In spite of the convincing systemic and theoretical considerations of someone like Minuchin (1974) or Watzlawick (1968), among others, we are forced to ask how these coded messages, these secret desires and yearnings, these tendencies to narcissistic seduction as described by Racamier, are to be interpreted from the standpoint of the participants' experience. I might add that, here, there appears to be a weak spot in the research on family dynamics in the case of schizophrenics. Of course we know all manner of things concerning the *hic et nunc* of the interreaction among a schizophrenic's relatives from family discussion and through the aid of such modern techniques as video. As I have already pointed out, the examples of behavior we are interested in are not recent ones, but old, ingrained ones – repetitions, in fact. Let me give you an example.

A 40-year-old mother told the therapist in the presence of her 20-year-old son that she had always given him the greatest possible freedom of decision and had never forced him to do anything. However, the therapist noted that, during that same session, she constantly dictated the strictest rules of behavior to her son, doubtless without being aware she was doing it. It is therefore justifiable to assume that the woman was unconscious of her own behavior. In spite of this frequently grotesque disparity between desire and reality, despite the existence of the most massive repressions, these parents do not regard themselves as ill. But what did this father and mother experience when the son who was later to become schizophrenic was a small child? Of this we know very little. Many questions still remain unanswered and it would be reasonable to hope that these young mothers and fathers might give us reports on their own emotional experiences. It is my opinion here that only the psychoanalytical approach can prove successful and that we must never stop hoping that the analyses of parents such as these will ultimately provide confirmation of our hypotheses. It is only on the basis of the most precise knowledge of the parents that we could say with more certainty that the pseudomutuality, the blurring of the generation boundaries as described by Lidz, the handing down of irrational thinking, the double bind, and the disturbance of the thought processes are really originally connected with the early disturbance of communication between parent and child. In other words, I believe that family therapy cannot manage without analytical research, just as the purely individual-based hypotheses concerning the genesis of schizophrenia as described, for example, by Freud (who analyzed the Schreber case) are not adequate. I should therefore simply like to recommend more intensive cooperation between psychoanalytical and systemic-theoretical thinking.

Let us now consider another aspect, namely that of the history of the schizophrenic within a family context. We shall attempt to follow all that happens in a schizophrenic family of this kind in the course of a generation.

First of all, it is necessary to differentiate between what Stierlin calls hard and soft reality. For the latter he has also coined the term "relational reality." Hard reality in a schizophrenic family can undergo change. A member of the family may die, parents may divorce, catastrophe can modify the social field, physical handicaps may affect the integrity of father or mother. There is also another hard reality: In spite of his disturbed emotional life, a schizophrenic is quite capable of building up a social position, of creating for himself a niche in society, just as – as a serious invalid – he can lead a marginal existence either inside or outside a clinic. The soft or relational reality, on the other hand, consists of everything present in the way of invisible links and myths, everything that is "delegated" (to use yet another of Stierlin's terms). All these elements of soft or relational reality care characterized by an obstinate and lifelong persistence, to the great misfortune of all concerned. Someone put it in this lapidary fashion: "Schizophrenics never completely break off family relations."

Thus, when we trace the history of the schizophrenic's family relations over a number of years, from adulthood right back to early childhood, we find a horrendously monotonous constancy in misinterpretation, misunderstanding, and disrupted family dialectics. In schizophrenic families it is possible for a clinch situation to exist for many years – another of Stierlin's terms, borrowed this time from boxing jargon. However, this clinch situation is not necessarily apparent to an outsider. On the contrary, misfortune and suffering are seldom openly discussed. We are acquainted with the pseudoidyll of a well-ordered, "harmonious" life in these families. So long as the schizophrenic and his parents can maintain the dream of undifferentiated and grandiose self-deception there will be no open crisis and a certain degree of stability is guaranteed. We are astonished to learn of families where sons and daughters have lived for years as if no oedipal problem existed at all, of families where mutual blindness reigns, and any genuine attempt at leading an autonomous life is speedily suppressed.

Crises occur and this pseudoequilibrium is shaken when hard, extrafamilial reality reaches such a massive degree of pressure that the carefully established balance collapses and a bottomless chasm opens at the feet of all concerned. The hero worshiped prince or the adored princess proves a failure in everyday life; the aggressive outside world attacks and there is a rude awakening from a sweet family dream. This is one version. The other version of the crisis is that we find ourselves at the end of a struggle lasting for years, a struggle that now reaches beyond the family. The ultimate inhibitions disappear and mutual aggression is given free and open rein, up to and including attempted murder or suicide on the part of one or the other member of the family. The psychiatrist now commences his therapy within the context of a crisis which is becoming progressively more acute.

He appears on the scene and, as I have already indicated, soon finds himself playing the role of mediator. When the person concerned becomes a case, a patient, a new chapter opens in his own life as well as in that of his family. But crisis also signifies hope, for it can frequently be salutary and it is no coincidence that successful therapy often commences when the situation is becoming acutely critical. It is not just a question of a rude awakening from a dream for many of those concerned: things have reached such an impasse that they can no longer be discussed within the family circle since the forces at work are beyond the family's combined abilities to deal with them. Someone now has to intervene in this situation of crisis, and everything that a psychiatric institution has to offer is mobilized during this period. There is a very good reason why I regard intervention during a crisis as the most central, indeed almost exclusive task of the psychiatric institution which cannot and should not at this time deny its medical character. There it will be seen whether it is possible to unblock the clinch situation, whether new patterns of relationship and behavior can be achieved.

What, however, is to be done if the crisis fails to lead to a relaxation of the situation and to new solutions, but proves a vain effort? What if the old, bogged-down positions are merely defended with renewed vigor, that is to say when paralysis is added to metaphoric blindness? At this point, clinically speaking, the disease now approaches chronicity. This signifies quite simply resignation, capitulation, a throwing in of the towel. The all-or-nothing positions become more immovable than ever. The sufferer, who has now irrevocably been labeled as sick, withdraws more and more into regressive spheres; the already meager dialogue dries up entirely. Schindler (1979) has outlined the phases leading up to chronicity and one of the notions he uses is the excellent term, "cocooning." The schizophrenic cocoons himself but processes of cocooning can also be observed in the family. And ultimately the third party, namely the doctor, and the institution and its staff that stands behind and beside him, are drawn into the cocooning process. The contacts and the mutual give and take in the institution – be it of asylum character or an ultramodern therapeutic community – become sparser, more meager, more stereotyped, and diluted. In the end neither side has anything more to say. There is no lack of outward evidence of this cocooning process and numerous studies have been devoted to this subject. Thus, we can demonstrate that it is precisely those chronic schizophrenics who are visited most rarely by their relatives who derive the least pleasure from the attentions of the nursing staff. From the subjective view of the schizophrenic himself, the results of a little study carried out are of significance. If a patient who has spent many years in an institution is asked to write a biographical report, it generally ends at the time the crisis set in, just as if life had ended at that point, as if the subsequent years were no longer life.

It becomes more and more important to create alibis. The sufferer hides behind the alibi of being a victim, that is to say it is not he who has failed but the wicked doctor, the wicked institution, the wicked family, or an, uncomprehending society that has forced him into his role. The alibi of the therapist is that everything has been done that was humanly possible, that one can withdraw to the standpoint of *ultra posse nemo obligatur* and, not least, that here, apparently, unknown biochemical brain processes are at work. But alibis are particularly rife in the family. The disease, medically certified, ultimately sanctions everything including increasing separation from the patient, the lifting of the load of guilt, the let's-keep-out-of-it attitude, the forgetting and burying of all unpleasantness.

This general retreat, which ends tragically enough in the frequently described and condemned institution syndrome, includes all the participants and when, today, so many cheaply furnished crusades are launched against the repressive, infantilizing institution, the contribution of alibis described here must never, ever be forgotten.

Everybody, all of us – the patient, the family, the nurses, the citizens, the State – are seeking an alibi; we need one and must repeatedly and at all costs find one.

You will say that here speaks an old, worn out, disillusioned institutional psychiatrist. I do not, however, regard myself as such. The thing that helps us is the fact that the terrible fate of complete withdrawal is reserved for a minutely small number of people who, at some time in their lives, were labeled schizophrenics. And surprises can happen even after years of permanent psychic invalidism. I have been able to demonstrate that, in some cases, even after 10 or more years of institutional life, it is possible for the patient to emerge from his withdrawal, to achieve a viable compromise and thus to approach a dignified level of life. Exactly what lies behind late, unexpected changes of this kind and just how far processes involving family dynamics play a role is largely unclear. Here and there we find quite apparent contextual evidence such as a change occurring after the death of a parent.

The last part of my reflections shall be devoted to therapy. The goal of therapy that we hope to achieve is that the schizophrenic is helped to a better understanding of himself, either in the context of family therapy or through individual therapy. We want to bring him to see that which is currently hidden from him. It is clear that this cannot be achieved on an intellectual level but, rather, within the framework of corrective emotional experiences. Please excuse this shockingly abbreviated and lapidary statement which must obviously be elaborated and supported. I should, however, like to stress that I have learned much from Stanton (1980) who, in a book dedicated to Lidz, has written about the limits of self-knowledge and clearly demonstrated that any notion of complete self-representation is utopian. "Self-representation is systematically incomplete," he writes. This is true and this realization prevents our overestimating our patients' capacity for self-discernment. All our efforts must inevitably bear the stamp of modesty. One thing is certain: The aim of both family therapy and individual psychoanalytical therapy is an expansion of self-representation. Both activities are addressed to the achievement of discernment and change brought about by corrective experience. It must, however, be explicitly stressed that the ways and means of achieving this goal are basically different. But when speaking of family versus individual therapy I must add that I am categorically opposed to playing off the one type of meeting with the schizophrenic against the other. There can be no doubt that the levels of experience of the schizophrenic vary considerably from case to case. I am also convinced that family therapy has opened – and will continue to open – new horizons in an extraordinarily fruitful manner. It is also beyond doubt that family interaction, with all its distortions within the context of the pathogenesis of schizophrenia, must be accorded priority. Nevertheless, I should like to take up the cudgels on behalf of the continuation of patient, analytically oriented individual therapy often lasting many years. I do this for the following reason: There is a potential in the dialogue with the therapist, in the confrontation with the long, lonely struggle to achieve new forms of identity which the systematic work with the family lacks. It is the uniqueness and unrepeatability of the "twosomeness" in the treatment of the schizophrenic that, for me, is still valid. We must not deprive the schizophrenic of this once-in-a-lifetime chance of meeting someone, in the person of the therapist, who invalidates the fossilized clichés, with whom discussion of a thus far unexperienced frankness is possible, who is long-suffering and loyal and not a partisan of any family myth. This is why I wish to stress that family therapy and analytical individual therapy are both feasible approaches and that we should be prepared to accept both today and in the future.

References

Benedetti G (1975) Ausgewählte Aufsätze zur Schizophrenielehre. Vandenhoeck & Ruprecht, Göttingen

Bleuler E (1911) Dementia praecox. In: Aschaffenburg G (ed) Handbuch der Psychiatrie. Special part, sect. 4, 1st half. Deuticke, Leipzig

Bleuler M (1968) A 23-year longitudinal study of 208 schizophrenics and impressions in regard to the nature of schizophrenia. In: Rosenthai D, Kety SS (eds) The transmission of schizophrenia. Pergamon Press, Oxford, pp 3–12

Conran MB (1976) Schizophrenia as incestuous failure. Theoretical implications, derived from transference observations of the young male schizophrenic and his mother, concerning the

mother-infant relationship. In: Jørstad J, Ugelstad E, (eds) Schizophrenia 75, Proceedings of the Vth international symposium on the psychotherapy of schizophrenia, Oslo 1975. Oslo, Universitetsforlaget, pp 203–210
Finzen A (ed) (1974) Hospitalisierungsschäden in psychiatrischen Krankenhäusern. Piper, München
Huber G, Gross G, Schüttler R (1979) Schizophrenie. Eine Verlaufs- und sozialpsychiatrische Langzeitstudie. Springer, Berlin Heidelberg New York
Kaufmann L (1975) Familientherapie. In: Kisker KP, Meyer JE, Müller C, Strömgren E (eds) Psychiatrie der Gegenwart, III. Springer, Berlin Heidelberg New York, pp 669–710
Langermann JG (1805) Über den gegenwärtigen Zustand der psychischen Heilmethoden der Geisteskrankheiten und über die erste zu Bayreuth errichtete psychische Heilanstalt. Med Chir Ztg, Salzburg 1805; reprinted in Allg Z Psychiat 2:601–605, 1845
Lidz T (1970) Das menschliche Leben. Die Persönlichkeitsentwicklung im Lebenszyklus. Suhrkamp, Frankfurt
Mann T (1936) Freud und die Zukunft. Bermann-Fischer, Wien
Minuchin S (1974) Families and family therapy. Harvard University Press, Cambridge
Müller C (1955) Über Psychotherapie bei einem chronischen Schizophrenen. Psyche 6(9):350–369
Müller C (1980) Der Psychiater und die Schizophrenie. Gedanken zu einer Umfrage unter Schweizer Psychiatern. Psychother Med Psychol 30(1):10–14
Müller C (1981) Psychiatrische Institutionen. Ihre Möglichkeiten und Grenzen. Springer, Berlin Heidelberg New York
Müller C (1981) Psychische Erkrankungen und ihr Verlauf sowie ihre Beeinflussung durch das Alter. Huber, Bern
Racamier PC (1980) Les schizophrènes. Payot, Paris
Reil JC (1803) Rhapsodieen über die Anwendung der psychischen Curmethode auf Geisteszerrüttungen. Halle
Riehl WH (1862) Die Familie. Gotta'scher, Stuttgart
Schindler R (1979) Psychotherapy for late-manifesting schizophrenics. In: Müller C (ed) Psychotherapy of schizophrenia. Proceedings of the 6th international symposium on psychotherapy of schizophrenia, Lausanne 1978. Excerpta Medica, Amsterdam, pp 39–46
Scott RD (1976) "Closure" in family relationships and the first official diagnosis. In: Jørstad J, Ugelstad E (eds) Schizophrenia 75, Proceedings of the Vth international symposium on the psychotherapy of schizophrenia, Oslo 1975. Universitetsforlaget, Oslo, pp 265–282
Searles HF (1965) Collected papers on schizophrenia and related subjects. Hogarth Press, London
Stanton AH (980) Insight and self-observation: their role in the analysis of the etiology of illness. In: Strauss JS, Bowers M, Downey TW, Fleck S, Jackson S, Levine I (eds) Psychotherapy of Schizophrenia. Plenum, New York, pp 131–144
Stierlin H (1981) Die „Beziehungsrealität“ Schizophrener. Psyche 35(1):49–65
Watzlawick P, Beavin JH, Jackson DD (1968) Pragmatics of human communications. Faber and Faber, London
Willis F: cited by Schrenk M (1973) Über den Umgang mit Geisteskranken. Springer, Berlin Heidelberg New York
Wynne L (1961) The study of intrafamilial alignments and splits in exploratory family therapy. In: Exploring the base for family therapy. Family Service Association of America, New York
Wyrsch J (1949) Die Person des Schizophrenen. Haupt Verlag, Bern

Reflections on the Family Therapy of Schizo-Present Families

Helm Stierlin

The Bertram family, consisting of the parents, both in their mid-fifties, and sons Karl (23) and Siegfried (20), came for a family interview one day after Karl's release from a psychiatric hospital. This had been Karl's third hospitalization within 2 years. According to the hospital records he suffered from schizophrenic episodes. He had been delusional and had alternated between being restless and withdrawn. At the beginning of the session Karl was stiff, distrustful, and uncommunicative. When he finally began to talk, he accused his parents of having tricked him into a pointless interview. The parents became defensive and proceeded to list examples of Karl's misbehavior over the last years: for example, playing truant from school, foolish giggling in the presence of outsiders, terroristically blowing the trumpet at night. All this could only be explained and excused by his illness. Karl answered his parents' accusations only with impertinent tittering. In contrast, Siefried, who kept himself in the background, seemed constrained and anxious. The parents conveyed total harmony and asserted their full agreement on all points. However, during the interview they exchanged hardly any feelings or ideas. Apparently they lived closely bound but nevertheless parallel to, not with, one another, even though they certainly had reason to communicate and seek one another's support. The mother appeared tired, listless, and prematurely old. She had often thought about taking her own life. The father seemed tough and energetic, but this toughness apparently overlay deep insecurity. We heard, more or less incidentally, that he had already had two heart attacks.

The Bertrams are rather typical of the "schizo-present" families who come into our outpatient service. They also showed two characteristics which have been repeatedly confirmed by various observers: massive communication deviances, as reported by Wynne and Singer (1963a, b; 1965a, b), and, particularly on the part of the parents, an extremely critical as well as intrusive attitude toward the index patient, which Vaughn and Leff (1976) have subsumed under the concept of "expressed emotions."

Disorders of Related Individuation

Communication deviances and high expressed emotions, along with other characteristics of a family such as the Bertrams, may also suggest typical relational or systems dynamics. To grasp them, the concept of related individuation [fully described by me elsewhere (Stierlin et al. 1980)] seems useful.

Related individuation means the ability and willingness of the members of a system to establish boundaries, while remaining related to each other, that is, they can and wish to articulate their own positions – their feelings, perceptions, expectations, ideas, rights, and obligations – while remaining able to concur in the positions of the others and share with them a common focus of attention. They can resolve conflicts, reach compromises, and work for reconciliation. They are able to negotiate their age-adequate balance between closeness and distance, and rights and obligations as appropriate within the phases of the family life cycle. At any point they are able to define their relationship, that is, they can express more or less clearly what they need from one another, who is more or less allied with whom (for example, forms a couple or a coalition), who receives more recognition from whom. They are able to establish a functional hierarchy and division of roles and tasks.

Members of schizo-present families do not share a common focus of attention; they do not define their important relationships; they straddle a precarious, rigid, but fragile balance between closeness and distance; they do not negotiate age-adequate changes; they lack a functional hierarchy; and they do not conduct a dialogue. We speak of stagnation and rigid homeostasis.

Also, such a disorder of related individuation appears the result and expression of a specific "relational epistemology" that is shared by all family members: a specific way of perceiving and judging the motives, behavior, and reactions of the others that forms the basis for one's personal behavior. Like in the armaments race between world powers such reciprocal, nonreflective perception programs a power struggle or rather a power game. However, the forces, rules, and moves in this game often remain opaque. The strongest weapon frequently lies, not with the one whose attacks are most massive and loudest, but rather with the one who through, for example, disqualifying or ambivalent statements arouses insecurity and feelings of guilt, while at the same time he blocks the definition of the relationship and parades his own helplessness, or physical or mental symptoms. Like the politics of nations such a family power game never ceases but frequently develops into a symmetrical escalation, in the sense of Bateson (1973), becoming a game of life and death. It leads finally to ever more rigidity in the relationships, to a "malign clinch," where in the long run there are no winners, only losers. The Bertram family showed all these characteristics.

The schizophrenic adolescent or young adult usually has a central part in such a rigidified system. He or she fulfills a cementing role, functioning as a massively bound delegate. The bound delegate, as shown elsewhere (Stierlin 1978), has to carry out certain contradictory missions which keep him captive in the family field. Thus, to play his part, he must often act as a source of overpowering anxiety and stimulation that diverts the parents from their own conflicts, deep-lying resentments, or wishes/fears of emotional outbursts; or perhaps he or she must act as a "garbage can," or projection screen, on which the parents can dispose of all the badness, meanness, and craziness whose destructive potential they fear within themselves, yet cannot own. Sometimes the delegate must be parent substitute and provide the flow of vital hope and affirmation that his or her parents never received. Typically, given these heavy and contradictory demands, the delegate's development suffers or becomes one-sided. But at the same time, he or she become important for the parents and the family. Our experience is that such a delegate is not immediately willing to give up this important role. On the contrary, he or she often persists in showing disturbing symptoms and madness, even when the other members of the family no longer need them and are trying hard to change their mutual relationships for the better.

Aims of the Therapy

This is not the place to go into the origins of these family dynamics (see Stierlin, 1974, 1975; Stierlin et al. 1980). I must limit myself to some consequences of this view for a theory of the therapy of schizophrenia.

It follows from the above that a central aim of therapy must be to promote and make possible related individuation, that is, the dialogue among the family members and between the family and the outside world. Among other things this requires the emotional and perhaps also physical mutual *unbinding* of the members of the family, above all the separation of generations (frequently three of them are involved), changing the relational rules and relational epistemology, breaking of rigid coalitions, whether open or concealed; progress in the definition of the relationship; when possible, repair of the parents' emotional divorce (or schism, as Ted Lidz called it), and the construction or reconstruction of a functioning hierarchy based on the parents' authority and cooperation. These steps are necessary in order to make possible new developments for each member and the family as a whole.

All these aspects are more or less interdependent. It is therefore necessary to set in motion a positive spiraling process, or positive mutuality, which eventually affects all parts of the system: separating the generations emotionally and physically, cracking rigidified, development–inhibiting coalitions (for example, between a parent and a child, or a parent and his or her mother); bringing the parents closer together, establishing parental authority and cooperation, and nullifying restrictive relational rules. We need to ask: How and at which point can this spiral start? How and where can the lever of change be used? By changing the rules? By separating the generations? By bringing the parents together? Also, how does the spiraling process work and how does it stay working? To answer these questions, we return once more to the concept of *related individuation.*

Relational Dynamics Versus Individuation Dynamics

The concept of related individuation, we saw, implies a reciprocal connection between on the one side relationships (or relational patterns) and on the other the dynamics of individuation. A closer look shows, however, that depending on whether we wish to understand and influence the relationship or the individuation dynamic, we need different settings for our observing telescope. In other words, we must employ differing perceptual or conceptual filters, as well as a different relational approach. Up to this point, I have focused on aspects of the members rigidified and constricted relationship.

However, these aspects give us almost no information about individuational dynamics. And these concern, above all, *motivation to individuation.* The therapist must ask himself: What is motivating or blocking this person most deeply, what old resentments, what inappropriate obligations, what open or concealed (conflictless or conflict-loaded) needs or wishes are driving him or her? And she or he must ask: How can I operate on this motivational matrix? How can I get him to behave in a new way so that he can contribute positively to the initiation and maintenance of a positively spiraling mutuality? Here the therapist observes and assesses events from the standpoint of motivation or individuation rather than from the standpoint of relationship and system. Such a view implies then a particular therapeutic approach geared essentially to the awakening of motivation. And for this approach we find probably the best model in the late Milton Erickson.

Erickson emphasized three sources of motivation to individuation: *curiosity,* the *striving for competence,* and *wish to belong to a desirable group or team.* He called these "intrinsic motivations," since they originate and are renewed internally. These intrinsic motivations he contrasted with "extrinsic motivations" which depend on a supply of external triggers. In his view it is the intrinsic motivations which are crucial and which the therapist must view as a person's foremost individuation potential.

This means that a therapist relying on the power of these motivations would by what he says and does try to awaken curiosity: for example, curiosity about new possibilities of living, of perceiving self and others differently, of shaping new and old relationships. Or, the therapist tries to mobilize the wish for competence, for example, in areas of professional or social life or in sports or the arts. Or, he might try to stimulate contact with or participation in a club, or peer group, a choir, a professional or political organization or new partnership.

It is, however, in just those families with schizophrenic members that overpowering binding forces threaten to squelch any such individuational dynamics that originate in and are supplied and renewed by awakened intrinsic motivations. Because if, for example, the curiosity of one or more members is awakened too strongly and enduringly, not only would alternative solutions to problems present themselves, but also sacrosanct family secrets and rules would be violated and the current meaning-providing epistemology, the homeostasis, the clinch and power games would be brought into question. If the efforts of individual members are mobilized too far towards competence, their mutual dependence must decrease and bindings would loosen, and there would be risk of envy, jealousy, and even worse, of uncontrollable or apparently uncontrollable aggression. Further, if one or other of the family members seems ready to leave the family in order to invest emotionally in a team, a new partnership, or new family this would imply the deepest disloyalty. Hence, the greater the fear that the family will break apart, the stronger will become the collective forces that rebind the individuating member into his old family.

It is therefore especially with these families that we need a continual dialectical change from a relational to a motivational perspective and vice versa. It follows that to work successfully with such families requires strategies which engender both change and the integration of various perspectives, in other words, a dialectical strategy.

A First Dialectical Strategy

Within the frame of a dialectical strategy the therapist has two jobs: first, to awake motivation to individuation in each individual member and thereby initiate and maintain a positive mutuality, and secondly, to locate and forestall possible systemic sources of resistance and to incorporate these into his therapeutic planning.

To awake motivation to individuation the therapist can point out educational and developmental opportunities which a schizophrenic adolescent apparently has not considered. Preferably, he does this indirectly. Thus, in the case of the Bertram family described above, the therapist mentioned rather casually that in other families with youngsters such as Karl he would recommend that the boy should move out of the parental house and live with his brother, should go back to school and prepare himself for the school leaving exam, should get to know some girls, should join a sport club, and so forth. Also, in those other families the adolescent and his parents could often reach an agreement in those matters. However, here he warned Karl not to expect any such possibilities, thereby removing sources of anticipated resistance from other members of the system. He warned that the parents with good reason would think it premature for their son to take such steps towards self-determination; after all, it had become quite clear that Karl had decided to vitalize his parents by providing them with anxieties and problems. Karl had well understood that without this source of vitalisation the suicidal intentions of the mother and the heart symptoms of the father would become more serious. It was therefore all for the best that he had decided to stay in the family in his role of problem provider for his parents. Thus dialectical strategy of necessity often results in paradoxes, or paradox-like meanings, recommendations, or prescriptions.

A Second Dialectical Strategy

Interwoven with the above dialectical strategy, which provides the impulse for change and at the same time forestalls resistance to it, is a second strategy that requires the therapist to become part of the family and at the same time continually reestablish distance from it.

Without establishing a trusted position within the system the therapist will not obtain informations about crucial relational dynamics, i.e., about Mr. Bertram's close and agonizing relationship to his own parents, and he (the therapist) is powerless to provide impulses that effect change. In other words, he has no leverage to awaken motivation. Unless he continually distances himself, he could be absorbed by the family and if he does become entangled and loses his perspective he will be unable to properly initiate such impulses in a goal-directed fashion.

According to their various theoretical orientations therapists accomplish the double task of simultaneously and alternately joining and maintaining distance from a family in different ways. For our Heidelberg team the process of obtaining a footing within a family means that the therapist develops an empathic, impartial, nonthreatening relationship with each member of the family; that he avoids even the softest, most covert criticism; that he poses no questions about whatever the members say or represent, that he rather accepts everything said without reserve and wherever possible gives it a positive connotation. At the same time, he uses the members' own turns of phrase, metaphors, arguments, and causal conceptions. Distance from the system is achieved by a specific, structuring, and reflective approach, which from the beginning is guided by certain hypotheses and which cools instead of inflaming conflicts and emotionality within the family. In this, the team which watches the interview through a one-way screen is helpful. They continually draw the therapist out of the family and help him or her to find a metaposition.

The Circular Method of Questioning Unifies the Two Dialectic Strategies

Present interview methods employ both of the two interconnected dialectical strategies; that is, the first strategy based on providing impulses for change and at the same time forestalling resistance, with the second that involves obtaining a foothold within the system while at the same time remaining outside the system. One excellent example is the interviewing method developed by the Milan team led by Mara Selvini-Palazzoli (1980), which is (with modifications) the preferred method of our Heidelberg team.

In this technique the interviewer calls on one member to speak about the relationship between two or more members. For example, in the Bertram family, he asked the younger sibling, Siegfried: How do you think your father takes it when your brother Karl is so involved with your mother? Which person in the family is best at cheering your father up then? and so on. The interviewer's questions stem from hypotheses about the family's dynamics, which arise and change continually as information is obtained by means of the circular questioning technique. The interviewer addresses himself to each member in turn and wherever possible uses positive, i.e., affirming and appreciative, questions. In its application of the first of the described strategies, such a procedure affronts existing taboos and rules and at the same time provides the members of the family with new viewpoints and information. It provides subliminal education, as it were. And while questioning the aims and motivations of the members the interviewer also expresses positive expectations and hope. In this way, he provides massive impulses for change via the motivation of individuation. Meanwhile, he uses the information newly obtained by the circular questioning process to convey warnings about change and thereby cuts off anticipated resistance to such change.

The circular questioning technique also forms the basis for the second strategy since it allows the therapist to obtain a foothold in the family and opens up for discussion subjects around which the fantasies and deepest fears of the family have long revolved. Everyone takes part in the discussion, is fascinated by it, and feels: Tua res agitur – your cause is at stake. At the same time, the interviewer again and again steps outside the system and thereby strengthens his metaposition, maintains control and perspective, structures events, and monitors (within limits) distance and closeness between the family members.

On the Way to an Integrative Theory of Therapy

The above shows that any theory of therapy of families with schizophrenic disorders is going to become complex. Every family starts from a unique basis that determines the factors that allow or effectively block change: for example, how acute or chronic the problem is, which phase of the therapeutic process and the family cycle is presenting, what resources exist outside the family, whether and to what extent the family physician or hospital staff are involved. But the first crucial step must always be: to unbind, to unlock the system while mobilizing motivation for individuation.

Thereafter we must ask: How far is the schizophrenic disorder of one member the expression and result of a stagnation and over-rigidity of the system, and how far expression and result of a deficit in social and interpersonal learning? Provided an initial necessary unbinding within and from the family has succeeded, cases of the last type can benefit from group therapy or psychoeducational programs as advocated, for example, by R. Liberman (1981) and C. Anderson (1981). The therapist must then be ready and capable of establishing a dialogue not only among members of a schizophrenic family, but also where necessary, with all other participants in the drama, such as family or clinic physicians, social workers, and so forth the aim always being to help these patients and their families.

References

Anderson CM (1981) A psycho-educational model of family treatment for schizophrenia. Paper read at the 7th International Symposium on the Psychotherapy of Schizophrenia, Heidelberg, 30 Sept.–3 Oct. This volume pp 227–235

Bateson G (1973) Steps to an ecology of mind. Paladin Books, Frogmore

Erickson M (1980) A seminar with Milton Erickson. Zeig J (ed). Brunner/Mazel, New York

Selvini-Palazzoli M et al. (1980) Hypothesizing-circularity-neutrality: Three guidelines for the conductor of the session. Fam Process 19:3–12

Stierlin H (1974) Separating parents and adolescents. Quadrangle, New York. Extended German edition (1980) Eltern und Kinder: Das Drama von Trennung und Versöhnung. Suhrkamp, Frankfurt. Extended English edition (1981) Aronson, New York

Stierlin H (1975) Von der Psychoanalyse zur Familientherapie. Klett, Stuttgart. English edition (1977) Psychoanalysis and family therapy. Aronson, New York

Stierlin H (1978) Delegation und Familie. Suhrkamp, Frankfurt

Stierlin H et al. (1980) Das erste Familiengespräch, 2nd rev edn. Klett, Stuttgart. English edition (1980) The first interview with the family. Brunner/Mazel, New York

Vaughn CE, Leff JP (1976) The measurement of expressed emotion in the families of psychiatric patients. Br J Soc Clin Psychol 15:157–165

Wallace CJ, Liberman RP (1981) Social skills training for schizophrenics. Paper read at the 7th International Symposium on the psychotherapy of Schizophrenia, Heidelberg, 30 Sept.–3 Oct.

Wynne LC, Singer MT (1963a) Thought disorder and family relations of schizophrenics: A research strategy. Arch Gen Psychiatry 9:191–198

Wynne LC, Singer MT (1963a) Thought disorder and family relations of schizophrenics: I. A research classification of forms of thinking. Arch Gen Psychiatry 9:199–206

Wynne LC, Singer MT (1965a) Thought disorder and family relations of schizophrenics: III. Methodology using projective techniques. Arch Gen Psychiatry 12:187–212

Wynne LC, Singer MT (1965b) Thought disorder and family relations of schizophrenics: IV. Results and implications. Arch Gen Psychiatry 12:201–212. German version: Denkstörung und Familienbeziehung bei Schizophrenen. Psyche 19:81–160

The Unconscious Transmission of Hidden Images and the Schizophrenic Process

Norman L. Paul

The puzzling phenomenon of the schizophrenic process and its treatment has been the focus of increasing investigative attention over the last half century. Yet despite the advance on two fronts, dynamic psychiatry and psychopharmacology, the schizophrenic patient still confronts the therapist with therapeutic disappointment. Although psychopharmacology has made the clinical management of these patients, both in and out of the hospital setting, considerably easier, the quality of improvement in their intrapersonal and interpersonal functioning, which dynamically oriented psychotherapy had hoped to achieve, leaves much to be desired.

In the search for improvement in interpersonal functioning of the schizophrenic, social psychiatry has also been drawn into the orbit of exploration. Efforts in this direction have concentrated both on the study of increased effectiveness of the hospital milieu and posthospital care, as well as on the therapeutic techniques in the area of group and family therapy. Impetus in the latter area stems not only from the interpersonal approach to schizophrenia from the Sullivan [1] / Frieda Fromm-Reichman (1950) School, but also from recent studies of family background and functioning of families with schizophrenic members by a variety of disciplines. Notable amongst these are Myers and Roberts (1959), Lidz [4], Bowen (1960), Wynne [6] and Jackson [7].

I, like many of the foregoing, have been impressed by a characteristic fixity of family equilibrium and role relationship in patient-family units designated as schizophrenic in nature. The features of this type of family include:

1. The existence of a pronounced denial of patient's illness, coupled with family behavior on the part of all family members designed unconsciously to reinforce patient pathology.
2. Definite evidence of a lack of ego boundaries of both patient and other family members, manifested by frequent use of projection, speaking for one another, speaking all together, and primary process thinking.
3. Defensive reactions against change in the patient and in other family members manifested by resistance and objection to therapeutic efforts.
4. The presence of an all-pervasive dread of abandonment or separation, coupled with high levels of reciprocal annihilation anxieties and fantasies. (Earlier pilot investigations have led me to recognize this factor as one of singular importance.)
5. The importance of the dread of abandonment in the families of schizophrenic patients is heightened by the recognition that the family members (usually the patient's parents) have suffered significant losses by death that have not been adquately acknowledged or grieved in the past. At times, such family members have considerable

---

Editorial Review by Betty Byfield Paul, L.I.C.S.W., Counseling Associates, Lexington, Massachusetts.

difficulty recognizing or remembering the reality of such losses. Focused confrontation of patient family units on such losses demonstrates the presence of residual grief responses, ambivalent affects, and a general reawakening of varied emotions related to loss.

A fundamental consideration at this point is whether, for whatever reasons, the schizophrenic individual is to be regarded as fundamentally capable of being rehabilitated to "normal" status, without stigma, or whether he is to be considered basically totally irremediably schizophrenic, irrespective of treatments tendered him. I take the position that until all experiential variables are explored, regardless of whether or not we, as therapists or investigators, find them appealing, it is inappropriate to regard the schizophrenic individual as totally irremediable.

The central hypothesis to be presented here is that the repressed mourning responses in family members (usually parents) are related to a fixity in family structure or equilibrium which precludes the formation of adequate ego boundaries on the part of family members. Thereby, both emotional maturation and the development of self-identity are inhibited. The fixity of this equilibrium also tends to counteract the patient's efforts to achieve a resolution of the schizophrenic process and the attainment of higher personality integration and functioning.

Presented here is a transgenerational perspective of the genesis of a schizophrenic process as it manifested itself in the life of a young adult in the Turner Family. The process I will describe never became available to the conscious experience of any member of this enmeshed family until we began our work together. This paper will demonstrate the emphasis on a transgenerational focus in the treatment of a schizophrenic process which bubbled beneath the surface in the Turner Family for over 25 years.

All sessions described herein were audiotaped for family review at home; segments thereof were also videotaped and played back to the family in my office. Various types of stressor tapes were used. Stressor stimuli are audiotapes or videotapes containing such universal emotionally charged experiences as repressed grief reactions, the exquisite pained existence of a schizophrenic person, or intense separation anxiety between a mother and child. In addition, letters, poems, and pieces of literature have been used as stressor stimuli. The rationale underlying the use of stressor material is to assist patients to grasp the idea that all feelings and fantasies are normal and that any designation of deviance is to be made exclusively on the basis of behavior. All adult participants had completed a family tree (including loss by death profile) according to the directions mailed to them before their first family session with me. Table 1 shows the family tree of Sally Kroner-Turner, the mother of the schizophrenic patient.

Over a period of almost 2 years, the family and I worked together to dislodge the reinforced fixity of the family relationships and equilibrium and to scan the losses over three generations. The critical loss was found to be the traumatic early death of the patient's aunt, Melanie, who died at age 7 in a shocking automobile accident in 1922. In November 1981 the family was to hold a belated memorial service for her at a cemetery not too far from the scene of the original accident, which was *felt* to be the site of her unmarked grave.

While every experience of the Turner Family treatment is based on actual episodes, the names, dates and ethnic origins have been changed to assure confidentiality. The following captures highlights of the work with this family.

Table 1. Sally Kroner-Turner's family tree

Kirsten Andreason married *Joseph Kroner* – 2 sisters – 1 brother

Kirsten Andreason: Born in Sweden 1872
Died 4/8/47

Joseph Kroner: Born in Sweden 1867
Died 7/3/59

1st child (infant) died after voyage to U.S.

Melanie	*Mary*	*Greta*	*Joseph*	*David*	*Elisabeth*	*Birgit*	*Sally*
B 11/18/14 Died 8/29/22 (auto accident)	B 7/26/1897 D 1/19/75	B 6/23/1899	B 1/17/01 D 9/9/64	B 8/7/02	B 11/11/04 D 5/29/75	B 12/30/06	B 12/26/10
	Unmarried	Married	Married	Married	Married 7/21/29	Married 10/6/29	Married 7/16/36
		Stephen Bergson	*Edith*	*Jean*	*David Svenson*	*Robert Stephens*	*Stanley Turner*
		Kathryn B 8/11/24 Susanne B 8/12/29	John B 7/31 Carl B 9/34	Andreas B 9/13/42	Greta B 4/29/30 Ingrid B 12/14/35	Heidi B 7/23/32 M – Curt Walden	Stillbirth B 11/4/38 Karla B 11/2/39 Jane and Judy B 7/24/43 Dean B 6/12/47

Table 2. Types and number of visits

Judy – 3 visits
Judy, Elizabeth, and Toby (daughters) – 4 visits
Judy, Jane, and Karla – 1 visit
Dean, Jane, and Karla – 1 visit
Jane – 5 visits
Jane and her husband – 10 visits
Jane's husband – 1 visit
Jane, her husband, and four children – 1 visit
Jane, her husband, and second daughter – 1 visit
Jane's second daughter – 1 visit
Jane's first child – 2 visits
Karla and her husband – 4 visits
Karla, her husband, and first child (daughter) – 1 visit
Karla's husband and his parents – 1 visit
Karla's husband and his father – 1 visit
Stanley and Sally (parents) – 4 visits
Stanley – 1 visit
Sally – 1 visit
Sally and Judy – 1 visit
Dean, Judy, Jane, Karla, Sally, and Stanley – 5 visits
Dean, Judy, Jane, Karla, and Stanley – 1 visit
Karla, Jane, and Dean – 6 visits
Karla and Jane – 1 visit

The Turner Family consists of the mother, Sally, 70; the father, Stanley, 71; a daughter, Karla, 42; twin daughters Jane and Judy, 39 (Judy was born 3 minutes after Jane); and a son, Dean, 33. At the time this chapter was prepared the family had been seen 57 times, in 23 different subsystem units (Table 2). They are all physically attractive, usually well dressed (except for Judy), of Swedish ethnic origin, and of the Lutheran faith. The family views itself as very close, though recognizing that there are a variety of communication problems present.

Before Karla was born there had been a stillbirth, a girl, who died at 7 months gestation. The parents recalled that *only* Stanley had been told by the obstetrician that the baby was dead before Sally delivered it 2 months later. At one of the meetings, Stanley recalled that after he had observed the dead baby, still obviously shaken and distressed, he went to visit his mother. His mother told him: "Forget about the baby; don't grieve. As long as there is an apple tree, there will be apples." So he had four apples after that.

My initial visit was with Judy Turner in October of 1979. She was the first member of the Turner Family to work with me. Judy is 5 feet tall, overweight, speaks softly and rapidly, and generally looks as if she is ready to explode. A divorced mother of two daughters, Elizabeth, 17, and Toby, 15, she appeared primarily concerned that her daughters might replicate toward her the chronic, intense, unforgiving, lifelong hatred that she had always had for her own mother. Judy, though an intelligent woman, had dropped out of college after 2 years because of terrifying, recurring, auditory hallucinations. She said that, since as far back as her early teens, she had had recurrent intense feelings of deadness, which, when associated with "strong" suicidal desires, had terrified her. Medication had generally kept these experiences under control, though much of the time only marginally. She had been hospitalized over the past 18 years in five different institutions, the longest stay having been for 18 months. From 1978 until the initial interview she had been seen on an outpatient basis, principally for medication surveillance. She had worked with six different psychiatrists in therapy since 1961. Most recently, she had been involved in an unresolved, excessive transference/countertransference episode with a psychiatrist at the Stonyhead Institute, whom, even though he had moved to Chicago in 1978, she continued to visit periodically for psychotherapy. She still viewed this relationship as very positive.

At the onset of Judy's illness in 1961, she had been diagnosed as having a "schizophrenic reaction, paranoid type, chronic, moderately severe." The hospitalizations had been triggered by attempted suicides with neuroleptic medication, excessive alcohol intake, and barbiturates. When first seen in October of 1979, she had been on 600 mg Mellaril and 200 mg Elavil daily, and she had just had lithium medication discontinued after 5 years, all for chronic, severe, suicidal depression. In addition, she had received four courses of electric shock treatment over the years.

In a letter to me prior to her first visit, she wrote: "My illness became very apparent at the age of 15 – however, it is obvious to me that it began promptly at birth."

First Interview with Judy

During the first interview, Judy claimed that she had never had a warm, tender moment with her mother. She regarded her father as erratic in his relationship with her. Though she had often regarded him as her only friend in the family, he had not spoken to her for the last 4 years, since an intense verbal battle. She viewed her "older" twin, Jane, as the stronger, more dominant one, whose job it was to pave the way for her in a variety of social activities over the years. More recently, and particularly since her divorce, Judy had been drinking to excess, her life was drifting aimlessly, and she was regarded as a conspicuous problem for her family. She also felt numbed with all the medication and terrified at her sense of deadness.

Of all the data presented during this first meeting, the most salient was the fact that her mother's (Sally) younger sister, Melanie, had been hit by a car at the age of 7 while chasing a ball that had been thrown by Sally, then age 11. Melanie died shortly thereafter. Judy wrote: "... this must be loaded with emotional repercussions. My mother never told me." She described her maternal grandmother, Kirsten, who died in 1947, as "the angry woman," juxtaposing this with her statement "... so is my mother still today," and so was Judy in my office that day. When speaking about her mother's stillbirth, Judy said: "My father never let her mourn the death of the child ... Because that's what he is ... no one in our family grieves for anyone. We just go on from where we are and keep on going. I never saw my parents cry or show anything."

At the end of that first session, I asked Judy about the existence of a picture of Melanie. She said that Sally had found one in a box of old family pictures and that Karla was startled when she first saw it because it looked so much like Judy. Judy added that she, herself, couldn't see the resemblance. I then asked her to bring in Melanie's picture to the next interview. I also asked her to bring in both her twin and her older sister, Karla, so that I could find out more about the family through their eyes.

Karla, Judy and Jane

Two weeks later, when the three women came to my office, they appeared like mannequins, as they were wooden in movement and posture. They revealed their intense struggle in coping with their parents. Karla, the oldest, reviewed her almost total cut off from both parents for the previous 8 years. She had been married for 20 years to a very hard driving business executive, who was in his father's electronics business, had two adopted daughters, Janice, 18, and Louise, 13, and a natural born son, Karl, 10. She and her husband, also a first child, had had a chronically turbulent marriage. They both had had intensive psychotherapy over the preceding 10 years. More recently, during the past 2 years, Janice had been involved in the drug scene with heroin and LSD. She had been incarcerated in a local private mental hospital for 8 months.

Karla described very poignantly her chronic frustration with Janice, who came to their home at 4 months of age, and with whom she could never establish a warm, hugging relationship. Janice resisted every attempt at physical closeness by Karla, and was always the subject of battles between her parents. Karla would try to curb or control her while her husband would side with Janice. At a later session, Karla wistfully looked back over her life and stated she could never remember being hugged or ever hugging her own mother. Though an attractive woman, she portrayed herself as both unlovable and unattractive.

Jane's marriage was also an unhappy tour de force. She looked chilly and said she felt cold toward her children. She mused about her perennial desire to be a teacher or a television producer, anything other than a mother. She was very envious of the manner in which her three daughters would gravitate toward their father, whom they viewed as being affectionate. Her husband was an easygoing man who distanced himself from his own controlling family, and who was only marginally interested in earning a living.

I sketched out to all three women present that I was interested in assisting this family in becoming more communicative and responsive to listening to one another. I added that it would be useful to allow me to share the videotape of this session with the parents in order to document some of the actual pain that had been concealed from the parents, and thereby enlist the parents' involvement.

I described the hypothesis about Melanie's death being a critical element, contributing to their seemingly numbed existential state. They were guardedly interested in pursuing the therapeutic program; each was concerned about being even more rejected by their parents. They added that they had had no relationship with their brother Dean since they went to college and that he was currently the father's favorite, a fact that made them very bitter. They took responsibility for initiating a session for the parents to meet with me.

The daughters contacted both parents, who subsequently called me from their home in Puerto Rico. They indicated in a lengthy phone conversation that they did not really want to be that involved with any of their daughters, including Judy. In fact, Stanley stated that he had arranged for Dean, who had been groomed to take over the father's business, to dispense funds to Judy and her children.

He added that he had also worked out a plan for a bookkeeper to take care of Judy's checkbooks. He concluded that he recognized Judy's profound incapacity to assume responsibility for her life, adding that he was doing the best he could.

First Interview with Stanley and Sally

In late January 1980, because of family inputs and concern about Judy's excessive drinking, Sally and Stanley flew to Boston for a joint interview with me. They looked strung out, appeared quite rigid, defensive, and distant. Shortly after arriving for the interview, Stanley revealed his terror of flying, stating that the had to take medication in order to come to this session. He then revealed the onset of this phobia to be related to when, at the age of 8, a small plane crashed 50 yards from him, burning up the pilot. Reviewing this traumatic occurrence provided Stanley with considerable relief. In a session 3 months later, he disclosed with pleasure his newfound ability to fly without any paralyzing anxiety.

I then had them view the videotape of their daughters. They were jarred into disbelief as they muttered repeatedly "... but we did everything to make them happy." Further discussion led to their agreement to plan for a meeting with their four children upon their return to the Boston area in early Spring. Stanley also agreed to assist in locating Melanie's grave site, as Sally seemed incapable of seizing any initiative to do so.

During the next few months, a variety of meetings were conducted to improve relationships among the siblings. Each daughter indicated an interest in expediting a resolution of the communicative difficulties in their own families with husbands and children. Dean was finally accepted as a peer, after a lengthy and bitter assault on him by his sisters. He rallied by sharing his distress at their exclusion of him.

Repairing relationships was going on as the family mission to find out all that could be made known about Melanie, living and dead, was being pursued. Nobody in Sally's family could remember where Melanie was buried. The only direct reference made to the children prior to the family therapy was to Karla at age 14, when her mother, Sally, had told her that, while she was in charge of Melanie, she was hit by a car and killed instantly while catching a ball thrown by Sally. At the time of Melanie's death, Sally had been reviled by her mother: "You are a murderer. You have killed your own sister." The family was apparently so traumatized by Melanie's death in August of 1922, that within the year they moved and never returned to that town.

So, the intial chore was to locate evidence of Melanie's death where she was buried, in fact, that she had existed at all. At times, Sally had indicated to her children that she was the youngest of seven, when actually there was an eighth child, Melanie.

Avenues to locating aspects of Melanie's death included an obscure newspaper account and the death certificate which was located in Concord, New Hampshire. None of the family members had any recollection of a funeral having taken place, other than a fragment of a memory that it may have taken place at home. There had been no grave site service according to all extended family members.

My hypothesis was that Judy, being both the youngest girl and the second youngest child, Sally's own sibling position, had been unconsciously created in the image of Melanie, and that the absence of any acknowledgement of Melanie's death and associated grief resulted in a spiraling reinforcement of this process. The therapeutic challenge was to help validate Melanie's existence, and at some point to see if some repressed grief could be stimulated so as to assist in finally completing this family's relationship with Melanie.

First Meeting With the Whole Family in May of 1980

In May of 1980 the entire family finally met. Present were the parents, Karla, Jane and Judy, and Dean. This was the first time all six were together in 21 years. The scene was very uncomfortable. It became clear that the parents' isolation from the children was quite intense. For example, Judy stated that she had not talked with her father in 4 years. Throughout the family meeting, Judy felt unfavorably compared to Jane.

When the focus shifted to the development of Judy's original difficulties, the tension and discomfort abated somewhat. It was apparent that all this was being reviewed for the first time in the presence of the whole family. Judy described how when she was 18 she had met a young man, Robert Janeway, with whom she fell in love. Subsequently, they became engaged. She recalled how she began to hear voices immediately after the engagement, threatening her, berating her, and telling her to "forget about Robert." The voices said that a marriage to him would be a "natural disaster," as she was not good enough for him, and that such a marriage "would hurt her mother." Frightened by these voices, Judy was seen by a psychiatrist, who diagnosed her as being schizophrenic.

The reviewing of this unhappy period of Judy's life made her siblings uncomfortable, as they were reminded of how chronic her problem had been. Judy recalled thinking of killing herself at that time. Family members remembered a serious auto accident that Judy had during that period. She suddenly revealed to the family that her intention in that accident had been to kill herself. As Judy was referring to her hoped-for mariage as "a natural disaster," Sally turned suddenly toward me, as if on cue, and asked me what went on in my head as Judy repeated this. (It was the first time mother had heard such "unusual phrases.") I said I was instantly reminded of an earlier disaster, namely Melanie's tragic death. I then urged Sally to review what had transpired when her younger sister was killed in 1922. She reluctantly did so and presented the details, as far as she could remember, that reflected her painful experience and her culpable role in the event. It was later, when the account by Sally was played back on videotape, that Judy interrupted the group to say that she was experiencing a strange feeling that was frightening and which she wanted to share with the whole family. With much hesitation she said that her body felt strange as she felt love for her mother for the first time. Both Judy and the mother began to cry and hug one another, obviously in a moment of deep tender, and mutual understanding. While this was going on, Stanley, the father, was so overcome with emotions that he bolted out of the room. Dean followed him and brought him back. Stanley said he had never been so shaken. His reserve was shattered as he indicated that he never expected to see Judy relate in this positive a way to her mother.

After this electrifying and exhausting 3-h meeting, there was a galvanized sense of purpose to locate Melanie's grave site. The search included the efforts of principally the four children, who talked with uncles, aunts, cousins, people who might have been present at the funeral, neighbors of where Sally's original family lived in the early 1920s, visits to various cemeteries, and phone calls to distant relatives, including cousins who had come for short visits from Sweden, and who might possibly have a bit of information about Melanie. All this yielded nothing. A search of Mount Pleasant Cemetery, which was mentioned in the death certificate, disclosed the presence of several small grave stones from the early 1920s, but no stone for Melanie Kroner was found. Mount Pleasant Cemetery was finally chosen as the site for the projected Memorial Service when Karla, after their search in several cemeteries, felt very strongly that Melanie was indeed buried there. At one point, thought was given to the unearthing of some of the unmarked graves of that period; however, the cemetery Association, after reviewing the situation, did not permit that.

The work in the summer of 1980 consisted in part of using a stressor tape of a schizophrenic young man and his brother and mother, wherein the young man reviewed his guilt and intense anguish about his sense of responsibility for having his schizophrenic father thrown out of the house into a hospital setting by his mother at the time when he himself was 6 and 16 years old. This stressor tape contained segments of sessions wherein the mother finally revealed to her son that the was conceived out of wedlock, and that her eight attempts to abort him had been unsuccessful. The emerging clear sense of this man's identity, coupled with his sense of joy about knowing the truth, concludes this stressor tape. The tape was first used with Dean, Jane, and Karla, to share with them what I thought was an approximation of Judy's lifelong experience of herself. It was then played to Judy and her sister Jane, and Judy confirmed that this was indeed the way she had always felt about herself. At a later date, this tape was played again for Judy and Sally, and Sally was very much impacted by both the tape and Judy's very positive response to it.

Later that summer, this tape was used with the whole family, and as a result of this, Judy felt increasingly acceptable to the family. In October of 1980, Sally was persuaded to take sensitivity training (EST) [8]. After that, she revealed that during one of the processes there, she was for the first time able to visualize her sister Melanie, and to cry, missing her, and for the first time since that accident felt conscious regret.

During the fall of 1980, Judy's medication requirements dictated that I refer her to a colleague who is expert in the use of medication with schizophrenics. As a result of this combination of family therapy sessions and a revised medication schedule, Judy began to curb her drinking and her relationship between her and her daughters, Elizabeth and Toby, began to improve.

In the spring of 1981, Judy's drug therapist suggested that Jane come in with Judy to see him in an attempt of getting Jane to assume responsibility for taking care of Judy. Concurrent with the meetings once every 3 weeks, Jane's daughter Kirsten, who had also displayed delinquent behavior together with Judy's daughter Elizabeth, settled down and became more responsive and better behaved with her mother. After 2 1/2 months of Jane's meeting with Judy's psychiatrist, Jane decided that she did not want to continue, and her daughter had reactivation of her delinquent behavior and rebelliousness, principally toward her mother. The tension at home was most intense, and it was resolved by having Kirsten live with a second cousin, where she is attending high school.

It has become very clear to Karla and Jane that residues of Judy's behavior have emerged in their respective daughters, and because of this, they actively pursued the belated memorial service with Dean. This was scheduled to take place in November 1981, with a Lutheran chaplain from a local college in charge, with increasing interest on the part of all. It was curious to observe how the family had been distracted briefly from this by a recent psychotic episode in Judy, which resulted in her moving in with her parents. There, she was unrelenting in confronting both parents, but especially

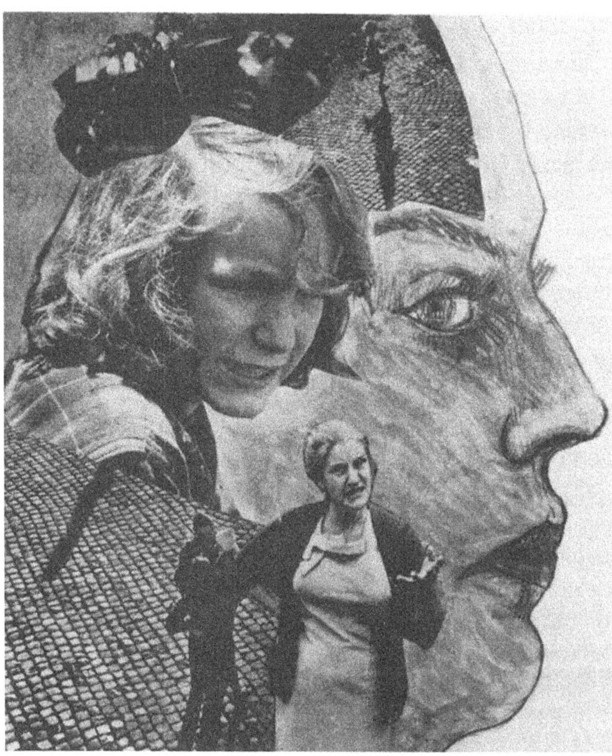

Fig. 1. The incident. This collage shows pictures of an angry mother, a frightened young girl, and a 1920 touring car moving toward a small, female child, Melanie. The lower part shows a picture oi parents holding an infant, recapturing a memory of Sally's parents' joy with her baby sister, Melanie

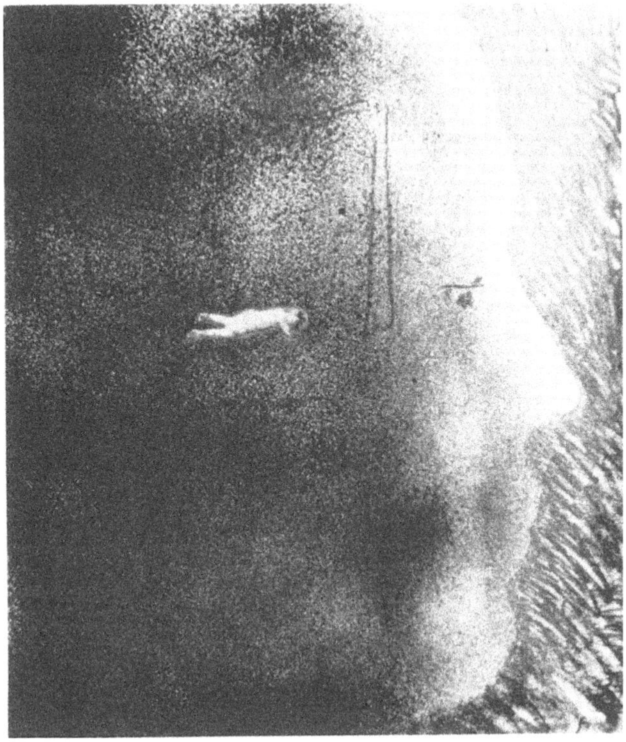

Fig. 2. The incident repressed. This represents only the image of Melanie lying presumably dead, as it existed in a dormant form in Sally's head.

her mother, about their shortcomings when she was a little girl. Mother's repeated apologies and agreement about her insensitivity and neglect of Judy resulted in Judy's convulsive sobbing, leading to her sleeping with Sally for a few nights in a manner suggesting that she was again a little girl. This evoked in me a fantasy of Kirsten's (the grandmother) comforting her dead little girl after the accident, as well as Sally's comforting herself by proxy in Judy.

In the context of the family moving in time toward the memorial service, the relationship between Jane and her husband has taken a dramatic turn toward the resolution of their prior intense enmeshment. They appear joyful with their newfound mutuality.

On September 22, 1981, Kirsten's individual therapist called me, surprised to have found Kirsten so responsive in treatment. She reported that Kirsten had told her, with a note of great joy: "My mother hugged me." The therapist added: "I don't know what's happening, but Jane is coming through with flying colors."

Following is a description of the collages by the artist Ray Langenbach (Figs. 1–3). The represent the inferred existence of images in the mind of Sally Turner since the incident of Melanie's death in 1922. *These images should be regarded as being completely unconscious.*

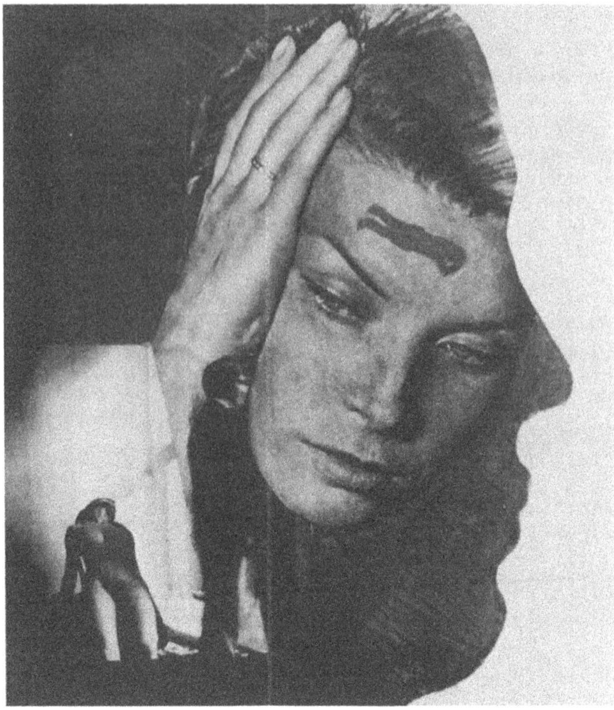

Fig. 3. The incident re-created. This collage captures the picture of Judy with the image of dead Melanie in her head, gazing upon a scene of herself in the nude, and feeling lifeless, with a man turning his back on her.

From the middle of life onward, only he remains vitally alive who is ready to die with life. For in the secret hour of life's midday the parabola is reversed, death is born. The second half of life does not signify ascent, unfolding, increase, exuberance, but death, since the end is its goal. The negation of life's fulfilment is synonymous with the refusal to accept its ending. Both mean not wanting to live; not wanting to live is identical with not wanting to die. Waxing and waning make one curve.

(Jung, The Meaning of Death)

Discussion

This case of the Turner Family provides a point of departure for reviewing the means by which images of a dead person are unconsciously transmitted and appear to generate the schizophrenic process in a child.

The basic problem in trying to discuss this has to do with using a language that is not process oriented in an attempt to convey a process, here the projection of the image of Melanie, dead, by Sally, onto Judy, who has introjected this image, all unconsciously. It is obvious in many ways that Sally was in a position to be scapegoated for her alleged role in her sister's death. It is of considerable interest to observe that nobody in the Turner Family knows to date whether a funeral actually took place or where this child is buried. As such, the experience of Melanie's death cannot help but remain alive, though unconsciously, in and through Sally and in her children, principally in Judy.

The impact of such unconscious images is enormous, generating a wide base of behavior, principally in the schizophrenic individual. For example, Judy felt that her mother had always hated her; it is obvious that Sally hated Melanie for dying and her own parents for accusing her of her alleged complicity in Melanie's death.

The planned family ritual, a memorial service, is designed to provide a means of repentance and mourning for, and commitment of, the dead, so that the images of the dead can be relaxed in their adverse impact on the living. It also affords a concurrent celebration for finally completing a transgenerational task. In addition, it commemorates and sanctions a dramatic shift to an animated expression of communication. Once a person's death and previous life have been acknowledged, permission is granted for the family to feel and be alive. A family transformation is thereby mandated where the conscious and unconscious focus of preoccupation about Melanie can be projected and resolved onto her final designated resting place, a grave site with a stone. This process of ritual mourning of deceased family members who had not previously been mourned is described by Robert McAll and Frances McAll (1980). They found this type of intervention to be effective in 15 out of 18 patients with anorexia nervosa, who had not shown improvement with conventional therapy, resulting in total cessation of symptoms. These authors include in their work reference to Maria Palazzoli's (1979) use of enforced mourning for a case of anorexia nervosa.

Enabling the individual and his family to mourn the dead through a long-neglected appropriate memorial service can provide exciting movement in a heretofore rigid and crippling family structure. It will remove the family's tendency to replace the living with the dead.

What must obviously happen in the context of a death such as Melanie's, when the event was completely forgotten, for whatever reasons, is that the energy related to the grief experience becomes dammed up and repressed. At the same time, it is seeking expression and will be represented in a myriad of forms, most of which have yet to be delineated. The absence of these themes in Paul F. Dell's (1980) article, "Researching the Family Theories of Schizophrenia: An Exercise in Epistemological Confusion," is astonishing and speaks eloquently for its silent power. Is it possible that, unwittingly, we may today have stumbled onto some stepping stone to a more complete understanding of the schizophrenic riddle?

Summary

This presentation consists of a description of the relationship between repressed grief and the schizophrenic process in a family. The Turner Family described herein lived through the re-creation in a child of an unacknowledged early death in the life of that family. This re-creative process is depicted via collages by artist Ray Langenbach. These collages represent the unconsciously generated images in Sally Turner's head after the death of her younger sister, Melanie, in 1922; they capture the artist's view of the original incident, the incident repressed, and the incident re-created in the life of Judy Turner, Sally's daughter. The rationale for a belated memorial service is discussed.

Bibliography

Aries P (1981) The hour of our death. Knopf, New York

Becker E (1973) The denial of death. Free Press, New York

Bellack L, Loeb L (1969) The schizophrenic Syndrome. Grune and Stratton, New York

Bowen M (1960) A family concept of schizophrenia. In: Jackson D (ed) The etiology of schizophrenia. Basic Books, New York, pp 346–372

Dell P (1980) Researching the family theories of schizophrenia: An exercise in epistemological confusion. Fam Process 19/4:321–335

Fromm-Reichman F (1950) Principles of intensive psychotherapy. University of Chicago Press, Chicago

Jackson DD (ed) (1960) Etiology of schizophrenia. Basic Books, New York

Jackson DD, Weakland JH (1961) Conjoint family therapy: Some considerations on theory, technique and results. Psychiatry 24:30–45

Lidz T, Cornelison A et al. (1958) Intrafamilial environment of the schizophrenic patient, Part 6: The transmission of irrationality. AMA Archives of Neurology and Psychiatry 79:305–316

Lidz T, Fleck S et al. (1963) Schizophrenic patients and their siblings. Psychiatry 26:1–18

Lidz T, Fleck S (1960) Schizophrenia, human integration, and the role of the family. In: Jackson D (ed) The etiologoy of schizophrenia. Basic Books, New York, pp 323–345

McAll RK, McAll FM (1980) Ritual mourning in anorexia nervosa. Lancet 368

Myers JL, Roberts BH (1959) Family and class dynamics in mental illness. John Wiley & Sons, New York

Palazzoli MS (1979) Family ritual, a powerful tool in family therapy. Lo Studio de la Famiglia, Milan

Paul NL (1967) The use of empathy in the resolution of grief. Perspect Biol Med 11:153–168

Paul NL, Grosser GH (1963) Operational mourning in family therapy. Unpublished research project

Paul NL, Grosser GH (1964) Family resistance to change in schizophrenic patients. Fam Process 3:377–401

Paul NL, Paul BB (1978) The use of EST as adjunctive therapy to family-focussed treatment. Journal of Marriage and Family Counseling 1/78:51–61

Riesman D (1955) The oral tradition, the written word, and the screen image. Antioch College Founders Day Lecture No. 1. Antioch Press, Yellow Springs, Ohio

Scott RD, Ashworth PL (1965) The "axis value" and the transfer of psychosis. Br J Med Psychol 38:87–116

Scott RD, Ashworth PL (1967) "Closure" at the first schizophrenic break-down: A family study. Br J Med Psychol 40:109–145

Scott RD, Ashworth PL (1969) The shadow of the ancestor: A historical factor in the transmission of schizophrenia. Br J Med Psychol 42:13–32

Shapiro A (1981) Contemporary theories of schizophrenia: Review and synthesis. McGraw-Hill, New York

Sheflen A (1981) Levels of schizphrenia. Brunner/Mazel, New York

Shershow JJ (ed) (1978) Schizophrenia: science and practice. Havard University Press, Cambridge, Massachusetts

Strauss JS et al (eds) (1980) The psychotherapy of schizophrenia. Plenum, New York

Sullivan HS (1953) The interpersonal theory of psychiatry. Norton, New York
Sullivan HS (1947) Therapeutic investigation in schizophrenia. Psychiatry 10:121
Walsh F (1978) Concurrent grandparent death and birth of schizophrenic offspring: An intriguing inding. Fam. Process 17:547–463
Welldon RMC (1971) The "shadow-of-death" and its implications in four families, each with a hospitalized schizophrenic member, Fam Process 10/3:281–302
Wynne LC, Rykoff I et al. (1958) Pseudo-mutuality in the family relations of schizophrenics. Psychiatry 21:205–220
Wynne LC, Singer M (1963a) Thought disorder and family relations of schizophrenics, Part 1: A research strategy. Arc Gen Psychiatry 9:191–198
Wynne LC, Singer M (1963b) Thought disorder and family relations of schizophrenics, Part 2: A classification of forms and thinking. Arc Gen Psychiatry 9:199–206

Brief Therapy of Schizophrenia

Paul Watzlawick

The juxtaposition of schizophrenia and brief therapy seems absurd, as it is generally agreed that schizophrenia is a severe mental disturbance whose treatment is long and of uncertain outcome. In this chapter an attempt will be made to show that the difficulties surrounding the treatment of schizophrenia are partly the result of the views held about the condition and not due to its intrinsic nature. This approach is based on the work of the Bateson group in the 1950s and on subsequent developments of this model by the staff of the Mental Research Institute in Palo Alto.

In his *Introduction to Cybernetics*, published in 1956, the famous cybernetician Ashby writes:

Suppose I am in a friend's house and, as a car goes past outside, his dog rushes to a corner of the room and cringes. To me the behaviour is causeless and inexplicable. Then my friend says, "He was run over by a car six months ago." The behaviour is now accounted for by reference of an event of six months ago. If we say that the dog shows "memory" we refer to much the same fact – that his behaviour can be explained, not by reference to his state now but to what his state was six months ago. If one is not careful one says that the dog "has" memory, and then thinks of the dog as having *something, as he might have a patch of black hair. One may then be tempted to start looking for the thing; and one may discover that this "thing" has some very curious properties.*

And Ashby then goes on to say:

Clearly, "memory" is not an objective something that a system either does or does not possess; it is a concept that the observer *invokes to fill in the gap caused when part of the system is unobservable. The fewer the observable variables, the more will the observer be forced to regard events of the past as playing a part in the system's behaviour. Thus "memory" in the brain is only partly objective. No wonder its properties have sometimes been found to be unusual or even paradoxical.*

And then, in one simple sentence, he draws the only logical conclusion:

Clearly the subject requires thorough examination from first principles (Ashby 1963, p. 117).

This sounds deceptively simple. In actual fact, scientists share with all higher animals an inability or unwillingness to reexamine their conceptual models "from first premises." If it were not so, there would be no such thing as an experimental neurosis in a laboratory animal whose "world view" is shattered when the experimenter turns the reward-and-punishment context upside down, or the fate of Galileo Galilei, with ether, phlogiston, the dilemmas of plane geometry, the inheritance of acquired characteristics, and a thousand other, similar "facts" lying somewhere between these extremes. Worse still, what is involved here is not just an inability to question one's assumptions, but to accept the possibility that one's "first premises" are just that: mere assumptions, paradigms in Kuhn's sense (1970), and not eternal truths discovered once and for all.

In the case of psychiatric theories this trend is, if anything, even more pronounced. The question of what is abnormal and what is normal, and how the former can be changed into the latter, is complicated by the fact that psychiatric theories are held by their authors and subscribers with much greater fervor than, say, those of the physicist or the economist. Since they do not involve merely impersonal issues but the human being as such (including, therefore, those who accept them), they are almost in the nature of religious beliefs. And the basic belief must not, may not, be wrong.

Take a book like *Freud or Jung*?, written by the eminent psychoanalyst Edward Glover (1956). The author painstakingly fills 195 pages in order to prove what can be said in one sentence: that Jung's ideas do not coincide with Freud's. In fact, this is what Glover does in his conclusion (p. 190): "As we have seen the most consistent trend of Jungian psychology is its negation of every important part of Freudian theory." A statement of this kind would not be worth making, if the authors and his readers did not believe Freud's ideas to be the basis of the final, true explanation of human behavior. Then *and only then* does it make sense to point to the fallacies of somebody else's thinking. (The same holds for Marxism or any other ideology which through political power *fiat* has been declared to be the scientific and therefore ultimate and eternally true explanation of the social and economic laws governing human existence and human values.)

If this is so and if actions taken in accordance with the theory are unsuccessful, the fault must be sought in the *applications* of the theory but not in the theory *itself*. This means further that in a very real sense the point of therapy may be to save the theory, not the patient. And it finally means also that within the framework of any theory, certain deductions are consistent with its premises and others must be ruled out as inconsistent. Symptom removal, for instance, is inconsistent and incompatible with the tenets of psychodynamic theory and must "therefore" not be attempted on pain of symptom substitution or exacerbation. But since as practitioners we are not trained as philosophers of science, we are likely to remain blind to the fact that this limitation is in the nature of the *theory* and not in the nature of the *human mind*. Hypnotherapy, behavior therapy, certain forms of family therapy, and a number of brief therapeutic techniques successfully practice what in the psychodynamic framework would be symptomatic treatment pure and simple. One is reminded of the fact that in the Ptolemaic, geocentric system some planets could be "seen" to perform weird dances, the so-called recessions, which contradicted everything that was already known about celestial mechanics, while in the heliocentric view of the solar system they do move in the smooth eliptical orbits that one would expect from any self-respecting planet. For the geocentric astronomer, however, the curlicues of Mercury and others were "facts" whose integration into his view of the universe created fantastic problems and called for ever more complicated refinements of his scientific model.

When in 1904 a panel of 13 eminent scientists certified that a stallion, since then known as Clever Hans (Pfungst 1965), was a genius, capable of the most amazing intellectual feats, the same mechanism seems to have been at work. What was involved in this weird miscarriage of scientific thinking was a simple process of nonverbal interaction between the horse and the experimenters. But nonverbal communication had no place in the scientific paradigm of that era and, therefore, exactly in Ashby's sense, the observers had to fall back on an absurd explanation "to fill the gap caused when part of the system is unobservable" – or, more to the point, when the observers are blind to that part. *If* a horse can do arithmetic and *if* deception can be ruled out, then this horse *is* a genius – this is how the panel of experts must have seen it.

In arriving at their fantastic but (for them) inevitable conclusion (which was led *ad absurdum* 3 months later by a graduate student who simply looked in the right direction) these scientists had actually committed the mistake which Molière had spoofed 250 years earlier in one of his comedies: He has a panel of learned doctors investigate the reason why opium makes people sleep. After careful consideration they arrive at the conclusion that this is so because opium contains a "dormitive principle." A word thus leads to a reification, i.e., is made into a thing (*res*) and – to quote Ashby once more – "one may then be tempted to start looking for the thing; and one may discover that this 'thing' has some very curious properties." For it seems naively obvious that if there exists a name, then the thing thus named *must* exist. That a disembodied name should flutter around in our conceptual universe, like those little bodiless angels in baroque paintings, is an almost intolerable thought, Alfred Korzybski notwithstanding. He never tired of insisting that the name is not the thing and the map not the territory (Korzybski 1933).

It should by now be fairly clear what all of this has to do with schizophrenia. When in 1911 Eugen Bleuler published his famous monograph, *Dementia Praecox, oder die Gruppe der Schizophrenien* (which was not translated into English until 1950 [Bleuler 1950]), he coined the term schizophrenia because he was dissatisfied with the then current name, *Dementia praecox*, which he considered misleading. In his *Textbook of Psychiatry* (Bleuler 1930) he explains: "As the disease need not progress as far as dementia and does not always appear *praecociter*, i.e., during puberty or soon after, I prefer the name *schizophrenia*."

As is known, the new name found rapid international acceptance. What was accepted together with the term was the unquestioned reification that it referred to a split or equivalent deficit of the mind. This was perfectly in keeping with the traditional, monadic approach in psychiatry. It did not, however, mean that there existed (or exists) consensus about the *thing* to which this name refers. To quote Arieti:

Although I admit that in what we call the schizophrenic syndrome there is still much that is indefinite, variable, inconstant, accessory, I feel nevertheless that there is a more or less homogeneous core which makes us recognize the schizophrenic person as such and leads us to some conclusions, some of which have pragmatic value. The fact that the nature of this core has not yet been fully or uncontroversially determined points to the incompleteness of the concept of schizophrenia but does not prove it is a fallacy. (Arieti 1959)

Since on the strength of available evidence little can be done to heal the supposed split of the mind, it is not surprising that a controversy continues to rage between the advocates of heredity or constitution, endocrine or cardiovascular causation, biochemistry or neuropathology, degenerative processes, and a large number of psychological and other hypotheses.

But every once in a while a case like the following, treated by the director of the Mental Research Institute, Carlos Sluzki, finds its way into the literature:

A 29-year-old man – diagnosed schizophrenic for the prior 6 years – is seen with his mother and two of his siblings. The family history includes the fact that his father left them when the patient was 6 years old. The patient, a very passive, mild-mannered man, was married, had three children and eventually had an affair that was discovered, and his wife expelled him – or he abandoned his family – over 6 years ago. A short time after this he began to produce delusional symptoms and hallucinations, and engaged in bizarre behavior such as masturbating in public and defecating in the living room of his house. From then on his history is a series of hospitalizations, remissions, releases, and relapses. In the course of the interview it becomes evident that when the patient behaves psychotically the family withdraws from him, but when not swamps him with infantilizing concern, only to withdrawn again as soon as he behaves symptomically. At the end of the interview the psychiatrist tells them: "It is evidently most important for you (the patient) and your family to differentiate clearly between your betraying, abandoning father and you yourself by declaring you insane and therefore not responsible for any action that may make you look like your father. Therefore, we shall suspend any attempt at curing you, for what you are doing is needed by you and your family." In fact, no further family meeting was proposed and the patient's individual therapy was discontinued. He was offered to request medication each day if he wished so, "for needing medication is as good a way of defining you insane as your symptoms."

About a month after this session he requested his discharge from the hospital and has so far remained free of symptoms for 12 months, a time span unheard of in his past. (Sluzki 1981, p. 278–279)

Clearly, this is an outcome for which none of the existing theories and therapies of schizophrenia, divergent as they may otherwise be from one another, can account. This being so, the claim of having achieved a long-term remission in a chronic schizophrenic in a single family session, is bound to be rejected in negative unison. The rejection is most likely to involve an *ex post facto* reasoning: Since it is *known* that schizophrenia is a serious mental illness of uncertain origin and difficult treatment, any condition that can be influenced by a brief intervention at the end of just one therapy session cannot, *for this reason*, be schizophrenia. This form of syllogism is well expressed by Salzman in his critique of a book dealing with the successful outcomes of behavior therapy with phobias: "(The author) defines the condition (i.e., phobias) in a way that is acceptable only to conditioning theorists and does not fulfill the criteria of the psychiatric condition of this disorder. Therefore, his statements should not apply to phobias, but to some other condition." (Salzman 1968)

The history of science is full of such mental acrobatics. "If the facts contradict the theory, so much the worse for the facts," Hegel is supposed to have said more than 150 years ago. In other words, once a theory has been accepted as "true," any facts contradicting its truth must be irrelevant or wrong, or – worse still – are likely to lead to a refinement of the theory, but not to its revision "from first premises." Only a "scientific revolution" in Kuhn's sense (1970) can make such a revision possible.

It is my contention that the controversy raging over the subject of schizophrenia or, for that matter, any functional disorder as well as over their treatment is of exactly the same kind. Endless time and tens of thousands of pages of learned books and journals are put into the service of establishing, once and for all, that one theory is right and the others therefore wrong. But the purpose of scientific investigation is not and cannot be the discovery of truth. Eternal truth has no place in science – least of all on a subject as intangible and self-reflexive as the human mind. The only sensible criterion is the greater *efficacy* of one approach rather than of another.

What relevance does all this have to the subject matter of this chapter? Apparently very little. Apparently this is nothing but a dilettantish excursion into epistemology rather than the description of a therapeutic technique that could be of some use to the clinician who has to deal with the stark manifestations of schizophrenia.

But this objection *is* the problem. It demands information on practical applications and it refuses to question the assumptions underlying these applications. In this sense it is analogous to the joke about the judge who asks the defendant: "Have you stopped beating your wife? Answer 'yes' or 'no'," and threatens him with contempt of court when he tries to explain that neither "yes" nor "no" applies, because he has *never* beaten his wife.

In other words: If it is assumed that the cause of schizophrenia is explained by one of the existing theories, then there is no need to look elsewhere and the unsatisfactory results of treatment are due to shortcomings of technique. If, on the other hand, all these theories were concepts "that the *observer* invokes to fill the gap when part of the system is unobservable" or – more likely – is observable but considered irrelevant to or inconsistent with the premises of a particular theory, then the theory *itself* is in need of revision.

A case like the one reported by Sluzki can be shrugged off as irrelevant in terms of existing theories; or it can be seen as the example of an outcome that becomes possible when observable facts are not *a priori* censored according to their theoretical relevance or irrelevance. Essentially this is an anthropological and not a psychiatric approach. As is known, the training in these two professions is different to the point of mutual exclusiveness. The psychiatrist typically attempts to unravel a patient's pathology on the strength of his knowledge of psychopathology. He tries to elucidate the *causes* of the psychiatric condition. Ideally, the anthropologist does the opposite: In studying an alien culture he tries to keep his mind as free from preconceived assumptions as possible, and he tries to understand that particular culture *on its own terms*, rather than in terms of its deviance from the norms of his own culture. He tries to understand the *effects* of these culture-specific patterns by observing them in the here and now, rather than by investigating their historic origin.

This approach was introduced into psychiatry by the anthropologist Gregory Bateson and his research group in 1956 through their by now classical paper, "Toward a Theory of Schizophrenia" (Bateson 1956), postulating the concept of the double bind. With hindsight wisdom it can indeed be called a reeximination from first premises. Space limitations do not permit to give here a detailed overview of this revision, but the conclusions of major relevance to this paper are the following:

1. In spite of its title the paper is not so much a theory of schizophrenia, as a basically new way of looking at the formation of human problems in general. Subsequent studies have not only shown the presence of double bind patterns in other major clinical pictures (Sluzki et al. 1971; Sluzki et al. 1976; Watzlawick 1969), but also the potentially therapeutic nature of these patterns (Berger 1978; Watzlawick et al. 1974).
2. The patterns are seen as existing in the here and now, as circular action-reaction processes between people, i.e., in human systems.

3. The circular causality of these patterns (with reaction feeding back into and thus modifying action) has a systemic nature of its own. It cannot be reduced to any one of the myriads of causes that went into its making in the course of time. In classical Gestalt terms, these patterns are more than and different from the sum of its parts.

4. This being so, the question as to *why* the so-called Identified Patient behaves the way he behaves (which is the question underlying the traditional reductionistic, linear, cause-effect approach to mental problems) is replaced by the question: "*What* is going on here and now?"

5. To ask *what*? instead of *why*? is a cybernic approach.

In dealing with the phenomenon of change and of the transformations involved in change, Ashby specifically points to the difference between these two questions:

Notice that the transformation is defined, not by any reference to what it "really" is, nor by any reference to the physical cause of the change, but by the giving of a set of operands and a statement of what each is changed to. The transformation is concerned with what *happens, not* why *it happens. (Ashby 1963, p. 11)*

There is another reason for the dwindling importance of the question *why*. Modern biology teaches us that the decisive element that can start a whole train of new, complex developments may be a chance event of the kind which comes about at the point of the fortuitous intersection of two independent causal chains. But once this chance event has occurred, the process set in motion by it usually is of an enormously complex, rule-governed nature. In view of this, the French biologist Jacques Monod (1970), for instance, speaks of Chance and Necessity as the two great interdependent principles of evolution. In fact, during the last 25 years intense interdisciplinary studies have been carried out in what is now known as *autopoiesis* (self-production), i.e., a "newly emerging category of paradigms addressing the issues of self-organization and spontaneous phenomena within physical, biological, and social systems" (Zeleny 1981). This as yet by no means unified approach to the processes of perseverance, change, and perturbations is linked with such names as Francisco Varela, Humberto Maturana, Ricardo Uribe, Ilya Prigogine, Henri Atlan, Gordon Pask, and many others.

As we study the immediate circumstance surrounding the outbreak of a psychotic crisis and as we resist the temptation of filling in the gaps in our understanding of the crisis by taking recourse in the "dormitive principles" of some existing theory, we may discover analogies to the findings of the researchers just mentioned, namely the effects of chance events on the eruption of seemingly monolithic crises.

This is the basis of the brief therapy approach not just to schizophrenia, but to any problem that may be termed a functional pathology: a careful investigation of the practical, concrete circumstances coinciding with the onset of the crisis. This search will yield a specific event or a set of connected events that either occurred for the first time and were mishandled or – more likely – will reveal the recurrence of particular events for which the same inappropriate and unsuccessful attempts at solving them were again applied, as already in the past. What is meant by just such a set of circumstances and how a chance event can further complicate them is illustrated by the following example:

A young woman in intensive psychotherapy develops the suspicion that her therapist has hired the services of a colleague to spy on her. It turns out that this colleague is a psychiatrist who occasionally substitutes for her therapist on weekends. She, therefore, knows his name (Dr. F.) but has never seen him. In a session she angrily reports that he again followed her around during a recent visit to a park. Her therapist suggests that she make an appointment with Dr. F. to see if this is indeed the man. She accepts the idea, but in order to save money decides that she will just sit in Dr. F's waiting room shortly before the full hour so that she can take a look at him when he dismisses one patient and asks the next one into his office.

It so happens that Dr. F. has an appointment with a new female patient whom *he* has not yet seen and who is late for her first visit. On finding the young woman waiting, he of course assumes her to be his new patient and in a matter-of-fact way says: "Oh, there you are already – I'll be with you in just a moment."

The patient realizes that, on the one hand, Dr. F. is not the man she saw in the park, but on the other hand his remark "proves" to her that he knows her and was expecting her. The suspicion of an ominous coalition between the two therapists is now much stronger, and is further compounded by both therapists' attempts to clarify the "innocent" nature of the complication.

The next example has very much the same structure, except that the chance event is replaced by a deliberate action undertaken with the best of intentions:

An elderly woman is in counseling for some rather minor, long-standing difficulties with her daugther and her daughter's husband in whose home she lives. She has the unpleasant impression (and many incidents to prove it) that the young couple is overprotective and intrusive. In particular she suspects that her son-in-law has recently installed hidden microphones in her part of the (rather large) house. She now feels invisibly surveilled even with doors and windows closed. When she complains and demands to know what is going on, she only gets evasive answers.

Rather than to interpret this idea as a well-documented part of many involutional complications, the psychiatrist decides to have a session with the young couple. Without being asked, they immediately express their concern for the old lady's failing health and their fear that she may fall, fracture a leg or a hip, and then lie helplessly in her part of the house, perhaps for several hours, without being discovered. Therefore the husband, who is an electronics engineer, decided to install microphones in her rooms, but in order to avoid worrying the old lady "unnecessarily," he and his wife decided not to tell her about these installations.

This example is nothing but a more flamboyant version of the numerous stories, known to every clinician, of medication being mixed into somebody's food who promptly develops "delusions" of being poisoned by his family, or of the supposedly "merciful" lies to trick somebody into hospitalization, to say nothing about what we now know about the famous Schreber case (Niederland 1974; Schatzmann 1973) and the starkly concrete external facts connected with it. Clearly, in all of these instances the attempt to look for the pathology in just one person in a system of relationships can be accomplished only at the price of attributing "dormitive principles" to that individual.

Of course, to all of this one may point out that an abnormal situation already existed before the trigger event occured, for otherwise, i.e., under "normal" circumstances, a human system would have no difficulty coping with the event. But by the same logic one might just as well argue that the crisis would never have arisen without the trigger event. This means further that the obvious goal of therapeutic intervention must be that particular event and its immediate consequences, so as to restore that human system to a level of adequate functioning. The purpose of responsible, realistic therapy cannot be a problem-free life, but adequate functioning – a term that embraces a wide gamut of more or less successful adaptations to the ups and downs of life, but is far from perfection.

Practical experience with these crisis teaches us that usually a difficult situation exists for a long time, but without any need for outside expert help, until a trigger event of the kind described above produces a crisis. The direct, practical consequences of this event are then typically dealt with by all concerned in a counterproductive, deviation-amplifying way. These attempted solutions then compound what started as a mere coincidence or a practical difficulty into a problem that is beyond the coping powers of the system, and snowball into dilemmas of bizarre proportions. Experience further teaches us that the difference between acute and chronic pathology is merely one of duration: chronic problems have been mishandled *longer*, but in very much the same way, than acute ones.

Taking these factors into account enables the therapist to intervene effectively and rapidly, as exemplified by the following case which was originally described elsewhere and in a different context (Fisch 1972, pp. 614–615):

A woman in her fifties came for help because her 25 year-old chronically schizophrenic son seemed on the verge of another psychotic break. Since the age of 15 he had spent most of his time in mental hospitals and had been in almost continuous intensive psychotherapy. He was asked to come in with his mother on her second visit. Although his statements were riddled with cryptic remarks, unlabelled metaphors, and other speech characteristics of schizophrenia, he did, when presses for a description of the *present* problem, explain his concrete dilemma: He was living a marginal existence in a rented room, financially supported by his parents. However, he could never be sure how much money he was going to receive from them and when. From the way the mother described the problem, it became clear that the parents found it unfeasible to give him a certain amount on a regular basis, because they were convinced that he would foolishly squander it within a few days and then demand more. It also seemed that their way of doling out money to him was determined by their judgement as to how sanely or how crazily he was behaving at any given time. The uncertainty created by this attempted solution contributed to his erratic behavior which, in turn, convinced the parents that another psychotic episode was imminent.

At this point the therapist made his intervention by instructing the son to *deliberately* utilize psychotic behavior, explaining that since the son felt helpless to contend with his parents' stubborn refusals to comply with his wish for a fixed weekly (or even monthly) living allowance, he had the right to defend himself by threatening to cause an even greater expenditure by his having to go to a mental hospital again. Therefore, the therapist suggested again, he should turn on psychotic behavior which the therapist described very much in terms of the eccentricities displayed by the patient in the course of the session. With this the session was terminated. The mother was seen individually for a few more times, during which she stated that she was now uncertain which of the son's behaviors were "really" crazy and which were feigned.

In the follow-up interview several months later it turned out that the mother had begun to feel much less threatened by her son's behavior and had been paying him a larger amount on a regular basis, making it clear that with this money he could sink or swim. The son, on the other hand, had managed to save enough of this money to buy an old car which in turn gave him much greater independence from his mother who until then had been acting as his chauffeuse.

This, of course, is not a "cure" of schizophrenia – but then, what is? The result is a significant, practical improvement of a situation which without the therapeutic intervention would probably have led to another hospitalization with all its additional economic, psychological, and social consequences. To many therapists a small, concrete, limited, and presumably not life-long improvement is not good enough. But he who operates with more grandiose designs may find himself with less grandiose results, or as Robert Ardrey (1970) once put it: "While we pursue the unattainable we make impossible the realizable".

The main ideas presented in this chapter were tested on a large scale not at the Mental Research Institute but independently by a group of clinicians and researchers who had arrived at similar practical conclusions. This work began in 1964 at the Family Treatment Unit of the Colorado Psychiatric Hospital in Denver under the direction of the psychiatrist Donald Langsley. Their main goal was the avoidance of hospitalization of acutely psychotic patients. They attempted this by means of an investigation of the circumstances of the precipitating crisis in the course of the first session in which all available family members were brought together as soon as the Identified Patient had been admitted to the Unit. For research and evaluation purposes these admittances were made on a random basis. To quote from one of their reports:

The request for hospitalization of one member of the family is assumed to evolve from a series of events. A hazardous event such as a death, maturation of a child, a job change or a host of other "usual problems of living," requires adjustment. Most families master these stresses without serious decompensation, but when the family includes a susceptible individual or when the family has become used to dealing with problems by using psychiatric hospitals, the stage may be set for symptoms of mental illness. (Langsley et al. 1968, p. 146)

In 1968 the Denver Group published the results of the first 75 (randomly assigned) cases treated by them and the comparison with a control group of 75 other patients who underwent routine psychiatric hospitalization at the same hospital. They reported:

Of the 75 family crisis cases, none *were hospitalized during the crisis treatment. Instead of being hospitalized they were treated by an average of 4.2 office sessions, 1.6 home visits, 4.5 telephone calls and 1.3 contacts with other social agencies. Of the 75 control cases, all were hospitalized. They were in the hospital a total of 1,959 days, an average of 26.1 days per case. In other words, none of the experimentals and 100 per cent of the controls became mental hospital patients as a result of the current problems and the treatment approach. (Langsley and Kaplan 1968, p. 161)*

The study also shows that the Denver group did not simply postpone hospitalization, but that the recidivism rate of their sample was much lower than that of the control group:

... For the controls (hospital cases) 13 (17%) of the sample were rehospitalized within a month after discharge. Over the next 5 months an additional three of the 75 cases were readmitted to a psychiatric hospital. By the end of six months, 21 per cent of the sample had been readmitted to a mental hospital. Of the 75 Family Treatment Unit cases, only five were admitted to a mental hospital during the first month. This

represents 7 per cent of the sample rather than 17 per cent. By the end of six months, a total of 14 patients had been hospitalized at one point or the other. This does not look enormously different for experimentals and controls. It would suggest that perhaps we have only delayed hospitalization rather than prevented it. If we had only delayed hospitalization, our subsequent hospitalization rate would be much higher than that of the controls. In fact it is lower. *(Langsley and Kaplan 1968, p. 162)*

The general approach described in this paper almost necessarily imposes certain departures from routine clinical practice. To conclude my presentation, I want to list some of them here without claiming this list to be complete or exhaustive:

1. If it is accepted that the very first contact with a new case is decisive, then it stands to reason that it must be made by the most experienced therapist available. Traditionally, the very opposite is the case: The intake interview is considered a lowly routine job and left to an intern or first-year resident. This practice is blind to the enormous therapeutic potential of this first contact for the entire course of treatment, to say nothing about the individual, familial, social, and economic consequences of being declared insane. For, as Rosenhan (1973) has shown, the diagnostic label routinely slapped on every case constructs a reality all of its own which by the nature of the ensuing interaction perpetuates itself. And once a schizophrenic, always a schizophrenic – because everybody "knows" what that is.

2. If diagnostic terms cannot be avoided altogether, they should at least be used as verbs and not as nouns. It is considerably less heuristic to think of *schizophrenia* as a thing, than to think in terms of *being* or *acting schizophrenic*, i.e., as the sum of behaviors in a specific context.

3. If it is accepted that the chance of intervening rapidly and decisively is lost by the routine application of some standardized intake procedure, it follows that only the immediate past must be concentrated on. What then matters are effects, not causes. Any attempt to explore the remote genesis of the problem in the Identified Patient's individual life is of little, if any, practical value. A detailed history makes sense in the linear model of intrapsychic treatment, but not in the interactional, system-oriented paradigm. One might even go so far as to suspect that the only effect of a well-taken history is to reduce the therapist to almost the same state of hopelessness and pessimism as his patients, and to blind him to the decisive facts and therapeutic potentialities inherent in the here and now.

4. In line with all of this, the question to be asked is not the time-honored *Why?* (i.e., why does the patient behave the way he is behaving?), but rather *What for?*. In other words, what specific purpose is served by that behavior in the interactional situation of which the patient is a part? This is another way of saying that his behavior may appear bizarre and pathological only when considered in monadic isolation, but when examined in its natural context reveals itself as the best possible – perhaps the *only* possible – adaptation to that context. It thus becomes the royal road towards the understanding of the pathogenic situation itself.

5. Once the dynamics of that situation are sufficiently understood, the task of therapy then consists in the introduction into this system of new behavior patterns which the system was unable to generate from within itself. As explained in detail elsewhere (Watzlawick 1978; Watzlawick et al. 1974), these interventions into a disturbed system are *active* ones and do not rely on the classic methods of explanation,

confrontation, interpretation, etc., but rather on direct behavior prescriptions, therapeutic double binds and positive connotations.

6. The goals of these interventions are concrete, practical, pragmatic changes and improvements, and not nebulous constructs like self-esteem, ego strength, emotional catharsis, consciousness raising, or the decoding of the deep, symbolic meaning of the patient's psychotic actions and verbalizations. Admittedly this is a radical departure from established practice which considers insight the precondition of change. But, as Heinz von Foerster once concluded: "If you desire to see, learn how to act" (Foerster 1973, p. 46).

References

Ardrey R (1970) The social contract. Atheneum, New York, p 3

Arieti S (1959) Schizophrenia: Other aspects; psychotherapy. In: Arieto S (ed) American Handbook of Psychiatry, vol 1. Basic Books, New York, p 501

Ashby W (1963) An introduction to cybernetics. John Wiley & Sons, New York

Bateson G et al. (1956) Toward a theory of schizophrenia. Behav Sci 1:251–264

Berger M (1978) Beyond the double bind. Brunner/Mazel, New York

Bleuler E (1930) Textbook of psychiatry. Macmillian, New York

Bleuler E (1950) Dementia praecox, or the group of schizophrenias. International Universities Press, New York

Fisch R et al. (1972) On unbecoming family therapists. In: Andrew Ferber et al. (eds) The book of family therapy. Science House, New York, pp 597–617

Foerster H von (1973) On constructing a reality. In: Preiser WFE (ed) Environmental research design, vol 2. Dowden, Hutchinson & Ross, Stroudsburg, pp 35–46

Glover E (1956) Freud or Jung? Meridian Books, New York

Korzybski A (1933) Science and sanity. Internat. Non-Aristotelian Library, New York

Kuhn TS (1970) The structure of scientific revolutions. University of Chicago Press, Chicago

Langsley DG et al. (1968) Family crisis therapy – results and implications. Fam Process 7:145–158

Langsley DG, Kaplan DM (1968) The treatment of families in crisis. Grune & Stratton, New York

Monod J (1970) Le hasard et la nécessité. Le Seuil, Paris

Niederland WG (1974) The Schreber case. Quadrangle Books, New York

Pfungst O (1965) Clever Hans. In: Rosenthal R (ed) Holt, Rinehart & Winston, New York

Rosenhan DL (1973) On being sane in insane places. Science 179:250–258

Salzman L (1968) Reply to critics. Int J Psychiatry 6:473–476

Schatzman M (1973) Soul murder. Random House, New York

Sluzki CE (1981) Process of symptom production and patterns of symptom maintenance. J Marit Fam Ther 7:273–280

Sluzki CE, Verón E (1971) The double bind as a universal pathogenic situation. Fam Process, 10: 397–410

Sluzki CE, Ransom DC (eds) (1976) Double bind. Grune & Stratton, New York

Watzlawick P (1969) Patterns of psychotic communication. In: Doucet P, Laurin C (eds) Problems of psychosis. Excerpta Medica Foundation, Amsterdam, pp 44–53

Watzlawick P (1978) The language of change. Basic Books, New York

Watzlawick P et al. (1974) Change. WW Norton, New York

Zeleny M (ed) (1981) Autopoiesis. Elsevier North Holland, New York, p xv

A Psychoeducational Model of Family Treatment for Schizophrenia

Carol M. Anderson

This chapter describes a model of family intervention that has been developed as one part of a research project which is investigating the impact of various strategies of intervention in the aftercare of patients with schizophrenia.[1] The larger research project screens patients to insure they meet research diagnostic criteria for schizophrenia, rates their family members on a measure of expressed emotion developed in Britain by Brown and his colleagues (Brown and Birley 1968; Brown et al. 1972; Vaughn and Leff 1976; Leff and Vaughn 1980), and randomly assigns patients with high expressed emotion families to one of four treatment cells: family therapy and medication, social skills training and medication, family therapy, social skills training and medication; or medication alone. Patients and their families are followed in these treatment modalities for 2 years with various measures of individual and family functioning taken at periodic intervals. This chapter will briefly note the assumptions and goals of the family program, describe its components and stages, present some preliminary findings about its effectiveness alone and in combination with social skills training, and list some of the insights gleaned from the first $2^1/2$ years of attempting to apply this model of family intervention.

Assumptions

We assume that whatever the "cause" of schizophrenia, two observations are extremely relevant to the development of treatment programs. First, patients with schizophrenia appear to have a "core psychological deficit" in which vulnerability to internal and external stimuli is increased (Broen and Storms 1966; Lang and Buss 1965; Payne et al. 1959; Rabin et al. 1979; Shakow 1962; Silverman 1972; Tecce and Cole 1976; Venables 1964, 1978). Second, some families of schizophrenics display a range of stimulating behaviors and emotions that are likely to negatively affect patients who are assumed to be vulnerable to such stimulation. Communication in families of schizophrenic patients is likely to include communicative behaviors that are intense, vague, unclear, amorphous, tangential, or lacking in acknowledgement (Goldstein and Rodnick 1975; Jacob 1975; Jones 1977; Jones et al 1977; Singer and Wynne 1966;

1 This research project, under the direction of Gerard Hogarty, is partially funded by Grant No. MH 30750 from the National Institute of Mental Health.

Singer and Wynne 1965; Wynne 1961). Whether or not these communication patterns predate the illness or contribute to its etiology, it would seem logical that a patient who has problems controlling and processing stimuli would have difficulty coping with these complicated and confusing family communications.

Furthermore, when a patient becomes acutely psychotic, the family usually reports feelings of anxiety, guilt, anger, and sadness (Hatfield 1978; Kreisman and Joy 1974). These emotions are likely to increase the intensity of family life, and since the illness is a chronic one, are likely to increase over time as family members are unable to find ways to help the patient. It might be hypothesized that family members in such chronic crises would come to respond to the patient in one of the two ways that Brown et al. (1972) have described as components of high expressed emotion: becoming overinvolved, with attempts to constantly monitor and protect the patient from himself or the environment, or becoming critical, frustrated, angry, rejecting, and withdrawn from both the patient and the systems that treat him. Either of these emotional responses would appear both to accentuate the family's inability to cope with the patient's behaviors, and to be problematic for a patient vulnerable to intense stimuli. In fact, the data from these British studies support the idea that these family emotional factors relate to the course of the patient's illness. They maintain that families manifesting high expressed emotion (EE), principally reflected in emotional overinvolvement and criticism, tend to have patient members with relapse rates of over 50% in the first 9 months after hospitalization as compared to relapse rates of 13% among patients from low EE households (Brown and Birley 1968; Brown et al. 1972).

In summary then, these two forces – the patient's vulnerability and the family turmoil – probably interact to the patient's disadvantage in a spiraling manner, the patient's vulnerability to stimuli causing symptoms which upset family members who in turn upset the patient and so on.

Because of this hypothesized relationship between patient vulnerability and family anxiety or behaviors, this family project was designed to accomplish two goals: (1) to decrease the patient's vulnerability to stimuli through a program of maintenance chemotherapy; and (2) to decrease the intensity of the family environment through a program which provided the family with support, information, structure, and specific coping mechanisms to use in dealing with a psychotic family member. The program was designed with the hope that a directive approach would increase the predictability and stability of the family environment by increasing their self-confidence and knowledge about the illness, thereby decreasing family anxiety about the patient and their ability to react helpfully to him.

The program has four basic overlapping phases, separated here for the sake of clarity. Since the entire program is discussed in more detail elsewhere (Anderson et al. 1980), only the major points will be stressed.

Phase I: Connecting with the Family

Based on the assumption that no intervention can succeed unless the family can hear or use it constructively, the first phase of treatment, which emphasizes the establishment of an alliance with the family, begins immediately after the patient's admission to the hospital. Since *all* families begin the program during a serious crisis, and *most* have had multiple unsuccessful contacts with other hospitals and professionals, special attention is given to the creation of an atmosphere which increases the family's receptivity to treatment interventions. Phase I interventions first involve joining the family, eliciting their reactions to the patient's illness and to past attempts to cope with it, as well as their perceptions of their own current needs and problems. Hopefully, these discussions communicate to the family that the therapist cares about what they have been through, is not critical about their role with the patient, and genuinely wants to know and learn about their ideas and views of what is helpful.

Once the family has begun to form a relationship with the therapist, he establishes himself as their ombudsman or representative in relationship to the hospital system. Since the inpatient hospital staff are primarily involved with the patient on a daily basis, it is easy for them to neglect families or fail to see the family's perspective. The creation of a family representative serves to balance this skewed perspective and prevent the alienation of families from the treatment team. Thus, the family ombudsman keeps the family informed of ward decisions about the patient, ensures the input of family concerns and needs into treatment planning, and provides the family with structure and concrete help in coping with the illness and the hospitalization. In this way, the therapist also begins to mobilize the family's concern and involvement into constructive attempts to help themselves and the patient. By the end of the hospitalization (which usually is less than 3–4 weeks), the family and therapist have arrived at a treatment contract which roughly specifies the goals, content, length, rules, and methods of the aftercare family program. This program, then, continues for 1–2 years after the patient's discharge from the hospital.

Phase II: The Survival Skills Workshop

Based on the assumption that people are more anxious about what they do not understand, the survival skills workshop seeks to provide the family with as much information as possible about the nature of schizophrenia. The workshop was designed as a multiple family enterprise in order to simultaneously promote de-isolation of the family and desensitization about the subject of mental illness. It is a day long event attended by all the members of four or five families new to the program. (The patient does not attend.) Every attempt is made to encourage an informal atmosphere in which families can question professionals and interact with one another. The workshop is held as early in the treatment process as possible because it also serves to establish the basic themes of the entire family program. The workshop focuses on the following categories of information.

Information About the Illness

The most recent data about the phenomenology, onset, treatment, course, and outcome of schizophrenic disorders is presented in clear, understandable language. Theories of etiology, ranging from genetic and biochemical to familial and cultural, are explained. What is known about the prognosis of the illness (including the risk of relapse on and off medication) is also outlined, as are various methods of treatment; psychotherapy, pharmacology, megavitamins, hemodialysis. Every attempt is made to discriminate between facts and theories or opinions about each of these issues. Because medication compliance is viewed as a crucial component of the program, the importance of antipsychotic medication is given special attention. Mechanisms of action, possible negative side effects, and the use of antiparkinsonian agents are explained. In particular, the critical importance of the family's support for and feedback about the medication program is stressed.

Information About Management of the Illness

Following the presentation of general facts and theories, the family is introduced to a series of techniques for managing the patient. Based on the assumption that families cannot accept staff suggestions unless they genuinely believe that staff know how hard it has been to cope with this illness, and the magnitude of the request the staff is making of them, this discussion begins with a description of what they have probably done over the years that has not worked.

Following this description, the family is told that while there is no evidence that families cause schizophrenia, there is reason to believe that families have the power to influence the course of the illness. They are helped to see the need to create barriers to overstimulation of the patient by establishing boundaries. Special attention is given to the patient's need for structure, modified expectations, and clear communication. The family is given permission and even encouragement to set limits on unacceptable behaviors. This theme is translated into specific suggestions for responding to the patient's fears, delusions, paranoid thoughts, obsessive rituals, or threats of violence. Finally, the family is strongly encouraged to avoid centering their lives around the patient. They are asked to attend to their own needs, the needs of other family members, and to mobilize a social support network to maintain their own abilities to cope and survive over time.

Phase III: Reentry and Application of Workshop Themes

Highly structured low-key individual family sessions are held as soon as the acute phase of the illness has been controlled sufficiently to enable the patient to attend. Once the patient has left the hospital, these sessions occur once every 2–3 weeks. The interventions of these sessions are based on the themes established in the survival skills workshop, and relate largely to the reinforcement of family boundaries and the gradual resumption of responsibility by the patient.

Three kinds of boundaries are stressed. The interpersonal boundaries between family members, the generational boundaries between parents and offspring, and the family boundary with the larger social community support system. The first two types of boundaries are reinforced, largely by encouraging families to establish clear expectations, rules, and limit setting processes. The third type of boundary, that between the family and the community, is weakened by stressing the family's need for the development of a support system beyond the nuclear family.

Over time, the patient is gradually encouraged to assume more responsibility for his life and functioning. Initially, the entire treatment focus is on the patient's survival outside of the hospital. As signs of change begin to occur in the patient, the sessions gradually emphasize a return to effective work and social functioning. This is initially accomplished by the assignment of small household tasks or tasks which involve a minimal amount of socialization with outsiders. Later, more ambitious tasks are assigned and the family is encouraged to increase their expectations of the patient. Since progress on these issues is exceedingly slow, a great deal of support is given to family members to enable them to tolerate inactivity, amotivation, and apathy.

Phase IV: Continued Treatment or Disengagement

Once the goals for effective functioning have been attained (and these goals differ depending on the patient's abilities, the length of his impairment, and the family's level of tolerance), the model calls for the family to be presented with two possible options for treatment: (1) more traditional, family-oriented treatment to resolve long-term family conflicts, or unfinished business; or (2) periodic supportive maintenance session of gradually decreasing frequency. The first three phases of this model of family intervention do not offer families the opportunity to deal with general family issues and problems. In fact, the model specifically discourages self-reflection and the discussion of upsetting topics. Nevertheless, some of these issues could interfere with the ongoing growth and development of family members, and once the crisis has passed, family members may wish to devote their energies to resolving them. Unless it is thought that the issues will have an immediate negative impact on the patient's progress, families are offered a choice about this phase of treatment, since contracting with the project to help the patient is not thought to give us the right to unilaterally determine the family's general goals or methods of coping with them.

Comments on the Method

Each of the phases of the program has presented its own issues or problems. Phase I, connecting with the family, has been difficult to operationalize as early as it should be because of the need for the research team to rate and assign patients before families can be assigned to the family clinician. It is our clinical impression that the longer the delay, the more difficult it is to form an alliance with family members.

Phase II, the survival skills workshop, has been the most exciting component of the program. In one day, resistant and skeptical families become interested and supportive of both the patient and the efforts of the treatment team. It is unclear why this workshop has such an enormous impact. One reason may be that actual information (the content) is useful in decreasing family anxiety. The information and concrete suggestions may give structure to the family's life in a time of uncertainty and crisis. Most families comment that although they do not feel that all of what they hear is positive, it is better than not knowing and feeling that professionals will not tell them the truth. Another possible reason for the impact of the workshop may be that the de-isolation of this multiple family experience positively influences a family's feelings about themselves, and provides them with the support of knowing others are attempting to cope with similar experiences. Certainly, the contact with other families seems important. In the original design of the program, the workshop was the only multiple family component. The plan involved primarily encouraging families to develop or use their own support network. Later, by popular demand, many families are still meeting together on a periodic basis. They seem to have formed an action-set network in which they help one another to cope. This special network appears to be useful in a way that general networks are not, since other families experiencing the illness understand what they are going through in a way that no one else does.

Finally, it may be that the metacommunication inherent in the workshop is the most useful component. Essentially, families are told that they are not to blame for the patient's illness, and are reassured that their attempts to cope have been normal responses to a difficult situation. This metamessage may enable families both to hear the suggestions of the staff and to develop their own coping mechanisms, since they have less of a need to defend against their own natural fears, responsibility, and guilt, and what they see as the implicit accusations of professionals.

During Phase III, reentry, the most serious problem encountered is that of coping with the patient's deficit (negative) symptoms of amotivation, apathy, and excessive sleep. During this phase of treatment, we have come to emphasize the need for patience and tolerance on the part of the family, while continuously pushing for the accomplishment of small tasks or small signs of effort on the part of the patient. This effort is made not only to prevent the patient's tendencies to become completely inactive or accepting of a permanently lowered level of functioning, but also to maintain family and staff morale.

The Phase IV plan of offering families a choice of an exploratory kind of family therapy or maintenance sessions has not materialized. While the family sessions tend to become a little more intense as time goes on, the length of time necessary to accomplish the initial goals of effective functioning has prevented a commitment to resolving more subtle or more general issues. In reality, this phase of treatment seems to continue the concentration on effective work and social functioning for the patient and support for the families in tolerating the slowness of the process of change.

Preliminary Results

This program has currently been in effect for a little over $2^1/_2$ years, and has involved 31 patients and their families. The patient group at this time consists of 23 males and 8 females, has a mean age of 29.1 years, has been ill for an average of 8.6 years, and hospitalized an average of 3.5 times. The results reported here are imcomplete and are based on small numbers in each group, but represent some interesting trends. A comparison is made of all those receiving family therapy with those being maintained on drugs and individual support alone. The relapse rates of this control group is consistent with most of the relapse rates reported in the literature, that is, about 48%. Combining the two groups that received family therapy with and without social skills training produces a relapse rate of about 16%, or one-third that of patients treated only by medication and individual support. Those patients in both family therapy and social skills training seem to do best of all, with no relapses having occured in this group over a period of 3 years.

Later reports will include a great deal of data about the quality of life for patients and families in each of the groups. At this point, it is only possible to say that there appear to be some qualitative differences for family members. For instance, measure of family distress pretreatment and a year later reveals that follow-up reports of family distress for those exposed to family therapy is significantly lower than those reported by high EE family controls.

Discussion

This program of aftercare for families and patients with schizophrenia appears to be effective in maintaining patients in their communities, avoiding the need for psychiatric hospitalization. The important components of the program seem to include the establishment of a collaborative relationship between therapist and family, the provision of information and support, and the creation of highly structured predictable environments in the treatment setting and in the home. These components appear to be present in similar projects, beginning with that of Goldstein and his colleagues (Goldstein et al. 1978; Goldstein and Kopeikin 1981) and including those of Liberman (Liberman et al. 1979; Snyder and Liberman 1981), Falloon (Falloon et al. 1981a, b), and Berkowitz (Berkowitz et al. 1981). Each of these programs appears to be reporting similar results.

While several of the other programs are explicitly behavioral in nature, this particular model of family intervention is not. While it does emphasize concrete tasks and observable behaviors, its goals for families are primarily structural in nature. Nevertheless, the model appears to be most effective when used in conjunction with a behavioral program of social skills training for individual patients. Because the social skills program appears to be so significant, it will be described briefly. (More detailed descriptions of this particular version of social skills training are in progress.)

The *social skills training* program attempts to decrease patient vulnerability to stress by increasing the patient's ability to deal with people effectively. Each patient is assessed individually to determine his or her level of interpersonal functioning. After the assessment is completed, patient and therapist choose specific behavioral goals on which they can agree. These goals always include attempts to increase desirable social interaction and decrease undesirable interaction by focusing on two issues: the patient's social perception and the patient's social behavior. In the category of social perception, the ability to perceive social cues accurately is stressed, helping patients to assess what is going on in social situations and to judge how others are responding to their behaviors. In the category of social behavior, patients are actually taught what to do, verbally and nonverbally, to get their messages across to others. Particular attention is given to helping patients decrease their vulnerability to stimulation by increasing their ability to limit the upsetting behaviors of those around them. Direct teaching of more effective social behavior is operationalized and practiced through the use of role play and the use of self-observation of videotaped sessions to increase the patient's awareness of his/her impact on others.

Summary

While the program has been in effect less than 3 years, the comparable results that seem to be emerging from similar programs would tend to indicate that psychoeducational family approaches can be applied in diverse ways and diverse settings. Practicing the model, however, does require a particular kind of training that often flies in the face of clinical instincts and learned therapeutic roles. This method of therapy requires that therapists not deal explicitly with interesting individual and family dynamics, and that they learn to be comfortable being directive, firm, and explicit with families. Certainly this role has less mystique and requires more activity than many other forms of therapeutic intervention. It is not surprising, therefore, that care must be taken to avoid the problem of slipping into more common passive therapeutic practices as therapist use this model over the long term with chronic patients and their families.

References

Anderson C, Hogarty G, Reiss D (1980) Family treatment of adult schizophrenic patients: A psycho-educational approach. Schizophr Bull 6(3):490–505

Berkowitz R, Kuipers L, Eberlein-Frief R, Leff J (1981) Lowering expressed emotion in relatives of schizophrenics. In: Goldstein MJ (ed) New developments in interventions with families of schizophrenics. Jossey-Bass, San Francisco

Broen WE, Storms LH (1966) Lawful disorganization: The process underlying a schizophrenic syndrome. Psychol Rev 73:265–279

Brown, GW, Birley JLT (1968) Crises and life change and the onset of schizophrenia. J Health and Soc Behav 9:203–214

Brown GW, Birley JLT, Wing JH (1972) The influence of family life on the course of schizophrenic disorders. A replication. Br J Psychol 121:241–258

Falloon I, Boyd JL, McGill C, Strang J, Moss H (1981a) Family management training in the community care of schizophrenia. In: Goldstein MJ (ed) New developments in interventions with families of schizophrenics. Jossey-Bass, San Francisco

Falloon I, Liberman R, Lillie F, Vaughn C (1981b) Family therapy for relapsing schizophrenics and their families: A pilot study. Fam Process 20:211–222

Goldstein M, Kopeikin H (1981) Short and long term effects of combining drug and family therapy. In: Goldstein MJ (ed) New developments in interventions with families of schizophrenics. Jossey-Bass, San Francisco

Goldstein M, Rodnick E (1975) The family's contribution to the etiology of schizophrenia: Current status. Schizophr Bull 1(14):48–63

Goldstein MJ, Rodnick EH, Evans JR, May PR, Steinberg M (1978) Drug and family therapy in the aftercare treatment of acute schizophrenia. Arch Gen Psychiatry 35(10):1169–1177

Hatfield AB (1978) Psychological costs of schizophrenia to the family. Social Work 23(5):355–359

Jacob T (1915) Family interaction in disturbed and normal families: A methodological and substantive review. Psychol Bull 82:33–65

Jones JE (1977) Patterns of transactional style deviance in the TAT's of parents of schizophrenics. Fam Process 16:327–337

Jones JE, Rodnick E, Goldstein M, McPherson S, West K (1977) Parental transactional style deviance as a possible indicator of risk for schizophrenia. Arch Gen Psychiatry 34:71–74

Kreisman DE, Joy VD (1974) Family response to the mental illness of a relative: A review of the literature. Schizophr Bull 1(10):34–54

Lang PJ, Buss AH (1965) Psychological deficit in schizophrenia: Interference and activation. J Abnorm Psychol 70:77–106

Leff J, Vaughn C (1980) The interaction of life events and relatives' expressed emotion in schizophrenia and depressive neurosis. Br J Psychiatry 136:146–153

Liberman R, Aitchison R, Falloon I (1979) Family therapy in schizophrenia: Syllabus for therapists. Mental Health Clinic Research Center for the Study of Schizophrenics, Box A, Camarillo, Calif. 93010

Payne RW, Mattussek P, George EI (1959) An experimental study of schizophrenic thought disorder. J Ment Sci 105:624–652

Rabin AI, Doneson SL, Jentons RL (1979) Studies of psychological functions in schizophrenia. In: Bellak L (ed) Disorders of the schizophrenic syndrome. Basic Books, New York, pp 181–231

Shakow D (1962) Segmental set: A theory of the formal psychological deficit in schizophrenia. Arch Gen Psychiatry 6:1–17

Silverman J (1972) Stimulus intensity modulation and psychological disease. Psychopharmacologia 24:42–80

Singer MT, Wynne LC (1966) Communication styles in parents of normals, neurotics, and schizophrenics. Psychiatric Research Reports 20:25–38

Singer MT, Wynne LC (1965) Thought disorder and family relations of schizophrenics. Arch Gen Psychiatry 12:187–212

Snyder K, Liberman R (1981) Family assessment and intervention with schizophrenics at risk for relapse. In: Goldstein MJ (ed) New developments in interventions with families of schizophrenics. Jossey-Bass, San Francisco

Tecce JJ, Cole JO (1976) The distraction-arousal hypothesis, CNV and schizophrenia. In: Mostofsky DI (ed) Behavior control and modification of physiological activity. Prentice-Hall, Englewood Cliffs, NJ

Vaughn CE, Leff JP (1976) The influence of family and social factors on the course of psychiatric illness. Br J Psychiatry 129:125–137

Venables PH (1978) Cognitive disorder. In: Wing JK (ed) Schizophrenia: Towards a new synthesis. Academic Press, New York, pp 117–137

Venables PH (1964) Input dysfunction in schizophrenia. In: Maher BA (ed) Progress in experimental personality research, vol. 1. Academic Press, New York, pp 1–47

Wynne L (1961) The study of intra-familial alignments and splits in exploratory family therapy. In: Ackerman N, Beatman F, Sherman S (eds) Exploring the base for family therapy. Family Service Association of America, New York, pp 95–115

A New Method for Therapy and Research in the Treatment of Schizophrenic Families

Mara Selvini-Palazzoli and Giuliana Prata

Introduction

In Oslo, in 1975, at the 5th Symposium on the Psychotherapy of Schizophrenia, the subject of our lecture focused on our book, *Paradox and Counterparadox*,[1] which had been published in Italian a few months earlier. The book conveyed the results of a therapeutic program developed at our Center between 1972 and 1975 with 15 families presenting patients diagnosed as schizophrenic. We use the Bleulerian term of schizophrenia, now universally employed, to signify a particular behavioral pattern inseparable from the pattern observable in the natural group in which it occurs: the family. This work was characterized by the attempt to operate with methodological rigor, devising therapeutic interventions which would be rigorously consistent with the conceptual model we had adopted, the systemic model, strongly influenced by Bateson's thinking. We devised four therapeutic tools: the positive connotation of all behaviors of each family member, family rituals, lengthy intervals between sessions, and paradoxical reframing. The effects of these tools were quite often astonishing and confirmed the validity of our model. Working along this line we definitely rejected any and all temptations to teach the family. It was no longer a question of showing, explaining, interpreting, or helping the family understand their situation rationally. It was, rather, a question of grasping – as quickly as possible – the game inside the family which maintained the symptomatic behavior. Once the game was understood our objective was to devise an intervention which would prevent its continuation.

Even those who have no direct experience with our work can easily perceive the extent of the effort required from the team when faced with the difficulty of discovering in each family, especially in the family with schizophrenic organization, the specific ongoing game. Families with schizophrenic organization are like chameleons; they have an unbelievable capacity for not supplying information while at the same time appearing to be giving a great deal. It takes a tremendous amount of effort as a therapist to discern the wide variety of masking games. When this effort fails – as it frequently does – it is a very bitter experience. Little has been learned. To shield themselves behind the stereotyped assumption that the family resists change is not only a poor consolation but also reveals insufficient comprehension of that family's organization.

---

1 At that time our research team was formed by the four authors of the book. Since 1979 our research team has been composed by the authors of this article and Maurizio Viaro, MD

The primary objective remains to devise a method to collect the largest amount of crucial information. Accordingly, since May 1979, we have devoted ourselves to a new research program with families presenting schizophrenic patients. This research is ongoing and is expected to continue for a long time. During this period we have treated, and are still treating, 19 families (six presenting patients with chronic infantile psychosis, ten presenting chronic schizophrenic patients, and three presenting acute delusional patients). All of these patients represented extremely serious, discouraging cases.

Method

One must keep in mind that, even though we are speaking of research, our primary goal is therapeutic change. Our primary objective is the improvement of the family. Our current method is radically different from our previous one. Previously our therapeutic interventions varied in accordance with the multifarious situations in the different families. Now all families are treated in an identical manner: they are given the same prescription.

The treatment process is as follows. On terminating the second session with the nuclear family, the therapist comes back to the family after the team discussion and announces: "This time we are able to tell you that according to the team's conclusion there is a precise indication for family therapy. The next session has been fixed for such and such a day at such and such a time. You (calling the sons and daughters by their names and in order of age) will be staying at home. Only you two, the parents, will be coming." Having said this, the therapist then leaves. The observers take note of the immediate verbal and nonverbal feedback from the various family members.

The following session, held with the parents only, is structured primarily around the following questions:

1. "Immediately after the session and on subsequent days, until today, how did the children A, B, C, ... (or the son or daughter, if there is only one) react to our inviting you two alone?" Each parent in turn responds.
2. Again asking the same question to each parent in turn: "And how did *you* react to our inviting you two alone? How did you understand it?"
3. Did the two of you talk about it?"

On terminating this session, after the team discussion, the therapist comes back to the parents and, speaking gravely and in an empathic tone says: "We've come to the conclusion that today it's necessary to give you a prescription. We've been talking about it for a long time because we've realized it's going to be very difficult for you to follow. Still it's necessary for you to do your best to follow it, because it's extremely important for the work we're doing together here. It's a complex prescription, which has to be carried out in four stages." The prescription we give them is as follows:

1. "You must keep everything about the session absolutely secret at home. If one or more of your children asks you what happened during the session, you'll have to

answer very gently exactly like this: 'Dr. X has prescribed that what has been said during the session *must* be kept a secret from everybody.' You must give the same answer to anybody asking you about the session (parents, relatives, family doctor, friends)."

2. "About a week after the session, you'll start to go out now and then in the evening. You'll do this a number of times; I'll tell you exactly how often. Your evenings out shall be organized as follows: After you two have agreed about the suitable date, you'll arrange to meet somewhere away from home, late in the afternoon, in any case earlier than your usual dinner time. At home, on the kitchen table, you'll just leave a note with the following words: 'Tonight we'll not be in.' This note will be written by each of you, Mr. the first time and Mrs. the second, and soon it should not be signed. You'll not come back earlier than 11. You'll not get dinner ready and you'll come home having dined (it's not important whether you have dinner 'Chez Maxim' or just have a sandwich). It's important not to go anywhere or with anybody who could explain your whereabouts. As well, you are not expected to tell me."

Having said this, the therapist will then prescribe precisely how many times the parents must go out in the evening. The number of the outings will have to be calculated in proportion to the interval between sessions. We consider it advisable that the interval should be at least 5 weeks.

3. "If, back home, your son/sons asks you where you've been and what you've been doing, you'll answer, in a very quiet tone: '*These things concern only the two of us*'."

4. "Finally, each of you will keep a notebook carefully hidden and out of reach of the children. In the notebook each of you, separately, will note the date and those verbal and nonverbal behaviors of each child, or other family members, which seem to be caused or connected with your following this prescription. We recommend diligence in taking these notes because it's extremely important not to forget anything. Next time the two of you will come again alone bringing with you your notebook and you will tell us what has happened in the meantime."

After this first "stage" of the prescription (if the couple, on coming back to us, has fulfilled it), a further stage follows including some weekends during which the parents will disappear from home for one or two nights, leaving a written, message: "We'll be back on ... after eleven."

The last stage consists of a prolongued disappearance – 10 days to 1 month – away from home, leaving only the usual written note, "We'll be back on ...," without supplying any other information or ever getting in touch with anybody during their absence.

Conceptual Observations on the Method

This prescription is an extraordinarily strong therapeutic context marker. It draws an unmistakable organizational chart, with the therapist in the staff position, and fixes a precise program to follow.

Now that we've presented the pragmatics of giving the presscription, the question is on what hypothesis is this new method based? Giving the schizophrenic families a fixed, invariable prescription structures for the therapists a repeatable context. A repeatable context supplies the optimal condition for learning about "schizophrenia."

This time again, as it so often happened in the history of our work, we were inspired by Gregory Bateson [2]. Here I am particularly referring to his essay "The Logical Categories of Learning and Communication". In this original theorization on the different logical levels of learning, Bateson maintains that the passage from learning level zero to learning level one is constituted by the appearance of the process of trial and error. This happens when a choice which has been shown to be wrong is substituted with a different choice. Wrong choices can thus become profitable errors inasmuch as they "provide information to the organism which might contribute to his future skill." He refers to this as a stochastic process. But, Bateson notes, in order to have this learning take place it is necessary to assume a repeatable context. Quoting Bateson, "Without the assumption of repeatable context ... it would follow that all learning would be of one type, namely would be zero learning." But that's not all.

Bateson also asserts that we think and know solely through differences and comparisons. So, the fact of giving one and the same prescription to different families allows us to compare their various reactions. It is evident that, in so doing, similarities and differences provide us with high quality information.

Observable Repetitive Phenomena

After these cursory, but very significant, conceptual comments, we would like to clarify some of the most interesting repetitive phenomena that we have observed.

Let us begin from what we observe when the parents faithfully keep the secret and the three progressive stages of the prescription. The identified patient shows an immediate improvement, and progressively abandons his symptomatic behaviors. *The prescription seems to break the ongoing game without it being necessary for the therapist to first understand what game has been going on.* The family Marsi was first seen in May 1979 and we devised for the first time this prescription. We realized at once its' powerful effect. The family presented a chronic anorectic daughter, aged 21, with repeated suicidal behaviors. Immediately after the parents had completed the first stage of the prescription (after the fourth session), the girl stopped her anorectic behavior. Later, while the parents completed the subsequent stages of the prescription, her behavior improved consistently until she moved away from home, started a relationship with a boy, and got involved in sports. At present she is doing well as a student at the University and has become a regional champion in one of her sports. All the relationships in the family have changed considerably.

There have been changes like these in 10 out of the 19 families we have treated or are now treating. One of the cases with which we were most pleased was that of the family with a 31-year-old, chronic schizophrenic, the only son of two elderly teachers. The son had suffered his first psychotic crisis shortly after having reached the age of 20, while he was in military service. He had been living for years at home under heavy medication. Hist most interesting activity seemed to be that of holding redhot political meetings behind the closed door of his room. He conversed at length with imaginary adversaries whom he attacked with a thundering voice, addressing himself to the wall. The parents, deeply motivated, faithfully fulfilled the prescription. There was immediately a noticeable improvement: the son got a job. However, the radical turning point was reached when the parents, summoning up all their courage, obeyed the last and most difficult stage of the prescription. They disappeared from home for longer than a month. When they came back they were met by a young man who not only had been able to organize himself, but had found a more important job and had even begun a romantic relationship. During the 10th and last session, which took place with the parents, we were told about a peculiar incident. Having quarreled with his girl friend, the former identified patient, on returning home, had tried to revive his psychotic behavior by attempting to stage a rather melodramatic suicide. But his attempt was not successful. Better said, it was so clumsy that he lacked credibility, so much so that the parents could not help but laugh.

However, we do not want to speak of only successful cases. We think it is highly interesting to list a number of other phenomena repeatedly observed with different families. We shall report the bare facts succinctly to avoid the temptation of adding interpretive comments.

One observation that has recurred with all 19 families: *It has never been the identified patient who shows the most dramatic reaction to the disappearance of the parents and later to their refusing to give any information about it*. Confronted with the disappearance of the couple and the laconic and impersonal written note "tonight we'll not be in," an unexpected character suddenly emerged from the juggler's hat of the schizophrenic family. Sometimes it was a son or a daughter who had been considered perfectly sane. In some other cases an unexpected and apparently insignificant type jumped out, or somebody whose existence had not even been mentioned before. Such is the magic informative power of this prescription of curs! I shall supply an example.

The following episode took place during the family therapy of a psychotic girl aged 7. Besides the members of the nuclear family we had invited an aunt, the mother's sister, to take part in the first session. We suspected the aunt to be an important character because, as she lived across the street, she often visited the family. However, despite my focused efforts she did not supply any information. Consequently we felt that the aunt was less significant as a member of the extended family system. We proceeded to work with the parents, prescribing their disappearances in the evening. The couple courageously fulfilled the prescription, leaving the two girls – that is the 7-year-old identified patient and her sister of 10 – alone. Well, it was that "insignificant" aunt who reacted dramatically to the disappearance of the parents, *not* the girls. When she came to her sister's home, at 9, her usual time, she found the two girls alone. Without any drama they had managed to prepare a simple dinner. Even though she had read the message left in the middle of the table, the aunt acted as though there had been tragedy. To do such a thing – without informing her beforehand! she decided that her sister must have planned a double suicide. She alarmed the village with dramatic phone calls and finally went downstairs into the basement looking for bodies. It had been necessary to give the prescription to learn that aunt was far from being an unimportant member of the extended family!

In some other cases, feedback providing high quality information is evident immediately following the prescription. In a session with parents of an obese and psychotic identified patient, the mother at once reacted to the prescription of disappearing in the evening, exclaiming: "But that's impossible! How can we avoid informing Emilia beforehand? She'd be terribly offended!" We thus discovered that the family, in compiling the telephone chart, had not even mentioned among its members this Emilia, an old but very important aunt who not only had always lived with the family, but who also held the keys to the pantry, ruled in the kitchen, cooked every meal. Since the identified patient was seriously obese, the presence in the home of a respected, nurturing aunt was important in the family system.

These two cases lead us to an important fact. We previously said that a key element in conducting a competent session using our approach is the gathering of significant information. During the first session we literally try to fascinate our families with our type of questions, with our competence. The families with schizophrenic members despise incompetent people; they get easily bored and drop out. But in spite of all the trouble we take, it is only the prescription which forces the schizophrenic families to give us information. This is a further proof, if proof should still be needed, of the effectivenes of making the family *act* instead of making the family *talk*.

Two further types of phenomena generated by the prescription are important and warrant comment. Four of the 19 couples have fulfilled only once the first stage of the prescription, that of disappearing in the evening. But all four stopped, either revealing the secret to one of the children, or keeping the secret but declaring in the following session their intention to stop the prescription. All four of these couples actually made the following unexpectedly sincere statement: "We don't want to risk losing the sane child (or children) in order to help the sick one." A statement like that throws at least some doubt on the so frequently alleged great love for the identified patient! The loss they feared evidently was that the healthy children, imitating the parents, would also disappear from home, profiting from the newly acquired liberty. But, compelled by the prescription to come out into the open, these families went so far as to offer the therapist to exchange the prescription against some other proposal made by themselves and meant to improve the conditions of the identified patient. We had a similar case with the parents of a chronic psychotic child, 18 years old, behaving as a mentally retarded boy. These parents got such a fright from the fulfilment of the first stage of the prescription that they jumped for safety by breaking the secret. Still they did come to the following session, with a proposal that would have been unthinkable at an earlier date, that of freeing the identified patient from a torturing and useless school attendance and finding him a job. The plan was carried out at once and produced very positive results. A fifth family, who had immediately broken the secret, was dismissed.

Last but not least, there are three cases about which we still have doubts. These parents faithfully followed the first stage of the prescription, reporting a definite improvement of the identified patient. But, on passing to the second stage, that is to the more prolonged disappearances, they stopped because of a sudden, sometimes dramatic relapse of the identified patient. We suspect, chiefly on account of the analogic behaviors, that the couple, or one of the parents, had broken the pact of secrecy, revealing everything – perhaps only by means of hints or tacit inferences – to some member of the nuclear or extended family. They do not confess to having done so. In our view, the sudden relapse of the identified patient is the pragmatic effect of the breach of secrecy. Once again, the patient becomes the one who does not know while the others know. Somehow feeling cheated, he reacts accordingly.

Our hypothesis – *the identified patient somehow feels cheated* – is the central point of our research. This hypothesis could explain the first explosion of the psychotic behavior as a dramatic protest and it could explain the relapse we had observed during the later stages of our prescription.

We use this hypothesis as Ariadne's thread with which we step forward in the labyrinth which is the organization of families presenting with a schizophrenic member.

Concluding Remarks

It would not be scientifically correct to draw conclusions from the results of only 2 years' work with 19 families. That is why we have deliberately restricted our statements to the bare description of the phenomena we have observed, fighting the temptation to influence the reader by interpretive comments. The phenomena appeared so clearly and were so stimulating that they were well worth this preliminary presentation.

Our research will continue until we have treated an extensive number of families – at least 50 – presenting with a schizophrenic child.

Consistent with the method we have devised, our research plan will also include the lapse of time required and the modality of the follow-up of the families treated.

References

Bateson G (1972) The logical categories of learning and communication. In: Steps to an ecology of mind. Chandler, S. Francisco

Selvini-Palazzoli M, Boscolo L, Cecchin G, Prata G (1978) Paradox and counterparadox. Aronson, New York

Final Discussion

Luigi Boscolo

One of my teachers in psychiatric and psychoanalytic training was an authority in the field of schizophrenia and the individual psychotherapy of schizophrenics. I refer to Professor Silvano Arieti of the New York Medical College, who, during the several hours of supervision he gave me, used to say that my enthusiasm of neophyte psychotherapist will in time be constrained by the reality of the therapeutic results. One of his favorite sentences was: "Of all the cases I have treated for years in individual psychotherapy, I don't believe I have cured anybody. I think I have helped many schizophrenics to reach what I can call a neurotic stage, that's all."

As I became a psychotherapist treating schizophrenics, I reluctantly had to admit that my teacher was right.

When, in 1972, I started treating families with a schizophrenic member, I often witnessed sudden, at times glamorous, results which I had not dreamed of before. The same impression was reported by Salvador Minuchin in an interview he gave to the magazine, *New Yorker*.

I have now been working many years with families following the systemic model. My general impression is that excellent results are often obtained in acute psychosis or schizophrenia while, in chronic cases, only a very limited number show satisfactory results.

I think we still have a long way to go in order to free ourselves from the pessimism related to the treatment of chronic schizophrenia.

A particular issue in the family therapy of chronic schizophrenia, which limits its effectiveness, is the following: Even if the family therapy is successful in changing the rigid repetitive communicational patterns characteristic of these systems and in freeing the family members towards individuation and separation, nevertheless, the designated patient is left with major learning gaps. For instance, a child or an adolescent schizophrenic who has been trapped for years in a web of pathological family communications, has not had the chance to develop those social and learning skills which are essential for a satisfactory maturation. For this reason, besides family therapy, adjunctive therapies such as individual or group therapy can be indicated.

Gianfranco Cecchin

Concerning the difference between the two ways of thinking, circular and linear thinking, I would say that it is impossible, in an experience, to make a systemic circular hypothesis if one has not made a series of linear causal observations.

The observer-therapist has to give himself many linear explanations, plausible, but often contradictory, and only then can he make a jump towards a more systemic circular description.

Our students are encouraged to make several linear punctuations before trying to think systemically. When the students work in teams, each of them is asked to make a hypothesis "blaming" a different member of the family. Soon afterwards it becomes obvious that "blaming" is not sufficient to explain, and a new systemic hypothesis usually emerges spontaneously from the team.

To move continuously back and forth from linear to circular thinking enhances creativity in the therapist, who is facilitated in finding original solutions and prescriptions.

Luc Kaufmann

I would like to make a statement about the Symposium: In "Mind and Nature", Bateson quotes William Blake as saying that truth can never be told so as to be understood and not to be believed. Now what shall we believe about the psychotherapy of schizophrenics? I was concerned about the feelings of the numerous participants, especially the younger ones, who did not talk but tried to integrate this enormous amount of information which was, as a whole, not very coherent. The participants are of course free to choose what seems to fit their background and their work in a given context. But what did they learn about differences between several epistemologies? I would think that the Symposium itself had some resemblance with a psychotic family: it was consensus-oriented (in the sense of David Reiss); there was quite a bit of pseudo-mutuality and conflict-avoidance behavior. There was keen competition for telling the "truth" about effective psychotherapy for a disease as mysterious as schizophrenia. Competition means sometimes hidden symmetrical escalation. We should have worked out our disparities of views, in order to grasp the differences.

Some of us "believe" in theoretical concepts such as "resistance" of patients and even whole families, or in the necessity of insight as a change-inducing agent. Other therapists do not "believe" in psychoanalytic hypotheses: they say one must induce change by changing the rules in family systems in order to make individual symptomatic behavior superfluous. The point is: there is no continuity between these two descriptions of therapeutic processes. "Two descriptions are better than one," said Bateson – but not always. We must know that these two descriptions entail different logical levels.

Psychoanalytic concepts may allow for descriptions of intrapsychic mental processes of several members of a family group including the psychotic patient. But one cannot correctly describe structures and processes of ongoing (circular) interactions in networks of relationships in psychodynamic terms. Psychoanalysis and system-oriented therapy do not directly fit in with each other. What we need is a theoretical model or metamodel sufficiently complex to allow for integration of several theories used in psychotherapy. Such a model should enable us to avoid a more or less polemic "either-or" thinking, but should also help us to overcome the confusion arising when psychoanalysis *and* so-called systemic approaches are used to define clinical situations and therapies. We should know more about what is therapeutic in which situation. When working with schizophrenics, we have to take into account at every moment the context – the family – and of course ourselves, as well as our institutions and other related agencies. As everybody is realizing, the context determines the choice of our therapeutic strategy. To apply counterparadox to families of schizophrenics during hospitalization, in parallel with drug treatment, can be a professional mistake.

We may perhaps also look more for common traits in as apparently different approaches in family therapy as those of Boszormenyi Nagy and the Milano group. Boscolo and Cecchin have given an illustration: their handing of the situation had apparently nothing to do with Boszormenyi-Nagy, but what they did in the end of the session fits in my opinion rather well with Boszormenyi Nagy's "contextual therapy." Working on blocked ledgers of merits and debts is not as far from paradoxical intervention as "system purists" believe: By extolling loyalties towards the family of origin, the therapist actually facilitates the emergence of the relative autonomy of the nuclear family. The nuance I am trying to show is the following: To work on ledgers and loyalties may be more *meaningful* for the family members than elegant system manipulations. This is, with regard to the nature of the relationship with the family, important under certain conditions, for instance when an institution is responsible for a catchment area. When treatment fails, or when the identified patient relapses month or years after therapy, or when other members of the family become symptomatic and one has to continue or to start treatment again, then it makes a difference as to which sort of relationship you have established 5 or 10 years before with the patient and the family.

This last point leads to the question: which time span is relevant for outcome studies of family therapy with schizophrenics? For how many years should we follow the evolution of the patient and the family in order to say something substantial about outcome?

Paul Watzlawick

Let me make a general point relating to what Dr. Kaufmann said about the impression he has had during these last days, and then a specific one.

The general point is that we have seen here a crash between two epistemologies. There can be no doubt that we are still caught in a dichotomy between the intrapsychic approach that is based mostly on a linear system of causality and therefore forces us to go back into the past to find out the reasons why the situation exists in the here and now; and the systemic approach that knows about the fantastic complexity of the interactions that make up the situation here and now. In this approach there is no room for the idea of an exploration of past causes. Instead, one looks at the situation here and now in order to grasp the system in its circular causality, in its repetitive patterns of behavior, and intervenes in these repetitive patterns. My colleagues and I in Palo Alto and, I am pretty sure, my colleagues in Milan do not believe in the compatibility and the final happy marriage between those two epistemologies. What is possible in one is not possible in the other; what is indicated in the one is taboo in the other. And parts of the discussions and the presentations I have been able to listen to over these past days have been dealing precisely with this kind of dichotomy.

The other point, I would like to make is about what we just saw, namely the use of language in psychotherapy. Did you notice how Boscolo – whether he knows it or not – (I don't believe for a moment it's just the question of how fluently he speaks English), did you notice the almost posthypnotic nature of his language? The repetitive, gradual approach of the final instruction or intervention, the branching off, the approaching of the same subject from yet another point, until eventually, just as a good hypnotherapist would probably do, there comes the intervention in its whole glory and its full penetrating power.

Martti Siirala

Luc Kaufmann is right, I think, when he maintains that here at this symposium we have been caught in pseudomutuality and conflict-avoidance, like a schizophrenic family. If transference from our subject matter, schizophrenia, has thus really taken hold of us, it is time to break with that pattern. By doing this I also am bringing to the plenary session a message from the workshop on "New Developments of the Psychotherapy of Schizophrenia in the Light of Philosophical Anthropology and Epistemology." My thesis there was that the Selvini team's interpretation of what they are doing and achieving far too centrally attributes the paradox-counterparadox procedure and process to systems theory.

As reaction to the present panel I want to argue against the statement Paul Watzlawick made just now. He spoke of a crash between two epistemologies, the systemic versus the causal approach. He also claimed that "the systemic approach knows about the enormous complexity" of the phenomena involved in the family therapy of schizophrenia. In my view, the claim that systems theory constitutes a new epistemology is sheer nonsense. Systems theory is a theory and no epistemology. Certainly, it does *not* possess the comprehensiveness, depth, meaningfulness, and differentiation needed to account for the human-inhuman situation "schizophrenia." It *has*, however, apparently given vital inspiration to the paradox-counterparadox method and even furnished the same with a temporary tool for profiling the characteristic family processes elicited thereby.

This significant and successful function exerted by systems theory – to my mind – rests with its capacity to account for the demonic circularities in the families manifesting schizophrenia. This it does in a way that simultaneously creates, so to speak, ironic distantiation from the hell of ruptured elementary reciprocity among us. Systems theory provides us therapists with distance from the pain that the schizophrenics and their families are in desperate flight from having to endure, and which would be intolerable for ourselves if we let ourselves be really exposed to it.

Systems theory, in such a function, appears anonymous enough not to scare the reductionist mind and not to threaten us therapists by opening up alarming perspectives of responsibility and of having a share in guilt. Concepts like "symmetrical" versus "complementary" furnish therapists with the protective illusion of being placed in a safe position of scientific neutrality outside the predicament of schizophrenia. In the "unreduced" situation "schizophrenia," however, such a pair of concepts keeps referring to the vicissitudes of human reciprocity. We are reminded of the failure of realization of reciprocity over the generations, and horizontally in present-day society. We are remined, further, of the pains to be suffered through on the way towards some restoration of elementary reciprocity.

In such reflections as the preceding ones, the dimension of epistemology (and, for that matter, also of philosophical anthropology) has become activated. I cannot see in what sense systems theory could be said to represent an epistemology, be it new or old. In the above-mentioned workshop it was Wolfgang Jacob who took up the central concept of reciprocity, referring to Viktor von Weizsäcker, who originally brought it to the fore and articulated its profound significance in medicine in general.

To my mind, the function of systems theory is first and foremost that of a strategic tool. Situating it epistemologically and in terms of philosophical anthropology is a task that lies ahead of us. That challenge is of vital importance lest we want just blindly to run the risk of being once again driven into commitment to a gradually self-exhausting manipulation of our patients and of the encountered whole predicament.

Stephen Fleck

Schizophrenia is not "something" that we should treat, but we should treat, and possibly cure, schizophrenics who suffer from certain developmental disorders. These difficulties should be addressed and/or treated through the context in which they lived and developed. As to the presentation of Mara Selvini, I would be interesed in knowing about follow-up data and the nature of the "cure" on which she reported.

John S. Kafka

I consider Dr. Selvini's prescription and claims dangerous from several points of view:

Those of us who have worked psychodynamically and/or psychoanalytically with schizophrenic patients for a long time know of the collapse of many claims of specific curative approaches. Particularly with this disorder very long and carefully documented follow-up studies are necessary before claims for improvement – yet alone cure – are justified. I have tried to show this in my presentation at this meeting of a 25-year study of a schizophrenic patient.

Claims such as those made by Dr. Selvini on the basis of evidence presented and the follow-up time involved are dangerous for our very standing and credibility in the scientific and professional community.

Dr. Selvini's prescription is more dangerous than other conceptualizations of therapeutic approaches. Seasoned therapists of all persuasions may make useful interventions based on preconsciously perceived cues which have nothing to do with the theoretical system to which they pledge public allegiance, but Dr. Selvini stresses uniformity. A charismatically presented *prescription* invites the suppression of subtle variations, independent of theory, especially since the uniformity and simplicity of a *prescription* invites its application by minimally trained individuals.

I do believe that Dr. Selvini's approach brings to the foreground the importance of secrets in the families of schizophrenic patients. We have noted in families observed for a long period that certain individuals avoided being alone with each other. Bringing those individuals together – and the careful management of the resistance to such encounters is essential – has proven to be one technique useful for therapeutically valuable exposure of such family secrets.

The secret-exposing contribution of Dr. Selvini's approach does not justify the introduction of the dangers inherent in her *prescription.*

Mara Selvini-Palazzoli

I disagree a little with what our friend Paul Watzlawick said, because I am not sure that there is here a crash of two epistemologies. I will explain what I mean. I do not see an opposition in the sense of systemic epistemology declaring war *on* intrapsychic epistemology or vice versa. In reality, we are in presence of two different logical levels, the individual – or intrapsychic – level and the systemic level. This is not equivalent to saying that I consider it possible to make an integration between psychoanalysis and systems theory. Of course not, because they belong to two different logical levels. One level is the level of the individual, and the other the level of the living natural group, that is of the system. But we must always remember that individuals are contained in the system. On the systemic level, therefore, observation is not focused upon the characteristics of the single individuals, but upon the way these individuals are organized. Consequently I don't see an opposition, but something contained in another something which is on another logical level.

Concerning Paul's observation that Luigi's way of concluding the session – repeating over and over, slowly, the same sentences – suggests a hypnotic effect, I radically disagree. This is Luigi's style, he is always very slow and goes on repeating and repeating. But I speak quickly, I never repeat, and yet I work on the same conceptual model and I get the same effects. The point I want to stress is essentially this: in our work there is absolutely no question of an hypnotic effect. The effect is brought about by the epistemology we use, which aims at striking the pathogenic organization of the family, compelling it to change its organization.

I should like to answer Dr. Fleck because, if I understood him correctly, he said that we cannot cure schizophrenics, since what we call schizophrenia is the expression of a particular learning context. This is true. What I think, exactly, is that we can cure schizophrenics by creating a different learning context. This is what we do by means of the prescription I have described today. We create a context in which the rules have changed and the game has changed, therefore there is no point any more in presenting a schizophrenic behavior. What we consider useless is trying to "teach" the schizophrenic's family. For instance: to teach the family how to communicate correctly. To communicate in a confusing way is part and parcel of the type of game of the schizophrenic's family. To teach this family to communicate correctly is therefore like endeavoring to cure the leaves of a tree which is suffering at its roots.

I'm grateful to Dr. Kafka for his remark on the possible risks inherent in our prescription, because it allows me to offer further clarifications. I'll say at once that this prescription of ours is difficult to handle, it is a tool that *cannot* be put into the hands of therapists who have not got much experience. It may in fact cause dramatic reactions which require the courage, the promptness, and the capacity of very experienced therapists. As to the danger represented by the secret, which Dr. Kafka is right in frequently detecting in the schizophrenic's family, I point out that the secret in our prescription is very different from the secret – or secrets – of the pathogenic families. Ours is an official secret, it is officially declared *urbi et orbi*. The parents accept a pact with the therapist: you must go home and declare that you must keep the secret with everybody. This is the contrary, absolutely the contrary, of what happens in the pathogenic family, where somebody tells something to somebody unknown to somebody else, and does not tell it to others, or tells it in a different way. It is exactly the contrary. Therefore our prescription is for the family a really *new* experience.

Monographien aus dem Gesamtgebiete der Psychiatrie/ Psychiatry Series

Herausgeber: H. Hippius, W. Janzarik, C. Müller

Volume 14

The Apallic Syndrome

Editors: G. Dalle Ore, F. Gerstenbrand, C. H. Lücking, G. Peters, U. H. Peters
With the editorial assistance of E. Rothemund

1977. 67 figures, 17 tables. XV, 259 pages (5 pages in German)
ISBN 3-540-08301-4

Volume 18

Transmethylations and the Central Nervous System

Editors: V. M. Andreoli, A. Agnoli, C. Fazio

1978. 45 figures, 44 tables. VI, 185 pages
ISBN 3-540-08693-5

Volume 20
R. M. Torack

The Pathologic Physiology of Dementia

With Indications for Diagnosis and Treatment

1978. 11 figures, 24 tables. VIII, 155 pages
ISBN 3-540-08904-7

Volume 22
G. Guntern

Social Change, Stress, and Mental Health in the Pearl of the Alps

A Systemic Study of a Village Process

1979. 45 figures, 36 tables. XX, 313 pages
ISBN 3-540-09631-0

Volume 28
H. B. M. Murphy

Comparative Psychiatry

The International and Intercultural Distribution of Mental Illness

1982. 28 figures. IX, 327 pages
ISBN 3-540-11057-7

Springer-Verlag
Berlin
Heidelberg
New York

www.ingramcontent.com/pod-product-compliance
Lightning Source LLC
Chambersburg PA
CBHW061204240926
51846CB00006B/1112
* 9 7 8 3 6 4 2 6 8 9 6 8 0 *